Principles and Practice of Perioperative Medicine

Principles and Practice of Perioperative Medicine

Edited by Bryson Cooper

hayle
medical

New York

Hayle Medical,
750 Third Avenue, 9th Floor,
New York, NY 10017, USA

Visit us on the World Wide Web at:
www.haylemedical.com

ISBN: 978-1-63241-746-6

Cataloging-in-Publication Data

Principles and practice of perioperative medicine / edited by Bryson Cooper.
    p. cm.
Includes bibliographical references and index.
ISBN 978-1-63241-746-6
1. Surgery, Operative. 2. Surgery--Complications--Prevention. 3. Therapeutics, Surgical. 4. Preoperative care.
5. Postoperative care. I. Cooper, Bryson.
RD54 .P75 2019
617--dc23

Table of Contents

Preface.. IX

Chapter 1   **Day of surgery cancellation rate after preoperative telephone nurse screening or comprehensive optimization visit**.. 1
Ronald P. Olson and Ishwori B. Dhakal

Chapter 2   **Potential return on investment for implementation of perioperative goal-directed fluid therapy in major surgery**.. 9
Frederic Michard, William K. Mountford, Michelle R. Krukas,
Frank R. Ernst and Sandy L. Fogel

Chapter 3   **Choice of anesthetic technique on plasma concentrations of interleukins and cell adhesion molecules**... 17
Daniela C Ionescu, Simona Claudia D Margarit, Adina Norica I Hadade,
Teodora N Mocan, Nicolae A Miron and Daniel I Sessler

Chapter 4   **Risk stratification by pre-operative cardiopulmonary exercise testing improves outcomes following elective abdominal aortic aneurysm surgery**...................... 25
Stephen J Goodyear, Heng Yow, Mahmud Saedon, Joanna Shakespeare,
Christopher E Hill, Duncan Watson, Colette Marshall, Asif Mahmood,
Daniel Higman and Christopher HE Imray

Chapter 5   **Coagulation during elective neurosurgery with hydroxyethyl starch fluid therapy: an observational study with thromboelastometry, fibrinogen and factor XIII** 38
Caroline Ulfsdotter Nilsson, Karin Strandberg, Martin Engström and Peter Reinstrup

Chapter 6   **A case management report: a collaborative perioperative surgical home paradigm and the reduction of total joint arthroplasty readmissions**.............................. 47
Navid Alem, Joseph Rinehart, Brian Lee, Doug Merrill, Safa Sobhanie, Kyle Ahn,
Ran Schwarzkopf, Maxime Cannesson and Zeev Kain

Chapter 7   **Implementation of goal-directed fluid therapy during hip revision arthroplasty: a matched cohort study** 56
Marit Habicher, Felix Balzer, Viktor Mezger, Jennifer Niclas, Michael Müller,
Carsten Perka, Michael Krämer and Michael Sander

Chapter 8   **Pre-operative anaemia is associated with total morbidity burden on days 3 and 5 after cardiac surgery**... 64
Julie Sanders, Jackie A. Cooper, Daniel Farrar, Simon Braithwaite,
Updeshbir Sandhu, Michael G. Mythen and Hugh E. Montgomery

Chapter 9   **Predictors of total morbidity burden on days 3, 5 and 8 after cardiac surgery**........................... 74
Julie Sanders, Jackie Cooper, Michael G. Mythen and Hugh E. Montgomery

Chapter 10   **Surgeons' views on preoperative medical evaluation**.. 85
Kevin R. Riggs, Zackary D. Berger, Martin A. Makary,
Eric B. Bass and Geetanjali Chander

Chapter 11   **Comparison of risk-scoring systems in the prediction of outcome after**
liver resection 94
S. Ulyett, G. Shahtahmassebi, S. Aroori, M. J. Bowles, C. D. Briggs, M. G. Wiggans,
G. Minto and D. A. Stell

Chapter 12   **Association of postoperative nausea/vomiting and pain with breastfeeding**
success.. 101
Ramon Abola, Jamie Romeiser, Suman Grewal, Sabeen Rizwan,
Rishimani Adsumelli, Ellen Steinberg and Elliott Bennett-Guerrero

Chapter 13   **Intraoperative oxygenation in adult patients undergoing surgery**
(iOPS).. 106
Clare M. Morkane, Helen McKenna, Andrew F. Cumpstey, Alex H. Oldman,
Michael P. W. Grocott and Daniel S. Martin

Chapter 14   **The sensitivity of the human thirst response to changes in plasma**
osmolality... 113
Fintan Hughes, Monty Mythen and Hugh Montgomery

Chapter 15   **Patient-reported outcomes 6 months after enhanced recovery after colorectal**
surgery 124
Thomas Deiss, Lee-lynn Chen, Ankit Sarin and Ramana K. Naidu

Chapter 16   **A systematic review and meta-analysis of perioperative oral decontamination**
in patients undergoing major elective surgery.. 130
Philip Spreadborough, Sarah Lort, Sandro Pasquali, Matthew Popplewell,
Andrew Owen, Irene Kreis, Olga Tucker and Ravinder S Vohra

Chapter 17   **Effects of different colloid infusions on ROTEM and Multiplate during elective**
brain tumour neurosurgery 137
N. Li, S. Statkevicius, B. Asgeirsson and U. Schött

Chapter 18   **Functional recovery is considered the most important target: a survey of**
dedicated professionals.. 147
Eirik K Aahlin, Maarten von Meyenfeldt, Cornelius HC Dejong, Olle Ljungqvist,
Kenneth C Fearon, Dileep N Lobo, Nicolas Demartines, Arthur Revhaug,
Stephen J Wigmore and Kristoffer Lassen

Chapter 19   **Incidence, outcome, and attributable resource use associated with pulmonary**
and cardiac complications after major small and large bowel procedures 152
Lee A Fleisher and Walter T Linde-Zwirble

Chapter 20   **How fast can glucose be infused in the perioperative setting?**................................... 159
Robert G. Hahn

Chapter 21   **Observational study of the effects of age, diabetes mellitus, cirrhosis and**
chronic kidney disease on sublingual microvascular flow 167
Toby Reynolds, Amanda Vivian-Smith, Shaman Jhanji and Rupert M Pearse

Chapter 22   **Perioperative acute kidney injury**... 172
Stacey Calvert and Andrew Shaw

Chapter 23   **Neither dynamic, static, nor volumetric variables can accurately predict fluid
responsiveness early after abdominothoracic esophagectomy** 183
Hironori Ishihara, Eiji Hashiba, Hirobumi Okawa, Junichi Saito,
Toshinori Kasai and Toshihito Tsubo

Chapter 24   **The cost-effectiveness of an outpatient anesthesia consultation clinic before
surgery**.. 191
Anna Lee, Po Tong Chui, Chun Hung Chiu, Tony Gin and Anthony MH Ho

Permissions

List of Contributors

Index

Preface

Perioperative medicine refers to the care of patients from the time of the contemplation of surgery till the time of the patient's full recovery, excluding the operation procedure. Such type of care is usually provided by an internal medicine generalist, intensivist or anesthesiologist. Perioperative medicine involves the care of the patients who are preparing for surgery, having a surgery, and recuperating from surgery. The knowledge about the patient specific risks, operative risks, and methods to reduce risk is closely related to this field. Preanesthetic assessment is highly crucial in ensuring the safety of the patient during perioperative care. This book is a valuable compilation of topics, ranging from the basic to the most complex advancements in the field of perioperative medicine. The various studies that are constantly contributing towards advancing technologies and evolution of this field are examined in detail. This book will prove to be immensely beneficial to students and researchers in this field.

Various studies have approached the subject by analyzing it with a single perspective, but the present book provides diverse methodologies and techniques to address this field. This book contains theories and applications needed for understanding the subject from different perspectives. The aim is to keep the readers informed about the progresses in the field; therefore, the contributions were carefully examined to compile novel researches by specialists from across the globe.

Indeed, the job of the editor is the most crucial and challenging in compiling all chapters into a single book. In the end, I would extend my sincere thanks to the chapter authors for their profound work. I am also thankful for the support provided by my family and colleagues during the compilation of this book.

Editor

Day of surgery cancellation rate after preoperative telephone nurse screening or comprehensive optimization visit

Ronald P. Olson[*] and Ishwori B. Dhakal

Abstract

Background: Structured preoperative assessment has been reported to improve operating room efficiency as measured by metrics such as day of surgery cancellations (DOSCs). However, not all patients require comprehensive assessment; routine full assessments can result in unnecessary duplication of tests and investigations. Selective nurse screening under the supervision of anesthesiology may provide adequate information gathering in lower risk patients. This study is undertaken to assess if DOSC rates vary with different assessment processes.

Methods: At a single academic tertiary care hospital, from Jan 2 to May 31, 2013, the consecutive patients undergoing comprehensive preoperative assessment (CPA) and nurse screening (NS), as well as the patients not assessed by the anesthesiology-supervised preoperative process, were followed for the occurrence and reason for DOSC. The operating room schedule of all elective surgery patients was analyzed to allow calculation of rates of DOSCs. Reasons for cancellations were documented as one of ten structured reasons by preoperative holding area clerical staff.

Results: Overall, there were 14,893 elective surgery patients in this time period, with 183 DOSCs, giving a rate of 1.23 % (95 % CI 1.06, 1.42). Patients who received CPA numbered 5980; 29 of them had a DOSC, giving a rate of 0.48 % (95 % CI 0.33–0.70) (P < 0.0001 vs. no assessment). Patients receiving NS numbered 1840; 11 of them had a DOSC, giving a rate of 0.60 % (95 % CI 0.30–1.10) (P < 0.0001 vs. no assessment). The most common reason for cancellation was new medical condition.

Conclusions: A very low DOSC rate can be achieved with a comprehensive preoperative process where some patients are selectively telephone screened by nurses, with complete assessment deferred to the anesthesiologist on the day of surgery.

Keywords: Preoperative assessment, Nurse screening, Day of surgery cancellation

Background

Day of surgery cancellations (DOSCs) are a source of inefficiency and frustration to patients and hospital staff alike. They may be a measure of operating room efficiency (Fixler and Wright 2013; Macario 2006). While some last-minute cancellations will always occur because of changes in medical conditions, many of the factors that result in DOSC can be detected in time to avoid gaps in the surgical schedule and inconvenience to patients. Reducing DOSCs requires knowing what

the causes are and whether the processes intended to reduce DOSC actually do reduce them.

One method proposed to minimize DOSC is a robust preoperative assessment process (Ferschl et al. 2005; Knox et al. 2009; Emanuel and Macpherseon 2013; Fischer 1996; Pollard et al. 1996; Bader et al. 2009; Xue et al. 2013). While traditionally this has been done directly by an anesthesiologist and/or consultants (Newman et al. 2013), in many cases it can be done at less cost by a nurse practitioner, physician assistant, or a registered nurse (Wittkugel and Varughese 2015), who is supervised by a department of anesthesiology (Kinley et al. 2002; van Klei et al. 2006). This observational study was undertaken to accurately determine the rate and reasons of

* Correspondence: ron.olson@duke.edu
Department of Anesthesiology, Duke University Medical Center, Box 309440 Duke Medicine Circle Dr, Durham, NC 27710, USA

DOSCs at a single academic tertiary care institution where the preoperative assessments are done primarily by non-physicians, as well as to observe the impact on DOSCs of the two complementary methods of preoperative assessment—a comprehensive clinical preoperative assessment by a nurse practitioner or physician assistant and a selective advanced nurse screening (NS) process, usually done by telephone, to see if there was a difference.

Methods

The study was approved by the Duke University Medical Center Institutional Review Board. It was determined that because information gathered did not include personal identifiers, individual consents were not required. At an academic tertiary care hospital, for the period Jan 2 to May 31, 2013, the operating room schedules, as published in the afternoon of the day before surgery, were collated to form the denominator of total elective cases. Emergency cases are not added to these schedules. Friday afternoon was used as the cutoff for Monday surgeries. Ambulatory surgery center cases, eye center cases, and electroconvulsive therapy cases were not included as documentation of reasons for cancellation was done by different staff, and thresholds for cancellation are different. Gastroenterology suite procedures done under anesthesiology care were similarly different but were included as there was special interest in the putative benefit of an extensive preoperative assessment in this generally low-risk situation.

The study period was begun when a consistent process for recording the date, time, and reason for DOSCs had been established. Previous observations suggested that preoperative area clerks were in the best position to record an unbiased reason for cancellation, although it was not done consistently. Therefore, they had been encouraged, empowered, and monitored over the previous 6 months by their supervisors and the study personnel, to be diligent and consistent in determining and documenting the reason for cancellation. The study period ended when implementation of a new electronic health record changed data-gathering methods and resource allocation.

The date and time of all cancellations were recorded in the electronic scheduling program. These cancellations were compared with the list of completed cases, to verify that no cancellation matched to a case that was ultimately started later that day. Those confirmed DOSCs were taken as the numerator for the rate calculation.

The reasons for DOSCs were noted as one of ten standardized categories. Where the reason was not noted, or if it was noted as unknown, the electronic medical record was examined retrospectively to determine a reason if possible.

At this institution, most patients scheduled for elective surgery are assessed by either telephone NS or comprehensive preoperative assessment. The surgical clinics utilize a published criteria list to determine which patients are lower risk and therefore eligible for the NS process (see Table 1). Some patients do bypass these two processes and are assessed by the perioperative team on the day of surgery. This occurs if they are very low risk or have had adequate outside assessment and documentation or late scheduling precluded earlier assessment.

Comprehensive preoperative assessment (CPA)

The comprehensive preoperative assessment (CPA) involves teaching by a nurse (described below), as well as assessment and management done by either a nurse practitioner or physician assistant. It includes a complete medical history, medication reconciliation, focused examination, securing outside records, and determining and arranging indicated tests and consultations. Limited medical management such as preemptive control of pain and nausea; smoking cessation; ordering and assessing echocardiography reports; and basic optimization of diabetes, asthma, simple infections, and hypertension is performed. Follow-up is instigated as needed. Preoperative medication instructions are given. Documentation is formatted in the institutional electronic record with anesthesiology in mind as the primary user, but the information can also provide the basis for the admission history and physical evaluation by surgeons and house staff.

Basic education on anesthesia options are given, and written anesthesia consent, separate from the surgical consent, is obtained.

CPAs are done in four locations and are supervised by one physician—either an anesthesiologist or a specifically trained family physician.

Nurse screening (NS)

A NS process entails reviewing health history, current health status, medication reconciliation, description of the logistics and expectations of the perioperative experience, and instruction on preoperative fluids. When indicated, specific instructions on bowel preparations and enhanced recovery after surgery protocols (Miller et al. 2014) are addressed. Instructions on preoperative medications are given, based on a protocol and in consultation with the attending physician. Documentation is in the same institutional electronic record as the CPA and can be used by other health care staff as appropriate.

Patients assessed by NS are intended to be a different, lower risk group of patients than those seen with CPA.

To determine the rate of DOSC for patients undergoing one of these encounters, the respective denominators were defined either by a compilation of the daily schedules of the preoperative assessment clinic or by

Table 1 Criteria for phone screening

Must be		
	-BMI < 40 and weight < 350 lbs (160 kg)	
	-Vital signs recorded within the last 60 days	
	-English speaking	
	-Age 14–65	
Acceptable co-morbidities include		
	-Allergies	< 5 food, drug, or other allergies Controlled seasonal allergies acceptable
	-Anemia	Only if from menorrhagia associated with planned surgery and Hct > 26 % (Hgb > 8 g/dl) documented <30 days
	-Seizures	Seizure-free >1 year
	-Depression	Stable on ≤ 2 meds
	-Endocrine	Stable hypothyroidism with no recent med changes
	-Diabetes	Controlled ≤ 1 oral med. Hgb A1C < 7.5 within the last 3 months
	-Hypertension	Controlled ≤ 3 meds (<170/<95)
	-Mitral valve prolapse	If asymptomatic
	-Neoplasms without organ metastasis	Head and neck, thyroid, soft tissue, orthopedic, breast, renal cell, melanoma
	-Smoker	No new productive cough, no severe COPD
Exclusions		
	-Severe systemic disease	
	-Coronary artery disease	
	-Scheduled for high-risk surgery	
	-Refuses blood transfusion (unless seen by a center for blood conservation)	

To be eligible for nurse screening, a patient must be all of the first group of criterion, may have any of the second group, but must not have any of the third group

the records of NS contacts. The numerators for rates were determined by scanning the list of all CPAs and NS encounters, with the dates, and matching forward to any DOSC occurring for that patient in the 30 days after the preoperative assessment. This is thus a cohort study of three groups: CPAs, NS, and other preoperative assessments.

Statistical analysis

DOSCs by cancellation reason and surgical service were presented as group frequencies and percentages. DOSC rate was calculated by dividing the number confirmed DOSC cases (numerator) by the total number of scheduled cases (denominator) in the corresponding category. Descriptive comparisons of rates between groups were made by using chi-square or Fisher's exact test, as appropriate. The proportions and 95 % confidence intervals (CI) were computed by employing the Clopper-Pearson exact method. Statistical significance was set at $P < 0.05$ (two-sided). The analyses were

performed with SAS statistical software (version 9.4, SAS institute Inc, Cary, NC).

Results

Rates of cancellations

From Jan 2 to May 31, 2013, the number of patients who were on the surgical schedule for the main operating rooms, offsite locations where anesthesiology care occurs, and the gastroenterology suite, as of the afternoon posting on the day before surgery, totaled 14,893. There were 183 DOSCs, giving an overall rate of 1.23 % (95 % CI 1.06, 1.42). The rate for medical reasons (inadequate investigation or optimization and new or changed medical condition) was 0.63 %.

In this time period, 62 % of the patients having elective surgery were assessed with one of the two preoperative processes—NS or CPA. The others were assessed by the perioperative team on the day of surgery.

Ninety-eight percent of elective cases were admitted on the day of surgery.

Patients who had no assessment by one of the structured preoperative processes numbered 7073; 143 of them had a DOSC, giving a rate of 2.02 % (95 % CI 1.71–2.38).

Patients who received CPA numbered 5980; 29 of them had a DOSC, giving a rate of 0.48 % (95 % CI 0.33–0.70) ($P < 0.0001$ vs. no assessment). Medical reasons (inadequate investigation or optimization and new or changed medical condition) accounted for 13 of these, giving a rate of 0.22 %.

Patients receiving NS numbered 1840; 11 of them had a DOSC, giving a rate of 0.60 % (95 % CI 0.30–1.10) ($P < 0.0001$ vs. no assessment). Eight of these were due to medical reasons giving a rate of 0.43 % (see Table 2). Of the preoperative assessments in this period, 23.5 % (12.5 % of the total scheduled cases) were done as a NS process. Application for NS was denied in 187 cases because the criteria were not met.

The overall DOSC rate for gastrointestinal cases was 0.69 %. Of the 385 cases seen by CPA or NS, there was only one DOSC (0.3 %).

Of the CPAs, 1982 were done on the day of or the day before surgery; 4 of these became DOSCs giving a rate of 0.20 % (95 % CI 1.71–2.38). Of the NS assessments, 385 were done on the day of or the day before surgery; 1 of these became DOSC giving a rate of 0.26 % (95 % CI 0.01–1.43). The absolute risk difference in DOSCs on the day of or the day before surgery between comprehensive assessments and NS was not statistically significant—0.06 % (95 % CI −0.60–0.49), $P = 0.59$.

Comparison of pediatric vs. adult patients showed no difference in the DOSC rates or the reasons. DOSC rates by surgical service are shown in Table 3. American Society of Anesthesiologists (ASA) Physical Classification Spectrum is shown in Table 4.

Table 3 Day of surgery cancellations by service

Service	DOSC	Cases	Rate (%)
Cardiac	9	2389	0.38
Dentistry	4	134	2.99
Dermatology	0	127	0.00
Gastrointestinal	6	1112	0.54
General	70	2372	2.95
Gynecology	4	558	0.72
Medicine	0	469	0.00
Neurosurgery	13	1475	0.88
Otolaryngology	11	839	1.31
Orthopedic	50	2175	2.30
Pediatric	16	498	3.21
Hematology	1	176	0.57
Plastic	12	556	2.16
Radiology	0	198	0.00
Thoracic	5	851	0.59
Urology	11	1101	1.00
Others < 50 cases per service	0	103	0.00
Grand total	212	15,133	1.40

Discussion

DOSC causes are multifactorial, as are solutions, but structured preoperative screening and assessment programs have been shown to reduce DOSCs (Ferschl et al. 2005; Knox et al. 2009; Emanuel and Macpherseon 2013; Pollard et al. 1996), as well as reduce operating room startup times, preoperative testing, postoperative complications, and workload for surgical clinic staff (van Klei et al. 2006). In a sometimes fragmented health care system, the preoperative assessment may be one of the few opportunities to identify long-term health issues (Kain et al. 2015) and initiate management. But while there is

Table 2 Reasons for day of surgery cancellations

Reasons for cancellation	Overall		Comprehensive preoperative assessment		Nurse screening	
	Number	%	Number	%	Number	%
Inadequate investigation or optimization	14	0.1	3	0.05	1	0.03
New or changed medical condition	91	0.6	14	0.24	2	0.06
NPO guidelines not met	7	0.05	2	0.03	1	0.03
OR or equipment unavailable, schedule changes	25	0.2	3	0.05	2	0.06
Patient-initiated cancellation	20	0.1	1	0.02	3	0.09
Pt transportation/logistics breakdown	7	0.05	1	0.02	2	0.06
Surgeon unavailable	3	0.02	0	0.00	0	0.00
Surgery no longer needed	27	0.2	2	0.03	0	0.00
Financial issues	2	0.01	1	0.02	0	0.00
Unknown/not stated	17	0.1	4	0.07	2	0.06
Grand total	212	1.4	31	0.5	13	0. 4

Table 4 American Society of Anesthesiologists (ASA) Physical Classification Spectrum

ASA classification	All surgery[a] (%)	CPA (%)	NS (%)
1	5.9	4.0	29.1
2	34.3	37.6	60.2
3	45.6	51.0	8.6
4	7.0	4.4	0.1
1–4E	7.3	3.0	2.1

[a]The dataset used to calculate "All surgery" was different than the denominator dataset in this study

good evidence to support such programs, they can be expensive (Qiu et al. 2006), and reimbursement for this process may increasingly become part of a global admission fee. Therefore, it is useful to analyze how these preoperative processes can be modified to reduce costs, duplication, and inconvenience but still to reliably triage unoptimized patients to more intensive investigation, to provide consistent assessment and documentation, and to minimize DOSCs. An increasingly common process is one where preoperative information gathering and education, in selected lower risk cases, are done by a nurse, often by telephone (Wittkugel and Varughese 2015; Kinley et al. 2002; Boudreau and Gibson 2011; Dexter et al. 2014). A previous study of these processes at this institution showed equally high patient satisfaction with NS and CPA (Olson and Bock 2011). Because of the success of this process, the thresholds are sometimes expanded to more complicated patients; as this happens, it is important to analyze whether downstream effects, such as DOSCs, are affected negatively.

Determining a rate of DOSCs is challenging (Dexter et al. 2005; Ehrenfeld et al. 2013) because cancellations and cases are increasingly electronic, changing, and difficult to capture after the fact. The iteration used in this study is similar to previous studies (Argo et al. 2009; Leslie et al. 2012; van Klei et al. 2002), being the schedule published in the afternoon of the day before surgery.

This study shows that the overall DOSC rate at this institution is only 1.23 %. That the preoperative process is driving at least part of the low rate is suggested by the fact that the CPA rate of 0.48 % and the NS rate of 0.60 % are both lower than the overall rate of 1.23 %.

Comparison with other studies

Comparison of DOSC rates between institutions and points in time must be done cautiously (Dexter et al. 2005) and in general terms only. But comparing the rate in this study to other studies does warrant some comment, as the rate in this study is one of the lowest published, with the methodology and numbers, though modest, are more substantial than most.

It has been suggested that a reasonable target for DOSC is a rate of less than 5 % (Macario 2006). Academic medical centers have been reported to have DOSC rates twice as high as private or smaller hospitals (Schuster et al. 2011). In all published cases of DOSC rates < 5 %, a significant part of the success has been attributed to a structured preoperative process (see Table 5).

Fischer described the lowest published rate (Fischer 1996). That study differed from others in that it enumerated only cancellations occurring just before the patient entered the operating room. The rate for medical reasons was 0.2 %, which is similar to the 0.22 % rate for similar reasons in this study.

van Klei reported a rate of 0.9 % for medical reasons. This study from the Netherlands in the late 1990s was at a hospital where, even after the introduction of the outpatient preoperative evaluation clinic, the average preoperative hospital stay was 1.5 days (van Klei et al. 2002). In our study, the DOSC for the comparable categories was lower—being 0.63 % overall, 0.22 % if assessed with CPA, and 0.43 % for selective NS.

Prospective studies tend to have higher DOSC rates than retrospective ones (Pollard and Olson 1999). In this study, while the list of scheduled cases, CPA, and NS was collated retrospectively, it was used in a prospective fashion to determine which of the cases assessed preoperatively became a DOSC.

Reasons for cancellation

Because causes of DOSC are often multifactorial (Leslie et al. 2012), statistical analysis of the causes is fraught with difficulty (Leslie et al. 2012). Fixing one cause may not result in an immediate improvement; nevertheless, it will be usually useful for each institution to determine the most common reasons for DOSC and tackle those first.

As a balance of ease of recording and amount of detail, we chose 10 categories similar to previous studies (Xue et al. 2013; Gillen et al. 2009; Trentman et al. 2010). Although the reason for cancellation may be described differently by different staff members, we previously observed that the preoperative area clerks were the most consistent and probably least biased source of cancellation documentation. The fact that "unknown" continued to be a common reason shows that it is still an imperfect source. There is currently no validated instrument for description of cancellations. Inter-observer or intra-observer reliability was not assessed.

The most common reason for cancellation was a new medical condition. This is consistent with many other studies (Emanuel and Macpherseon 2013; Pollard et al. 1996; Trentman et al. 2010; Garg et al. 2009).

In this study, there was no clinically significant difference in the DOSC rate between services. Other studies

Table 5 Comparable published studies of DOSC rates

Study	Year	Subjects	DOSC rate (%)	Most common		Preop assess	Notes
				Reason	Absolute rate (%)		
Fischer (Fischer 1996)	1996	7485	0.2	Medical reasons	0.2	Yes	Cancellations after patient in operating suite
van Klei (van Klei et al. 2002)	2002	8466	4.6	Logistical reasons	2.7	Yes	Patients admitted preoperatively, mean 1.5 days
			0.9	Medical reasons	0.9	Yes	4.6 % is overall DOSC rate, 0.9 % for medical reasons
Trentman (Trentman et al. 2010)	2010	12,176	2.0	New condition	0.7	Yes	Expandable block time scheduled
Hussein (Hussain and Khan 2005)	2005	8526	4.0	Not stated	4.2	Yes	Pakistan
Hovlid (Hovlid et al. 2012)	2012	3021	4.9	Schedule overrun	Not stated	Yes	Norwegian community hospital
Gillen (Gillen et al. 2009)	2009	27,632	5.0	New/unknown medical condition	Not stated	Not stated	
Xue (Xue et al. 2013)	2013	2751	7.5	Inadequate preop preparation	2.2	No	
Pollard (Pollard et al. 1996)	1996	561	6.6	Medical reasons	2.2	Yes	Outpatient surgery
Leslie (Leslie et al. 2012)	2012	19,141	8.1	Process	4.7	Not stated	Canada, urological procedures
Argo (Argo et al. 2009)	2009	329,784	12.4	Patient related	4.3	Yes	Administrative data VA hospitals
Pollard (Pollard and Olson 1999)	1999	529	13.2	Insufficient OR time	2.8	Yes	Prospective

Studies at Ambulatory Surgery Centers are not included. The most common reason is expressed as a percent of total cases
Preop assess Institutional Preoperative Assessment Process, *VA* Veterans Administration

have reported higher relative rates for general surgery (Argo et al. 2009).

Anecdotally, doing a preoperative assessment the day before surgery is considered suboptimal as the opportunity to optimize is limited. However, this study does not show an increased rate of DOSCs for patients assessed the day before or the day of surgery. At this institution, there are staff and resources available to coordinate last-minute assessments and investigations if needed. At some institutions, these resources may not be available, and cancellation would be necessary. A recent study of cancellations of inpatients also suggested that late assessments were not a major contributor to DOSCs (Dexter et al. 2014).

Patients undergoing gastroenterology endoscopy procedures had a low rate of DOSC. One of these DOSCs had been assessed by NS on the scheduled day of surgery and cancelled because surgery was no longer needed. So while this study suggests that there is room for improvement, possibly with preoperative assessments, the rate is already so low that justification of preoperative assessments in this group will need to include reasons other than prevention of DOSC—such as preventing delay of surgical start time. Further study on the effect of preoperative assessments on delay of surgery start time is needed.

ASA classification
The threshold for NS was fairly inclusive—60 % were ASA 2 and 9 % were ASA 3 classification. The mix of ASA

classification of patients assessed with CPA was of slightly higher complexity than other studies which describe the classification (Ferschl et al. 2005) (see Table 4).

Shortcomings
This is a cohort study with subgroups; therefore, comparison of rates can only be done in a very general, observational fashion. The demographics and preoperative morbidity of the CPA, NS, and non-assessed groups were not compared.

The denominators of this study are snapshots of a constantly changing number. The posted schedule the afternoon before surgery will differ from the completed case list, not only by the DOSCs and by add-ons but also by cases moved to other sites. Cases that were known to be cancelled by the surgeon and the patient more than 24 h before scheduled time, but not known to the scheduling staff, will have been included as DOSCs.

It is not possible to determine how many DOSCs, potentially a result of inadequate preoperative process, were averted by cooperative schedule adjustments or urgent arrangement of medical investigations that satisfied concerns and allowed a postponed start. The study did not capture who made the decision to cancel the case.

The study included primarily outpatients. In the time period of the study, 98 % of elective cases where admitted the day of surgery. Emergency cases from either the emergency department or the wards were not included.

Thus, it cannot be compared to studies that concentrate on inpatients (Epstein and Dexter 2015).

Some authors have described that cancellation rates should be compared in batches, because one cancellation may result in others (Dexter et al. 2005). In this study however, there was rarely more than one cancellation per day, so such interactions were not likely a common issue.

Cost of DOSC
Calculating the financial impact of cancellations is challenging, as cancellations actually decrease some variable costs, and the potential lost income varies by the contribution margin of the procedure (Macario et al. 2001).

The value of a low DOSC also includes patient satisfaction, less delays in the preoperative holding area, and less staff frustration (Bader et al. 2009). It is difficult to assign a monetary value to these issues.

A low DOSC rate is perhaps more a marker of medical optimization and efficiency than a determinant of those factors. As long as the rate of cancellations is relatively predictable, it is possible to plan for it and thus not impact operating room efficiency. Therefore, a more practical goal is to maintain a low DOSC rate commensurate with the efficiency of other aspects of a particular institution's operating room management but with the least resources and patient inconvenience required to produce safe and efficient perioperative care.

Outside referral vs. surgical home model of care
Many facilities operate without a comprehensive preoperative process by deferring the preoperative process to clinicians outside the institution. This will minimize the inconvenience and cost of such preparation from the institution's perspective but not necessarily reduce inconvenience and cost from the perspective of patients or insurers.

However, it is likely that in other systems—such as single payer or Accountable Care Organizations—a coordinated, comprehensive perioperative care would prove to be a more cost-effective and patient-centered approach (Song et al. 2014). Studies are needed which compare overall charges in the perioperative period in a system with comprehensive coordinated perioperative care (surgical home model) vs. overall charges in a more traditional system with routine protocols for testing, and outside consultations are needed. The increase of all-payer claims databases should allow assessment of this (Peters et al. 2014). The state where this study was conducted does not yet have such a database.

There is much recent interest in anesthesiology involvement in the perioperative surgical home (Dexter and Wachtel 2014), but anesthesiologists are probably best utilized as directors of protocols and care as opposed to the actual delivery. This study shows that such

information gathering and basic medical management can be done effectively and efficiently by advanced care clinicians and nurses, albeit with strong support, backup, and continual education from anesthesiology.

Conclusions
A DOSC rate for all causes of less than 2 % is achievable at a tertiary care academic hospital where a CPA and management process are in place, supervised by the department of anesthesiology, but where a significant proportion of those assessments are done by a selective NS process.

Abbreviations
CI: confidence interval; CPA: comprehensive preoperative assessment; DOSCs: day of surgery cancellations; NS: nurse screening.

Competing interests
The authors declare that they have no competing interests.

Authors' contributions
RO conceived the study, participated in the design and coordination of the study, and drafted and wrote the manuscript. ID performed the statistical analysis and assisted with the drafting of the manuscript. Both authors read and approved the final manuscript.

Acknowledgements
The author gratefully acknowledges the assistance of Anthony Basil and Mildred Perry in data collection.

Funding
There were no funding sources for this project.

References
Argo JL, Vick CC, Graham LA, Itani KM, Bishop MJ, Hawn MT. Elective surgical case cancellation in the Veterans Health Administration system: identifying areas for improvement. Am J Surg. 2009;198(5):600–6.
Bader AM, Sweitzer B, Kumar A. Nuts and bolts of preoperative clinics: the view from three institutions. Clev Clin J Med. 2009;76 Suppl 4:S104–11.
Boudreau SA, Gibson MJ. Surgical cancellations: a review of elective surgery cancellations in a tertiary care pediatric institution. J Perianesth Nurs. 2011; 26(5):315–22.
Dexter F, Wachtel RE. Strategies for net cost reductions with the expanded role and expertise of anesthesiologists in the perioperative surgical home. Anesth Analg. 2014;118(5):1062–71.
Dexter F, Marcon E, Epstein RH, Ledolter J. Validation of statistical methods to compare cancellation rates on the day of surgery. Anesth Analg. 2005;101(2):465–73.
Dexter F, Maxbauer T, Stout C, Archbold L, Epstein RH. Relative influence on total cancelled operating room time from patients who are inpatients or outpatients preoperatively. Anesth Analg. 2014;118(5):1072–80.
Ehrenfeld JM, Dexter F, Rothman BS, Johnson AM, Epstein RH. Case cancellation rates measured by surgical service differ whether based on the number of cases or the number of minutes cancelled. Anesth Analg. 2013;117(3):711–6.
Emanuel A, Macpherseon R. The anaesthetic pre-admission clinic is effective in minimising surgical cancellation rates. Anaesth Intensive Care. 2013;41(1):90–4.
Epstein RH, Dexter F. Management implications for the perioperative surgical home related to inpatient case cancellations and add-on case scheduling on the day of surgery. Anesth Analg. 2015;121(1):206–18.
Ferschl MB, Tung A, Sweitzer B, Huo D, Glick DB. Preoperative clinic visits reduce operating room cancellations and delays. Anesthesiology. 2005;103(4):855–9.
Fischer SP. Development and effectiveness of an anesthesia preoperative evaluation clinic in a teaching hospital. Anesthesiology. 1996;85(1):196–206.
Fixler T, Wright JG. Identification and use of operating room efficiency indicators: the problem of definition. Can J Surg. 2013;56(4):224–6.
Garg R, Bhalotra AR, Bhadoria P, Gupta N, Anand R. Reasons for cancellation of cases on the day of surgery-a prospective study. Indian J Anaesth. 2009;53(1):35–9.

Gillen SM, Catchings K, Edney L, Prescott R, Andrews SM. What's all the fuss about? Day-of-surgery cancellations and the role of perianesthesia nurses in prevention. J Perianesth Nurs. 2009;24(6):396–8.

Hovlid E, Bukve O, Haug K, Aslaksen A, von Plessen C. A new pathway for elective surgery to reduce cancellation rates. BMC Health Serv Res. 2012; 12(1):1–9.

Hussain AM, Khan FA. Anaesthetic reasons for cancellation of elective surgical inpatients on the day of surgery in a teaching hospital. J Pak Med Assoc. 2005;55(9):374–8.

Kain ZN, Hwang J, Warner MA. Disruptive innovation and the specialty of anesthesiology: the case for the perioperative surgical home. Anesthesia Analgesia. 2015;120(5):1155–7.

Kinley H, Czoski-Murray C, George S, McCabe C, Primrose J, Reilly C, et al. Effectiveness of appropriately trained nurses in preoperative assessment: randomised controlled equivalence/non-inferiority trial. BMJ. 2002; 325(7376):1323.

Knox M, Myers E, Hurley M. The impact of pre-operative assessment clinics on elective surgical case cancellations. Surgeon. 2009;7(2):76–8.

Leslie RJ, Beiko D, Van Vlymen J, Siemens DR. Day of surgery cancellation rates in urology: identification of modifiable factors. Can Urol Assoc J. 2013;7(5-6): 167–173.

Macario A. Are your hospital operating rooms "efficient"? A scoring system with eight performance indicators. Anesthesiology. 2006;105(2):237–40.

Macario A, Dexter F, Traub RD. Hospital profitability per hour of operating room time can vary among surgeons. Anesth Analg. 2001;93(3):669–75.

Miller TE, Thacker JK, White WD, Mantyh C, Migaly J, Jin J, et al. Reduced length of hospital stay in colorectal surgery after implementation of an enhanced recovery protocol. Anesth Analg. 2014;118(5):1052–61.

Newman MF, Mathew JP, Aronson S. The evolution of anesthesiology and perioperative medicine. Anesthesiology. 2013;118(5):1005–7.

Olson R, Bock K. Assessment of patient satisfaction of nurse screening vs complete preoperative assessment. Clev Clin J Med. 2011;78 Suppl 1:eS30.

Peters A, Sachs J, Porter J, Love D, Costello A. The value of all-payer claims databases to states. NC Med J. 2014;75(3):211–3.

Pollard JB, Olson L. Early outpatient preoperative anesthesia assessment: does it help to reduce operating room cancellations? Anesth Analg. 1999;89(2):502–5.

Pollard JB, Zboray AL, Mazze RI. Economic benefits attributed to opening a preoperative evaluation clinic for outpatients. Anesth Analg. 1996;83(2):407–10.

Qiu C, Macvay MA, Sanchez AF. Anesthesia preoperative medicine clinic: beyond surgery cancellations. Anesthesiology. 2006;105(1):224–5.

Schuster M, Neumann C, Neumann K, Braun J, Geldner G, Martin J, et al. The effect of hospital size and surgical service on case cancellation in elective surgery: results from a prospective multicenter study. Anesth Analg. 2011; 113(3):578–85.

Song Z, Sequist TD, Barnett ML. Patient referrals: a linchpin for increasing the value of care. JAMA. 2014;312(6):597–8.

Trentman T, Mueller JT, Fassett SL, Dormer CL, Weinmeister KP. Day of surgery cancellations in a tertiary care hospital: a one year review. J Anesthe Clinic Res. 2010;1:109. doi:10.4172/2155-6148.1000109.

van Klei WA, Moons KG, Rutten CL, Schuurhuis A, Knape JT, Kalkman CJ, et al. The effect of outpatient preoperative evaluation of hospital inpatients on cancellation of surgery and length of hospital stay. Anesth Analg. 2002;94(3): 644–9. table of contents.

van Klei WA, Kalkman CJ, Moons KG. Effects of an anesthesia preoperative medicine clinic. Anesthesiology. 2006;105(1):224.

Wittkugel E, Varughese A. Development of a nurse-assisted preanesthesia evaluation program for pediatric outpatient anesthesia. Paediatr Anaesth. 2015;25(7):719–26.

Xue W, Yan Z, Barnett R, Fleisher L, Liu R. Dynamics of elective case cancellation for inpatient and outpatient in an academic center. J Anesth Clin Res. 2013;4(5):314.

Potential return on investment for implementation of perioperative goal-directed fluid therapy in major surgery: a nationwide database study

Frederic Michard[1*], William K. Mountford[2,3], Michelle R. Krukas[2,4], Frank R. Ernst[2,5] and Sandy L. Fogel[6]

Abstract

Background: Preventable postsurgical complications are increasingly recognized as a major clinical and economic burden. A recent meta-analysis showed a 17–29 % decrease in postoperative morbidity with goal-directed fluid therapy. Our objective was to estimate the potential economic impact of perioperative goal-directed fluid therapy.

Methods: We studied 204,680 adult patients from 541 US hospitals who had a major non-cardiac surgical procedure between January 2011 and June 2013. Hospital costs (including 30-day readmission costs) in patients with and without complications were extracted from the Premier Inc. research database, and potential cost-savings associated with a 17–29 % decrease in postoperative morbidity were estimated.

Results: A total of 76,807 patients developed one or more postsurgical complications (morbidity rate 37.5 %). In patients with and without complications, hospital costs were US$27,607 ± 32,788 and US$15,783 ± 12,282 ($p < 0.0001$), respectively. Morbidity rate was anticipated to decrease to 26.6–31.1 % with goal-directed fluid therapy, yielding potential gross cost-savings of US$153–263 million for the study period, US$61–105 million per year, or US$754–1286 per patient. Potential savings per patient were highly variable from one surgical procedure to the other, ranging from US$354–604 for femur and hip-fracture repair to US$3515–5996 for esophagectomies. When taking into account the volume of procedures, the total potential savings per year were the most significant (US$32–55 million) for colectomies.

Conclusions: Postsurgical complications occurred in more than one third of our study population and had a dramatic impact on hospital costs. With goal-directed fluid therapy, potential cost-savings per patient were US$754–1286. The highest cost-savings per year were observed for colectomies. These projections should help hospitals estimate the return on investment when considering the implementation of goal-directed fluid therapy.

Keywords: Surgery, Complications, Costs, Goal-directed fluid therapy, Savings, Return on investment

Background

Preventable postoperative complications are increasingly recognized as a major healthcare burden (Birkmeyer et al. 2012; Dimick et al. 2006). After major operations, especially in patients with co-morbidities, complications are not exceptions (Ghaferi et al. 2009) and have adverse effects on long-term quality of life and survival (Khuri et al. 2005; Brown et al. 2014; Artinyan et al. 2015). They are

also responsible for a significant increase in hospital length of stay (LOS) (Eappen et al. 2013), readmission rates (Lawson et al. 2013; Merkow et al. 2015), and costs (Eappen et al. 2013; Dimick et al. 2004; Wick et al. 2011).

Perioperative fluid management is a key determinant of postoperative outcome. Both hypovolemia and fluid overload are associated with an increase in complications after surgery (Bellamy 2006). For a given surgical procedure, studies have shown a large intra- and inter-practitioner variability in the amount of fluid administered during the perioperative period (Lilot et al. 2015). Goal-directed fluid therapy (GDFT) consists of assessing

* Correspondence: frederic.michard@bluewin.ch
[1]Department of Critical Care, Edwards Lifesciences, 1 Edwards Way, Irvine, CA, USA
Full list of author information is available at the end of the article

individual fluid needs during and/or after surgery by monitoring flow parameters such as stroke volume and cardiac output (Pearse et al. 2014). A recent meta-analysis of 38 randomized controlled trials showed that the use of GDFT decreases the rate of patients developing one or more complications by 17–29 % (Pearse et al. 2014). Fuelled by this body of evidence, consensus statements (Mythen et al. 2012; Navarro et al. 2015) and guidelines (Vallet et al. 2013; Gustafsson et al. 2013) have been published, and GDFT has been integrated into the Enhanced Recovery in NSQIP (ERIN) collaborative. But today, the adoption of GDFT is still very limited in the USA (Cannesson et al. 2011; Miller et al. 2011). One of the barriers to the hospital adoption of GDFT may be the short-term financial investment necessary to acquire cardiac output-monitoring technologies. To ensure a fair economic evaluation, this investment must be balanced with the economic benefits related to the decrease in complications that is expected from the implementation of GDFT.

The goals of our study were twofold: describe the economic consequences of postoperative complications in a nationwide population of patients undergoing major non-cardiac surgery and estimate the economic impact of the reduction in postoperative morbidity expected from GDFT. This estimation should help hospitals to estimate the return on investment when considering the implementation of GDFT.

Methods
Data source
De-identified data from all adult inpatients, who had major non-cardiac surgery between January 2011 and June 2013, were selected from the Premier research database. The Premier research database contains patient data from over 600 US hospitals spanning all geographic regions, containing teaching and non-teaching as well as urban and rural hospitals of all sizes. Examination of the database allows the determination of patients' characteristics, postsurgical complications, and costs of care. The database complies with the Health Insurance Portability and Accountability Act of 1996 (HIPAA) and other related regulations. Any institutional review board approval was not sought because of the pre-existing, retrospective, and de-identified nature of the data.

Patient selection
Ten major surgical procedures were selected based on previous studies showing positive outcomes associated with the use of GDFT (Benes et al. 2010; Bisgaard et al. 2013; Boyd et al. 1993; Gan et al. 2002; Kuper et al. 2011; Lobo et al. 2000; Noblett et al. 2006; Pearse et al. 2005; Pillai et al. 2011; Ramsingh et al. 2013; Sinclair et al. 1997; Ueno et al. 1998; Venn et al. 2002; Wakeling et al. 2005; Wilson et al. 1999). Corresponding International

Classification of Diseases, Ninth Revision, Clinical Modification (ICD-9) codes were used to search specific procedures in the Premier research database (see Additional file 1: Table S1). Because GDFT has thus far been shown to be effective only in adults, those under 18 years of age were excluded. Patients in whom cardiac output was monitored on the day of surgery were also excluded, since they may have received GDFT.

Patient characteristic data collection
Patients' characteristics, including gender, age, and co-morbidities (based on ICD-9 diagnosis codes) were tabulated. The Charlson Co-morbidity Index (CCI) was calculated as previously described (Charlson et al. 1994). Twenty six infectious, gastro-intestinal, respiratory, renal, cardiovascular, neurologic, and hematologic in-hospital postoperative complications were identified using ICD-9 diagnosis codes, ensuring that the diagnosis was not determined to be present at admission (see Additional file 2: Table S2). Morbidity rate was defined as the proportion of patients developing one or more complications during the index hospital stay. Patients were sorted into two groups: those with one or more complications and those without any complications. For each group, hospital length of stay and readmission rates at 30 days were studied.

Cost data collection and cost-savings projection
Costs related to the in-hospital treatment and readmission up to 30 days after discharge were obtained from the Premier database and compared in patients with and without complications. Costs are those associated with the actual procedures, as determined by the hospital using its accounting systems, and include both fixed and variable components.

The recently published JAMA meta-analysis by Pearse et al. (Pearse et al. 2014) was used to estimate the potential reduction in postoperative morbidity with GDFT. This meta-analysis reported an average 23 % reduction in odds of a postoperative complication (odds ratio 0.77, 95 % CI 0.71 to 0.83, $p < 0.05$) associated with the use of GDFT. Potential cost-savings were determined by using the projected number of patients developing one or more complications and the estimated related costs. This analysis was performed for the entire cohort, as well as for each surgical procedure. The analysis assumes a complete, new implementation of GDFT.

Statistical analysis
Hospital LOS, readmission rates, and costs were compared between patients with and without complications. Readmission rates (%) were compared using chi-squared tests and hospital LOS (median ± interquartiles), and costs (mean ± SD) were compared using Wilcoxon rank-

sum and *t* tests, respectively. All statistical comparisons were considered statistically significant assuming a two-tailed alpha level of 0.05.

Total costs were further analyzed using multivariable generalized linear models. The models utilized a gamma distribution and log link to account for the skewness in the outcome data. The model estimated the least-squares mean total costs while controlling for potential confounding variables including patient age, gender, co-morbidities (as measured by the CCI), and elective/non-elective admission. An additional model was performed as a sensitivity analysis and added the type of surgery to the other potential confounders.

Results

A total of 204,680 patients from 541 medical centers met the search criteria. Among these centers, 86.6 % were urban, 58.3 % were non-teaching hospitals, and 65.7 % had 300 or more beds. Patients' characteristics are summarized in Table 1. Numbers of patients per surgery group are reported in Table 2. A total of 76,807 patients developed one

or more postsurgical complications (average morbidity rate 37.5 %). Complication rates ≥1 % are shown in Fig. 1. Morbidity rates for each surgery group are presented in Table 3.

Impact of postsurgical complications on hospital length of stay and readmission rate

In patients with one or more complications and in patients without any complications, 30-day readmission rates were 17.2 and 11.9 % (*p* < 0.001), respectively. Median hospital length of stay was 7 [4, 10] (25th–75th percentiles) and 4 [3, 5] days (*p* < 0.001), respectively. The impact of postoperative complications on hospital length of stay and 30-day readmission rates for each surgery group is presented in Table 2.

Economic impact of postsurgical complications

Average unadjusted costs (index hospitalization + 30-day readmission costs when applicable) were US\$27,607 ± 32,788 per patient with one or more complications (*n* = 73,108) and US\$15,783 ± 12,282 (*p* < 0.001) per patient with no complications (*n* = 127,398).

Table 1 Characteristics of the study population

	All	With complications	Without complications
	n = 204,680	*n* = 76,807	*n* = 127,873
Age (years)	64.8 ± 17.2	68.8 ± 16.0	62.4 ± 17.4
Gender (% female)	58.8	58.4	59.0
Elective surgery (%)	54.8	45.2	60.5
ICU admission (%)	22.4	36.2	14.1
Mortality (%)	1.9	4.6	0.2
Myocardial infarction (%)	6.2	8.8	4.6
Congestive heart failure (%)	7.5	12.3	4.6
Peripheral vascular disease (%)	7.3	9.0	6.2
Cerebrovascular disease (%)	2.0	3.2	1.4
Hemiplegia or paraplegia (%)	0.4	0.7	0.2
Dementia (%)	0.8	1.1	0.5
Chronic pulmonary disease (%)	19.3	23.8	16.6
Rheumatologic disease (%)	2.6	3.0	2.3
Peptic ulcer disease (%)	1.3	1.9	0.9
Mild liver disease (%)	1.0	1.3	0.8
Moderate or severe liver disease (%)	0.4	0.6	0.2
Diabetes (%)	19.9	21.1	19.2
Diabetes with complications (%)	2.2	2.8	1.9
Renal disease (%)	9.3	14.1	6.3
Any malignancy (%)	22.1	24.1	20.8
Metastatic solid tumor (%)	6.6	7.7	6.0
AIDS (%)	0.1	0.1	0.1
Charlson Co-morbidity Index	1.8 ± 2.3	2.2 ± 2.5	1.5 ± 2.2

All comparisons "with complications vs. without complications" were statistically significant with *p* < 0.0001, with the exception of gender (*p* = 0.0386) and AIDS (*p* = 0.2912)

Table 2 Hospital length of stay (HLOS), 30-day readmission rate, and costs in patients with one or more complications (with) and in patients without any complications (without)

Surgery	HLOS, days, median [IQR]		Readmission rate, %		Cost, dollar[a], mean ± SD	
n	With	Without	With	Without	With	Without
All	7 [4–10]	4 [3–5]	17.2	11.9	27,607 ± 32,788	15,783 ± 12,282
204,680						
AAA open repair	8 [6–14]	6 [4–7]	16.5	8.7	48,002 ± 48,841	24,619 ± 14,543
2328						
Vascular bypass	6 [4–9]	3 [2–5]	21.3	14.1	31,979 ± 30,386	16,849 ± 12,543
16,336						
Esophagectomy	13 [9–20]	9 [8–11]	18.5	15.4	67,924 ± 65,377	37,382 ± 17,973
690						
Gastrectomy	4 [2–10]	2 [1, 2]	12.7	5.2	27,794 ± 33,530	12,641 ± 9,452
25,118						
Colectomy	8 [5–11]	4 [3–6]	15.2	9.0	27,851 ± 29,286	14,755 ± 10,524
75,121						
Resection of rectum	7 [5–11]	5 [3–6]	15.2	10.4	26,916 ± 24,466	15,979 ± 18,855
10,753						
Hepatectomy	7 [5–11]	5 [3–6]	17.9	9.4	37,315 ± 38,100	20,272 ± 13,566
2362						
Pancreatectomy	11 [8–18]	7 [5–9]	26.1	18.6	50,559 ± 46,784	27,488 ± 19,653
3569						
Cystectomy	10 [7–14]	7 [6–8]	29.2	21.9	41,128 ± 38,293	25,978 ± 15,061
2552						
F&H fracture repair	5 [4–7]	4 [3–5]	18.9	17.4	22,218 ± 32,644	16,805 ± 12,167
65,851						

All comparisons "with vs. without" were statistically significant with $p < 0.0001$

AAA abdominal aortic aneurysm, *F&H* femur and hip

[a]For patients with valid cost data, unadjusted

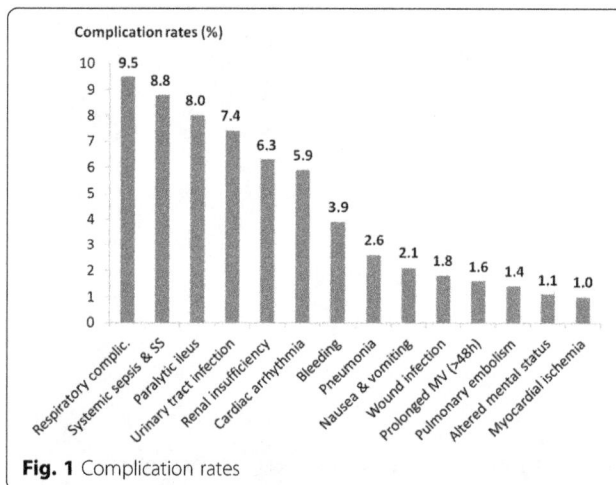

Fig. 1 Complication rates

In other words, patients with one or more complications were on average US$11,824 more costly than patients with no complications. Thus, from January 2011 to June 2013, the 541 hospitals whose data were used in these analyses spent an estimated total of more than US$908 million (US$11,824 × 76,807 patients) to treat postsurgical complications in the study population (US$363 million per year). The economic impact of postoperative complications for each surgery group is presented in Table 2.

Results from the multivariable model were directionally consistent with the descriptive analysis. The average estimated costs after controlling for confounders were significantly different, US$25,390 vs. US$14,841 ($p < 0.001$, cost difference US$10,549) per patient with one or more complications and per patient with no complications, respectively. Furthermore, when the model also controlled for the type of surgery, the estimated costs remained significantly different (US$32,182 vs. $19,803; $p < 0.001$, cost difference US$12,379).

Table 3 Morbidity rate, cost difference between patients with and without complications, and expected savings per patient receiving goal-directed fluid therapy (GDFT)

Surgery	Morbidity rate, %	Cost difference between patients with and without complications, dollar	Potential savings per patient with GDFT, dollar[a]
All	37.5	11,824	754–1286
AAA open repair	64.9	23,383	2580–4401
Vascular bypass	26.3	15,130	676–1154
Esophagectomy	67.7	30,542	3515–5996
Gastrectomy	20.2	15,153	520–888
Colectomy	43.3	13,096	964–1644
Resection of rectum	33.6	10,937	625–1066
Hepatectomy	34.3	17,043	994–1695
Pancreatectomy	47.5	23,071	1863–3178
Cystectomy	58.9	15,150	1517–2588
F&H fracture repair	38.5	5413	354–604

AAA abdominal aortic aneurysm, F&H femur and hip
[a]For patients with valid cost data, unadjusted

Projected cost-savings with implementation of GDFT

The projected number of patients developing one or more complications, assuming an odds ratio ranging between 0.71 and 0.83, was 54,533–63,750 (morbidity rate 26.6–31.1 %). Thus, after implementation of GDFT, projected gross savings were US$153–263 million for the study period, US$61–105 million per year, or US$754–1286 per patient (Table 3). Projected cost-savings per year for each surgery group are presented in Fig. 2.

Discussion

In our large patient population who underwent major non-cardiac surgery, postoperative complications were observed in more than one third of the cases and increased costs on average by US$11,824 per patient (+75 %). These findings are consistent with those reported by previous and smaller studies. In 1008 patients who underwent general and vascular surgery, Dimick et al. (Dimick et al. 2006) reported a US$10,178 cost difference between patients with and without complications. In a similar surgical population, Boltz et al. (Boltz et al. 2012) showed in 2250 patients that the excess costs were US$6358, US$12,802, and US$42,790 for patients developing 1, 2, 3 or more complications, respectively. In the present study, the occurrence of postoperative complications was also associated with prolonged length of stay (+3 days) and increased hospital readmission rates at 30 days (+5.3 % absolute increase, +44 % relative increase). These findings are consistent with previous reports (Eappen et al. 2013; Lawson et al. 2013)

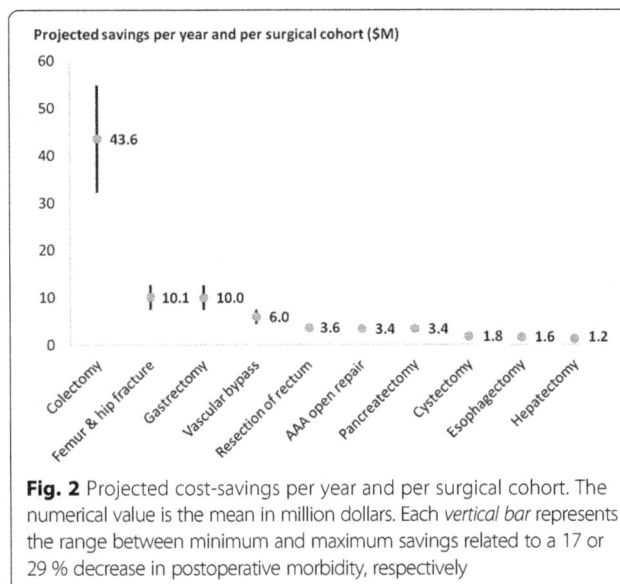

Fig. 2 Projected cost-savings per year and per surgical cohort. The numerical value is the mean in million dollars. Each *vertical bar* represents the range between minimum and maximum savings related to a 17 or 29 % decrease in postoperative morbidity, respectively

emphasizing the dramatic impact of complications on length of stay and readmission rates. This highlights a relevant savings capacity for major surgical procedures.

According to a recent meta-analysis of 38 randomized controlled trials, GDFT has the potential to decrease postoperative morbidity by 17–29 % (Pearse et al. 2014). In our study population, such a decrease in postoperative morbidity would translate into cost-savings ranging between US$754 and US$1286 per patient. Interestingly, potential savings were highly variable from one surgical procedure to the other (Table 3). Two factors affect savings per patient: the actual morbidity rate (the higher the morbidity rate, the higher the savings when all patients receive GDFT) and the cost of complications (the higher the cost, the higher the savings). The actual morbidity rates ranged from 20.2 % for gastrectomies to 67.7 % for esophagectomies (Table 3), and cost of complications ranged from US$5413 for femur and hip-fracture repair to US$30,542 for esophagectomies (Table 3). This large range in morbidity rates and costs of complications explain why the range of potential savings with GDFT was also wide, from US$354–604/patient for femur and hip-fracture repair to US$3515–5996/patient for esophagectomies (Table 3). A third factor affects savings at the hospital level: the volume of surgeries. When taking into account the volume of procedures, the total potential savings per year were the most significant (US$32–55 million), for colectomies, by far (Fig. 2). This finding supports the notion that GDFT should be implemented as a priority in this surgical population.

Three recent studies tried to estimate potential savings related to the use of GDFT. The first study (Bartha et al. 2012) from Sweden is a decision analytic model where assumptions were made regarding morbidity rates before and after GDFT implementation, as well as on hospital costs. This study focused on elderly hip-fracture patients, and the model estimated a 1882 € (around US$2000) cost reduction per patient with GDFT. The second study from the UK was based on a small population of 122 patients who underwent major surgery (Ebm et al. 2014). Morbidity rates before and after GDFT implementation were real, but assumptions were made regarding hospital costs. This study suggested a cost reduction of £2631 (around US$4000) per patient with GDFT. Differences between US and European healthcare systems and costs, as well as the fact that costs were not real but estimated in the Swedish and the UK study, may explain why they both reported potential savings higher than our projections. In the third study, Manecke et al. (Manecke et al. 2014) used real morbidity rates and real costs extracted from the UHC database, which is a large administrative database containing clinical and economic data from over 120 US academic hospitals. As in our study, the only assumption made was related to the reduction in postoperative morbidity with GDFT. Manecke et al. (Manecke et al. 2014) reported potential cost-savings ranging from US$569 to US$970 per patient, i.e., slightly lower than ours. The UHC database contains only 11 possible postoperative complications and is known to underestimate postoperative morbidity rates (Steinberg et al. 2008). For instance, they did not take into account postoperative paralytic ileus, which is not a major complication but a frequent one (Fig. 1), known to have a significant impact on hospital length of stay and costs (Iyer et al. 2009). Finally, the economic evaluation of Manecke et al. (Manecke et al. 2014) did not include 30-day readmission costs, and was limited to academic hospitals. Our analysis was based on a larger number of patients and considered 26 different postoperative complications (including paralytic ileus). We took into account 30-day readmission costs, and 58.2 % of our study population came from non academic centers. For these reasons, we believe that our study provides a more accurate estimation of potential savings associated with the implementation of GDFT at a national level.

To assess a return of investment, our projected savings must be balanced with costs related to GDFT implementation. Assuming average cardiac output-monitoring-related costs of US$300 per patient (US$250 for disposable sensor + US$48 for the amortization of a US$15,000 monitor used two times a week over 3 years), our findings suggest that for each dollar spent to implement GDFT, hospitals should save in return between US$2.5 and US$4. GDFT implementation costs may vary from one hospital to the other, but each hospital could easily forecast the return on investment using its own costs and our model.

Another major burden of complications is the opportunity cost of lost beds for increased length of stay and re-admissions in patients with complications. In busy hospitals, these are beds not taken by new patients with new DRGs and the accompanying payments. With an increased length of stay of 3 days for patients with complications (Table 2), the 76,807 patients with complications represent 230,421 ($3 \times 76,807$) days lost. With the assumption that GDFT would decrease the number of patients with one or more complications to 54,533–63,750 (a 17 to 29 % decrease), it would now represent only 163,599–191,250 days lost. In other words, GDFT has the potential to save between 39,171 and 66,822 days. With the average hospital length of stay across all studied surgical cohorts being 5 days, the implementation of GDFT could result in 7834–13,364 (39,171 and 66,822 divided by 5) new patients admitted in our 541 hospitals over the 2.5-year study period, or 3134–5346 new patients per year. Since payments to hospitals vary so widely, each hospital can use this approach to calculate the increased payment and profit to the bottom line. This is the lost opportunity cost of having patients with complications take up hospital beds needed for other patients and represents the potential additional profit to the hospital. This may easily outweigh the savings from decreased complications.

Our study has certain limitations that should be considered. The analysis was limited to specific major surgeries in which outcome has already conclusively been shown to be improved by the use of GDFT. There are other surgeries, such as major spine and gynecologic surgeries, in which this approach would likely be associated with fewer complications (Mythen et al. 2012; Gan et al. 2002). Our study assumes complete implementation of GDFT, which may be an unrealistic goal. Also, we considered the same postsurgical morbidity reduction with GDFT for all surgical procedures, which may not always be the case. However, previous meta-analysis (Pearse et al. 2014; Hamilton et al. 2011) did not find any interaction between the type of surgery and the effect of GDFT. The article by Pearse et al. (Pearse et al. 2014) was chosen to estimate the effect of GDFT on postoperative morbidity because it is the most recent meta-analysis on the topic. It is important to note that it included studies published many years ago. Because both anesthesia and surgical practices changed over time, the assumption that GDFT would reduce postoperative morbidity by 17–29 % may be questioned in 2015. A meta-analysis by Hamilton et al. (Hamilton et al. 2011) studied the clinical effects of GDFT over time. If GDFT had no effect on mortality in studies published after 2000, the reduction in postoperative morbidity was still highly significant, ranging between 50 and 71 % (average odds ratio 0.38, CI 0.29 to 0.50). Interestingly, if we had used these odds ratios for our calculations, the projected savings with GDFT would have been much higher than those we have reported. Having said that, we must acknowledge that enhanced recovery programs have gained acceptance only recently, as well as changes in the type of fluid administered during the perioperative period (starches and unbalanced crystalloid solutions are used less often). Therefore, the clinical effects of GDFT in this new perioperative medicine era remain to be evaluated by large studies. Finally, we did not have access to reimbursement data, so we were unable to study the effects of morbidity reduction on hospital profit or profit margin, another very important economic driver for the hospital adoption of any new therapeutic strategy (Dimick et al. 2006; Flynn et al. 2014).

Conclusions

In patients who underwent major non-cardiac surgery, our study demonstrates that postsurgical complications are frequent and have a significant impact on hospital length of stay, readmission rates, and costs. It also suggests significant savings with GDFT; for each dollar spent to implement GDFT, our projections suggest that hospitals should save in return between US$2.5 and US$4. Projected cost-savings were the highest for the colectomy cohort, suggesting that priority should be given to the implementation of GDFT in this patient population.

Abbreviations
GDFT: Goal-directed fluid therapy; CCI: Charlson co-morbidity Index.

Competing interests
FM is an employee of Edwards Lifesciences, and SLF received consulting fees from Edwards Lifesciences. However, this manuscript does not support the use of any specific medical device for GDFT. MRK, WKM and FRE were employees of Premier, Inc. at the time of the analyses.

Authors' contributions
FM designed the study, participated in the interpretation of data, drafted the manuscript, and revised it critically for important intellectual content. WKM, MRK, and FRE participated in data analysis and revised the manuscript critically for important intellectual content. SLF has been involved in the interpretation of data and revised the manuscript critically for important intellectual content. All authors read and approved the final manuscript.

Acknowledgements
The study was sponsored by Edwards Lifesciences, and the analysis was performed by Premier Inc.

Author details
[1]Department of Critical Care, Edwards Lifesciences, 1 Edwards Way, Irvine, CA, USA. [2]Premier Inc., Charlotte, NC, USA. [3]Current address: Quintiles, Durham, NC, USA. [4]Current address: Quintiles, Cambridge, MA, USA. [5]Current address: Indegene Total Therapeutic Management, Kennesaw, GA, USA. [6]Virginia Tech Carilion School of Medicine, Roanoke, VA, USA.

References
Artinyan A, Orcutt ST, Anaya DA. Infectious postoperative complications decrease long-term survival in patients undergoing curative surgery for colorectal cancer: a study of 12,075 patients. Ann Surg. 2015;261:497–505.

Bartha E, Davidson T, Hommel A. Cost effectiveness analysis of goal-directed hemodynamic treatment of elderly hip fracture patients. Anesthesiology. 2012;117:519–30.

Bellamy MC. Wet, dry, or something else? Br J Anaesth. 2006;97:755–7.

Benes J, Chytra I, Altmann P. Intraoperative fluid optimization using stroke volume variation in high risk surgical patients: results of prospective randomized study. Crit Care. 2010;14:R118.

Birkmeyer JD, Gust C, Dimick JB. Hospital quality and the cost of inpatient surgery in the United States. Ann Surg. 2012;255:1–5.

Bisgaard J, Gilsaa T, Ronholm E. Haemodynamic optimisation in lower limb arterial surgery: room for improvement? Acta Anaesthesiol Scand. 2013;57:189–98.

Boltz MM, Hollenbeak CS, Ortenzi G. Synergistic implications of multiple postoperative outcomes. Am J Med Qual. 2012;27:383–90.

Boyd O, Grounds RM, Bennett ED. A randomized clinical trial of the effect of deliberate perioperative increase of oxygen delivery on mortality in high-risk surgical patients. JAMA. 1993;270:2699–707.

Brown SR, Mathew R, Keding A. The impact of postoperative complications on long-term quality of life after curative colorectal cancer surgery. Ann Surg. 2014;259:916–23.

Cannesson M, Pestel G, Ricks C. Hemodynamic monitoring and management in patients undergoing high risk surgery: a survey among North American and European anesthesiologists. Crit Care. 2011;15:R197.

Charlson M, Szatrowski TP, Peterson J. Validation of a combined comorbidity index. J Clin Epidemiol. 1994;47:1245–51.

Dimick JB, Chen SL, Taheri PA. Hospital costs associated with surgical complications: a report from the private-sector national surgical improvement program. J Am Coll Surg. 2004;199:531–7.

Dimick JB, Weeks WB, Karia RJ. Who pays for poor surgical quality? Building a business case for quality improvement. J Am Coll Surg. 2006;202:933–7.

Eappen S, Lane BH, Rosenberg B. Relationship between occurrence of surgical complications and hospital finances. JAMA. 2013;309:1599–606.

Ebm C, Cecconi M, Sutton L. A cost-effectiveness analysis of postoperative goal directed therapy for high-risk surgical patients. Crit Care Med. 2014;42:1194–203.

Flynn DN, Speck RM, Mahmoud NN. The impact of complications following open colectomy on hospital finances: a retrospective cohort study. Perioper Med. 2014;3:1.

Gan TJ, Soppitt A, Maroof M. Goal-directed intraoperative fluid administration reduces length of hospital stay after major surgery. Anesthesiology. 2002;97:820–6.

Ghaferi AA, Birkmeyer JD, Dimick JB. Variation in hospital mortality associated with inpatient surgery. N Engl J Med. 2009;361:1368–75.

Gustafsson UO, Scott MJ, Schwenk W. Guidelines for perioperative care in elective colonic surgery: enhanced recovery after surgery (ERAS) society. World J Surg. 2013;37:259–84.

Hamilton M, Cecconi M, Rhodes A. A systematic review and meta-analysis on the use of preemptive hemodynamic intervention to improve outcomes in moderate and high-risk surgery. Anesth Analg. 2011;112:1392–402.

Iyer S, Saunders WB, Stemkowski S. Economic burden of postoperative ileus associated with colectomy in the United States. J Manag Care Pharm. 2009;15:485–94.

Khuri SF, Henderson WG, DePalma RG. Determinants of long-term survival after major surgery and the adverse effect of postoperative complications. Ann Surg. 2005;242:326–43.

Kuper M, Gold SJ, Callow C. Intraoperative fluid management guided by oesophageal Doppler monitoring. BMJ. 2011;342:d3016.

Lawson EH, Hall BL, Louie R. Association between occurrence of a postoperative complication and readmission. Ann Surg. 2013;258:10–8.

Lilot M, Erhenfeld JM, Lee C. Variability in practice and factors predictive of total crystalloid administration during abdominal surgery: retrospective two-centre analysis. Br J Anaesth. 2015;114:767–76.

Lobo SMA, Salgado PF, Castillo VGT. Effects of maximizing oxygen delivery on morbidity and mortality in high-risk surgical patients. Crit Care Med. 2000;28:3396–404.

Manecke G, Asemota A, Michard F. Tackling the economic burden of postsurgical complications: would goal directed fluid therapy help? Crit Care. 2014;18:566.

Merkow RP, Ju MH, Chung JW. Underlying reasons associated with hospital readmission following surgery in the United States. JAMA. 2015;315:483–95.

Miller TE, Roche AM, Gan TJ. Poor adoption of hemodynamic optimization during major surgery: are we practicing substandard care? Anesth Analg. 2011;112:1274–6.

Mythen MG, Swart M, Acheson N. Perioperative fluid management: consensus statement from the enhanced recovery partnership. Perioper Med. 2012;1:2.

Navarro LHC, Bloomstone JA, Auler Jr JOC. Perioperative fluid theory: a statement from the international Fluid Optimization Group. Perioper Med. 2015;4:3.

Noblett SE, Snowden CP, Shenton BK. Randomized clinical trial assessing the effect of Doppler-optimized fluid management on outcome after elective colorectal resection. Br J Surg. 2006;93:1069–76.

Pearse R, Dawson D, Fawcett J. Early goal-directed therapy after major surgery reduces complications and duration of hospital stay. A randomised, controlled trial [ISRCTN38797445]. Crit Care. 2005;9:R687–93.

Pearse RM, Harrison DA, McDonald N. Effect of a perioperative, cardiac output-guided, hemodynamic therapy algorithm on outcomes following major gastrointestinal surgery: a randomized clinical trial and updated systematic review. JAMA. 2014;311:2181–90.

Pillai P, McEleavy I, Gaughan M. A double-blind randomized controlled clinical trial to assess the effect of Doppler optimized intraoperative fluid management on outcome following radical cystectomy. J Urol. 2011;186:2201–6.

Ramsingh DS, Sanghvi C, Gamboa J. Outcome impact of goal directed fluid therapy during high risk abdominal surgery in low to moderate risk patients: a randomized controlled trial. J Clin Monit Comput. 2013;27:249–57.

Sinclair S, James S, Singer M. Intraoperative intravascular volume optimisation and length of hospital stay after repair of proximal femoral fracture: randomised controlled trial. BMJ. 1997;315:909–12.

Steinberg SM, Popa MR, Michalek JA. Comparison of risk adjustment methodologies in surgical quality improvement. Surgery. 2008;144:662–9.

Ueno S, Tanabe G, Yamada H. Response of patients with cirrhosis who have undergone partial hepatectomy to treatment aimed at achieving supranormal oxygen delivery and consumption. Surgery. 1998;123:278–86.

Vallet B, Blanloeil Y, Cholley B. Guidelines for perioperative haemodynamic optimization. Ann Fr Anesth Reanim. 2013;32:454–62.

Venn R, Steele A, Richardson P, Poloniecki J. Randomized controlled trial to investigate influence of the fluid challenge on duration of hospital stay and perioperative morbidity in patients with hip fractures. Br J Anaesth. 2002;88:65–71.

Wakeling HG, McFall MR, Jenkins CS. Intraoperative oesophageal Doppler guided fluid management shortens postoperative hospital stay after major bowel surgery. Br J Anaesth. 2005;95:634–42.

Wick EC, Shore AD, Hirose K. Readmission rates and cost following colorectal surgery. Dis Colon Rectum. 2011;54:1475–9.

Wilson J, Woods I, Fawcett J. Reducing the risk of major elective surgery: randomised controlled trial of preoperative optimisation of oxygen delivery. BMJ. 1999;318:1099–103.

Choice of anesthetic technique on plasma concentrations of interleukins and cell adhesion molecules

Daniela C Ionescu[1,2]*, Simona Claudia D Margarit[1], Adina Norica I Hadade[3], Teodora N Mocan[4], Nicolae A Miron[5] and Daniel I Sessler[6]

Abstract

Background: Whether inflammatory responses to surgery are comparably activated during total intravenous anesthesia (TIVA) and during volatile anesthesia remains unclear. We thus compared the perioperative effects of TIVA and isoflurane anesthesia on plasma concentrations of proinflammatory and anti-inflammatory interleukins and cell adhesion molecules.

Methods: Patients having laparoscopic cholecystectomies were randomly allocated to two groups: 44 were assigned to TIVA and 44 to isoflurane anesthesia. IL-1β, IL-6, IL-8, IL-10, IL-13, and the cellular adhesion molecules intercellular adhesion molecule-1 and vascular cell adhesion molecule-1 were determined preoperatively, before incision, and at 2 and 24 hours postoperatively. Our primary outcomes were area-under-the-curve cytokine and adhesion molecule concentrations over 24 postoperative hours.

Results: The only statistically significant difference in area-under-the-curve concentrations was for IL-6, which was greater in patients given isoflurane:78 (95% confidence interval (CI): 52 to 109) pg/ml versus 33 (22 to 50) pg/ml, $P= 0.006$. Two hours after surgery, IL-6 was significantly greater than baseline in patients assigned to isoflurane: 47 (95% CI: 4 to 216, $P<0.001$) pg/ml versus 18 (95%CI: 4 to 374, $P<0.001$) pg/ml in the TIVA group. In contrast, IL-10 was significantly greater in patients assigned to TIVA: 20 (95% CI: 2 to 140, $P<0.001$) pg/ml versus 12 (95% CI: 3 to 126, $P<0.001$) pg/ml. By 24 hours after surgery, concentrations were generally similar between study groups and similar to baseline values.

Conclusion: The only biomarker whose postoperative area-under-the-curve concentrations differed significantly as a function of anesthetic management was IL-6. Two hours after surgery, IL-6 concentrations were significantly greater in patients given isoflurane than TIVA. However, the differences were modest and seem unlikely to prove clinically important. Further studies are needed.

Keywords: Inhalation anesthetics, Intravenous anesthetics, Propofol, Cell adhesion molecules, Interleukins

Background

Surgery provokes hemodynamic, metabolic, and inflammatory responses; it also provokes a complex immune reaction [1] that includes activation of the interleukin network [2]. For example, surgery and anesthesia provoke an increase in proinflammatory interleukins and adhesion molecules, and a subsequent increase in countervailing anti-inflammatory interleukins [3-5]. The most important proinflammatory interleukin is IL-6, while the most potent anti-inflammatory interleukin is IL-10.

Cell adhesion molecules (CAMs) are members of the immunoglobulin family and are regulated by the inflammatory interleukins [6]. CAMs promote wound healing [7,8] and can also promote tumor progression and metastasis [9,10], either directly or by promoting overproduction of inflammatory interleukins. The mechanisms of action differ for intercellular adhesion molecule

* Correspondence: dionescuati@yahoo.com
[1]Department of Anesthesia and Intensive Care I, 'Iuliu Hatieganu' University of Medicine and Pharmacy, Croitorilor, nr. 19-21, Cluj-Napoca 400162, Romania
[2]Outcomes Research Consortium, Cleveland, OH, USA
Full list of author information is available at the end of the article

(ICAM)-1 and vascular cell adhesion molecule (VCAM)-1. ICAM-1 produces its effects by promoting recruitment and adhesion of leukocytes to the activated endothelium via bonds with integrins, thus promoting migration through endothelial cells [11]; VCAM-1, produced mainly by the endothelial cells after interleukin-mediated stimulation, promotes adhesion of inflammatory cells to the vascular wall and subsequent migration [12]. Reduced plasma ICAM-1 concentration may facilitate tumor cell movement across vessels into surrounding tissues, thus promoting metastasis. Some tumor cells may also use VCAM-1 to adhere to the vascular walls and to migrate [13,14]. CAMs are influenced by the surgery [15] and may influence outcome after oncological surgery [14-17].

The two major approaches to general anesthesia are volatile anesthetics such as isoflurane and intravenous anesthesia such as propofol. General anesthesia may impair immune function directly by affecting immunocompetent cells such as natural killer (NK) cells and macrophages, cytokine responses, and adhesion molecules. Alternatively, anesthesia may indirectly influence the stress response to surgery [1,5,18,19].

There appear to be substantial differences between intravenous and volatile anesthetics in their effects on various immune functions [20-22]. While isoflurane inhibits interferon stimulation of NK cell cytotoxicity and sevoflurane alters the release of cytokines by NK, propofol does not significantly suppress NK cell activity [19]. Propofol alone increased apoptosis and cell adhesion and did not significantly influenced cell migration in breast cancer cells, while propofol conjugates significantly increased apoptosis and decreased migration and adhesion in breast cancer cells [23]. Propofol down-regulates proinflammatory interleukins [24,25]. Although some studies suggest that total intravenous anesthesia (TIVA) suppresses inflammatory responses and promotes release of anti-inflammatory cytokines [18,20,21], the reported results are inconsistent [26]. The few studies that evaluated the effects of anesthesia on cellular adhesion molecules report that both inhalation agents and propofol blunt the increase in ICAM and VCAM expression [27,28]. Whether interleukins and other inflammatory molecules are comparably activated during TIVA and volatile anesthesia thus remains unclear.

Our study was designed to compare the effects of TIVA and volatile anesthesia on plasma concentrations of proinflammatory and anti-inflammatory interleukins and on CAMs during laparoscopic surgery. Specifically, we tested the hypothesis that TIVA blunts the inflammatory response to laparoscopic cholecystectomy more than isoflurane anesthesia. Laparoscopic surgery was chosen because the amount of tissue injury is small and similar from case to case, thus reducing the impact of surgery *per se* on immune responses.

Methods

After obtaining university Ethics Committee approval (Comisia de Etica a Universitatii de Medicina si Famacie 'Iuliu Hatieganu', Cluj-Napoca, No. 178A/2007) and written informed consent, we enrolled 88 patients with American Society of Anesthesiologists physical status scores 1 or 2 who were scheduled for laparoscopic cholecystectomy. We excluded patients with known inflammatory diseases (including acute cholecystitis) or immune system disorders, asthma, obesity (body mass index ≥ 30 kg/m^2), diabetes, gastric ulcers, and allergies. We also excluded patients who currently or recently used steroid or anti-inflammatory medication, or who had white blood cell counts $>10^4/\mu l$ or a preoperative core temperature $>37°C$.

Protocol

Midazolam, 7.5 mg orally, was given 1 hour before surgery. Dexamethasone, 4 mg intravenously, was given shortly before induction of anesthesia as prophylaxis against postoperative nausea and vomiting [29]. Then 500 ml crystalloid was infused during anesthetic induction, and thereafter as clinically indicated.

Patients were randomized into two study groups using a computer-generated sequence: one-half were assigned to target-controlled infusion TIVA with propofol, and one-half to isoflurane volatile anesthesia. Allocation was concealed in sequentially numbered sealed envelopes, with assignments revealed when patients were arriving in the operating theater. Laboratory staff were blinded to group assignments and anesthetic management.

TIVA was induced and maintained with a target-controlled infusion of propofol with an initial target plasma concentration of 4 µg/ml (Orchestra, Base Primea; Fresenius Kabi, Fresenius Vial SAS, Brézins, France). The propofol infusion was adjusted to target a Bispectral Index between 40 and 55 (Covidien, Dublin, Ireland). Isoflurane anesthesia was induced with propofol 1.5 to 2 mg/kg and maintained with isoflurane 1 to 1.5 minimum alveolar concentration titrated to Bispectral Index 40 to 55 and hemodynamic parameters.

Patients were ventilated with 70% oxygen in air and a positive end-expiratory pressure of 3 to 4 cmH$_2$O. The respiratory rate and inspiratory pressure were adjusted to maintain an end-tidal carbon dioxide partial pressure of 35 to 45 mmHg (Drager-Vamos, Lubeck, Germany). Remifentanil was infused under manual control with an initial dose of 0.5 µg/kg/minute in the first minute and 0.25 µg/kg/minute thereafter; the remifentanil dose was adjusted in 0.05 to µg/kg/minute increments as clinically necessary. Atracurium 0.6 mg/kg was initially given to provide paralysis for intubation; subsequently, 10 mg boluses were given as clinically needed. Hypotension (defined as a decrease in blood pressure >30% from baseline) was corrected with additional fluids and/or ephedrine. At the end of surgery, anesthesia was discontinued and muscle relaxation antagonized with neostigmine and atropine.

Postoperative analgesia was provided by oral paracetamol 1 g every 8 hours and intravenous meperidine 0.3 to 0.4 mg/kg upon patient request or when verbal response pain scores exceeded 3 (on a 5-point scale with 0 = no pain and 5 = worst pain possible). Nonsteroidal agents (nonsteroidal anti-inflammatory drugs) were not given. Metoclopramide,10 mg intravenously, was the initial treatment for postoperative nausea and vomiting; 4 mg ondansetron was added if necessary.

Measurements

Routine anesthetic monitoring was used as recommended by the American Society of Anesthesiologists.

Venous blood (7 ml) was sampled immediately after inserting the first peripheral cannula (T1), after intubation but before incision (T2), 2 hours after emergence (T3) and 24 hours (T4) after anesthesia. Samples were collected and centrifuged at 2,500×g for 10 minutes at room temperature; the resulting 3 to 4 ml plasma samples were stored at less than −20°C until assayed.

Plasma concentrations of interleukins and the CAMs soluble ICAM-1 and soluble VCAM-1 were measured by an ELISA technique using commercially available kits (Quantikine; R&D Systems, Minneapolis, MN, USA) as per the manufacturer's instructions. Laboratory staff were unaware of study groups and were not involved in anesthetic management.

Detection limits for interleukins as given by the manufacturer were as follows: IL-1, typically <1 pg/ml; IL-6, <0.7 pg/ml; IL-8,<1.5 pg/ml; IL-10,<3.9 pg/ml; and IL-13 ,<32 pg/ml. Intra-assay and inter-assay coefficients of variation were both <10%. The detection limits for soluble VCAM-1 ranged from 0.2 to 1.3 (mean =0.6) ng/ml and the limits for soluble ICAM-1 ranged from 0.05 to 0.25 (mean = 0.10) ng/ml, with intra-assay and inter-assay variation coefficients both <8% (Quantikine; R&D Systems).

Normal plasma concentrations of interleukins, as given by the manufacturer, are: IL-1β,1 to 4 pg/ml; IL-6, 0.7 to12 pg/ml; IL-8,4to 31 pg/ml; IL-13,32 to 62 pg/ml; and IL-10,4 to 8 pg/ml. Normal plasma concentrations of CAMs, as given by the manufacturer, are 349 to 991 ng/ml for soluble VCAM-1 and 99 to 320 ng/ml for soluble ICAM-1.

Statistical analysis

Sample size was estimated from a pilot study with 22 patients per group. Calculated area-under-the-curve (AUC) values for IL-6 showed a 46 pg·hour/ml difference between the two groups (standard deviation = 60 and 62, respectively). Using a two-tailed α error of 0.01, we estimated that 41 patients per group would provide an 80% power. Anticipating some inadequate samples, we enrolled 44 patients in each study group.

Chi-square tests were used to assess correlations between dichotomous data. The distribution for continuous data was evaluated using the Kolmogorov–Smirnov test, with subsequent comparison by t test or Mann–Whitney U test as appropriate. AUC values over 24 hours and values at each measurement time were determined in individual patients using the preoperative concentration as the baseline; between-group AUC differences were subsequently determined using Mann–Whitney U tests.

Data are expressed as either mean ± standard deviation or median (95% confidence interval (CI)). *Post-hoc* comparisons with baseline values of biomarker concentrations recorded at two different postoperative time intervals were performed using the Wilcoxon test. A Bonferroni correction was used with a consequent reduction of the α threshold to 0.01.

Data analyses were performed using SPSS 17.0 (SPSS Inc., Chicago, IL, USA) and Medcalc 8.3.1.1 (MedCalc Software, Mariakerke, Belgium) statistical packages.

Results

Ninety-one patients were enrolled in the study and were randomized (46 to isoflurane and 45 to TIVA). Three patients were excluded from analysis because they were discharged within 24 hours or acute inflammation of the gallbladder was identified intraoperatively; we thus present data from the remaining 88 patients (44 per group) who completed the study. Demographic data were similar in each anesthetic group, as were anesthetic and surgical management (Table 1).

Propofol targeted plasma concentrations in the target-controlled infusion TIVA group averaged 2.4 ± 0.5 µg/ml. The mean end-tidal isoflurane level in patients assigned to volatile anesthesia was 1.1 ± 0.3%.

None of the patients became hypothermic during operation. The mean intraoperative temperature was 36.6 ± 0.2°C.

Pre-induction plasma cytokine and adhesion molecule concentrations were similar in the two study groups (Table 2).

Plasma concentrations for IL-1β, IL-6, IL-8, IL-10, IL-13, soluble ICAM-1, and soluble VCAM-1are shown in Figures 1, 2, 3, 4, 5, 6, and 7, respectively. The largest cytokine responses to surgery were observed for IL-6 and IL-10, each with significant peak concentrations 2 hours after surgery. IL-6 was significantly greater in patients assigned to isoflurane: 46.4 (95% CI: 34.3 to 70.7) pg/ml versus 17.6 (95% CI: 11.9

Table 1 Demographic data of the study groups

	Total intravenous anesthesia (*n*= 44)	Isoflurane (*n*= 44)	*P* value
Age (years)	52 ±12	46 ±14	0.19
Weight (kg)	74 ± 16	75 ± 16	0.72
Gender (female/male)	34/10	38/6	0.40
American Society of Anesthesiologists I/II	20/24	25/19	0.39
Anesthesia time (minutes)	54 ± 15	54 ± 14	0.90
Intraoperative Bispectral Index	43 ± 4	44 ± 4	0.22
Intraoperative mean arterial pressure (mmHg)	84 ± 17	78 ± 16	0.07
Intraoperative heart rate (beats/minute)	76 ± 14	74 ± 14	0.44
Intraoperative core temperature (°C)	36.5 ± 0.3	36.6 ± 0.3	0.13
Intraoperative intravenous fluids (l)	1.2 ± 0.2	1.3 ± 0.2	0.47
Intraoperative remifentanil (µg/kg/minute)	0.3 ± 0.06	0.3 ± 0.05	1.00

Data expressed as mean ± standard deviation or number of patients.

to 20.7) pg/ml (*P*<0.01). In contrast IL-10 was greater in patients assigned to TIVA: 20.1 (95% CI:14.2 to 32.4) pg/ml versus 12.4 (95%CI:8.8 to 18.7) pg/ml (*P* = 0.03). By 24 hours after surgery, concentrations were similar in each group and similar to baseline values, except for IL-6 that remained significantly increased in both groups (*P*<0.001) and for IL-10 that remained significantly increased in patients given isoflurane (*P*= 0.009). IL-4 concentrations were below the detection limits of our assay at all times and are therefore not reported.

Between-group comparisons of the cytokine plasma concentration AUC for every measured parameter in the study groups are showed in Table 3; the only significant difference was for IL-6 (*P* = 0.006), with values being greater in patients assigned to isoflurane anesthesia.

Discussion

The possibility that anesthetic management influences long-term outcomes in surgical patients is intriguing, but remains largely speculative. Nonetheless, there is

Table 2 Pre-induction interleukin and cell adhesion molecules plasma concentrations

	Total intravenous anesthesia (*n*= 44)	Isoflurane (*n*= 44)
Il-1β (pg/ml)	1.0 (1.02 to 1.18)	1.0 (0.99 to 1.31)
IL-6 (pg/ml)	3.4 (2.6 to 5.5)	2.2 (1.2 to 2.7)
IL-8 (pg/ml)	19.3 (12.4 to 34.6)	16.7 (12.1 to 24.0)
IL-10 (pg/ml)	6.1 (5.1 to 6.9)	4.8 (4.1 to 6.0)
IL-13 (pg/ml)	30.6 (27.2 to 34.0)	33.7 (28.8 to 35.8)
Soluble ICAM-1 (ng/ml)	69.0 (65.2 to 76.6)	66.1 (60.74 to 74.7)
Soluble VCAM-1 (ng/ml)	383 (349.03 to 408)	362 (335 to 402)

Data expressed as median (95% confidence interval). ICAM, intracellular adhesion molecule; VCAM, vascular cell adhesion molecule.

limited (and often controversial) evidence – or at least plausible mechanisms – to suggest that anesthetic management might influence diverse outcomes including wound infection [30-32], major cardiac complications and strokes [33], brain development [34], cancer recurrence [35-37], and mortality [30,38]. Because the inflammatory response to surgery seems likely to be an important potential mechanism, and possibly even a common pathway for many outcomes, we evaluated the cytokine responses in patients randomly assigned to TIVA or volatile anesthesia.

Based on our primary AUC analysis, the only cytokine that differed significantly as a function of anesthetic approach was IL-6, and the increase was only marginally statistically significant (*P*= 0.006 with an α threshold of 0.01 because of multiple comparisons). Furthermore, the factor of two increase – which is small by the standards of cytokines – seems unlikely to be clinically important. Judging by cytokine responses, our results thus suggest that the choice of TIVA versus volatile anesthesia only slightly alters the inflammatory response to surgery.

Within-group comparisons showed that IL-6 increased significantly at 2 hours postoperatively in both groups, but that the increase was significantly greater in patients assigned to isoflurane anesthesia. IL-10 was also significantly increased in both groups after 2 postoperative hours, but with greater plasma concentrations in patients given TIVA [3]. At 24 hours postoperatively, IL-6 remained increased in both study groups while IL-10 remained increased only in the inhalation group, probably to counteract the increase in IL-6; however, the increases were marginal.

Our results are generally consistent with previous reports by Ke and colleagues, Gililand and colleagues, and Crozier and colleagues [20-22]. For example, Ke and colleagues reported similar responses for IL-6 and IL-10 during laparoscopic cholecystectomy. Results reported

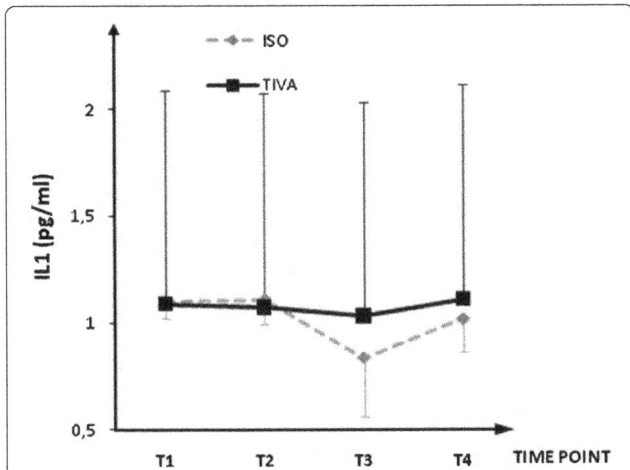

Figure 1 Plasma IL-1β concentrations. Data expressed as median (95% confidence interval). T1 = before induction; T2 = immediately after induction; T3 = at 2 hours after skin closure; T4 = at 24 hours after skin closure. Area under the curve: isoflurane (ISO) = 3.3, total intravenous anesthesia (TIVA) = 3.4.P= 0.428.

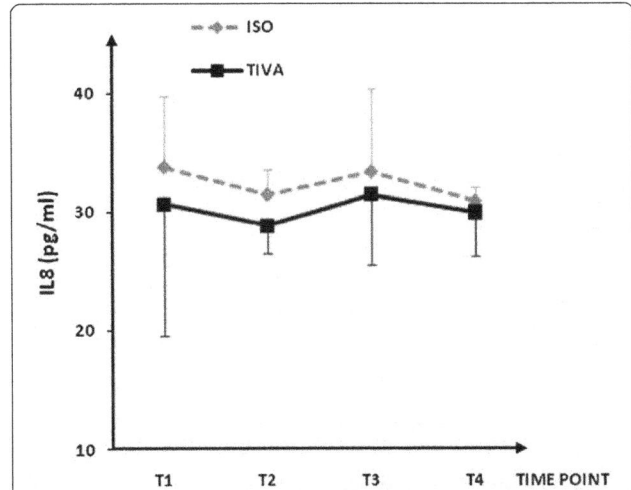

Figure 3 Plasma IL-8 concentrations. Data expressed as median (95% confidence interval). T1 = before induction; T2 = immediately after induction; T3 = at 2 hours after skin closure; T4 = at 24 hours after skin closure. Area-under-the- curve: isoflurane (ISO) = 54, total intravenous anesthesia (TIVA) = 49. P = 0.285.

by Gililand and colleagues in abdominal surgery and by Crozier and colleagues after abdominal hysterectomy were also generally similar. In contrast, Helmy and colleagues reported that IL-6 does not increase after laparoscopic cholecystectomy [39]. Potential explanations include use of a different kit for interleukin assays and variations in surgical technique.

Although there were differences in anesthetic protocols and type of surgery, Deegan and coworkers observed IL-10, IL-8, and IL-13 responses similar to ours when propofol and paravertebral anesthesia was compared with volatile

anesthesia [35]. However, they also found that IL-6 concentrations did not much differ as a function of anesthetic dose. Potential explanations include their use of regional anesthesia rather than TIVA, breast surgery rather than abdominal surgery, and the fact that all their patients had cancer, which *per se* can depress immune responses. Furthermore, in our study neither soluble ICAM-1 nor soluble VCAM-1 differed significantly as an effect of anesthetic technique.

A possible explanation for the results on interleukins may consist of the antioxidants and anti-inflammatory

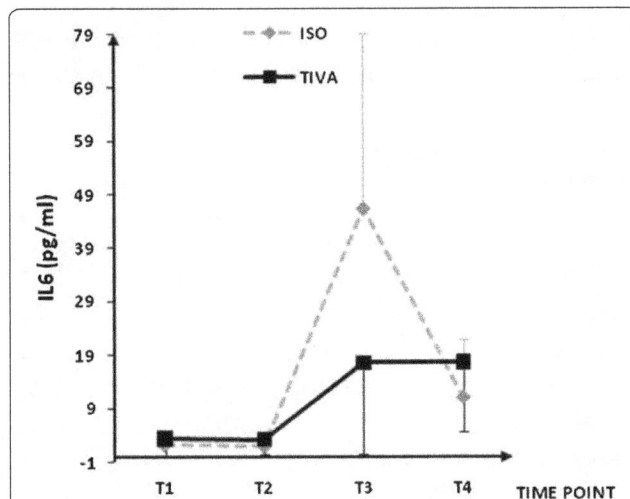

Figure 2 Plasma IL-6 concentrations. Data expressed as median (95% confidence interval).T1 = before induction; T2 = immediately after induction; T3 = at 2 hours after skin closure; T4 = at 24 hours after skin closure. Area-under-the-curve: isoflurane (ISO) = 78, total intravenous anesthesia (TIVA)= 33. P = 0.006.

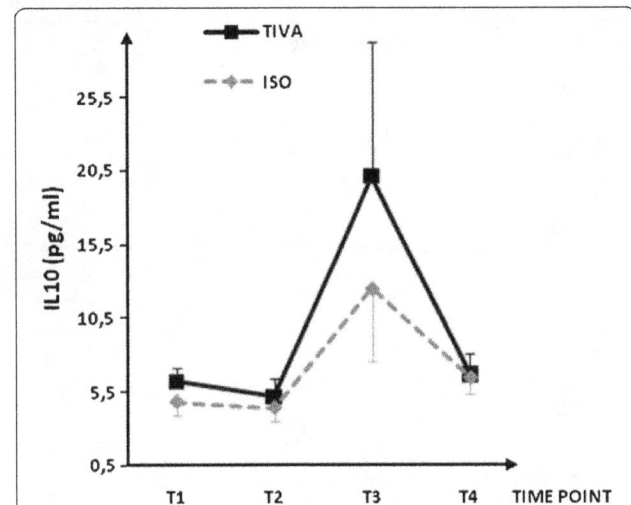

Figure 4 Plasma IL-10 concentrations. Data expressed as median (95% confidence interval). T1 = before induction; T2 = immediately after induction; T3 = at 2 hours after skin closure; T4 = at 24 hours after skin closure. Area-under-the-curve: isoflurane (ISO) = 26, total intravenous anesthesia (TIVA) = 37. P = 0.151.

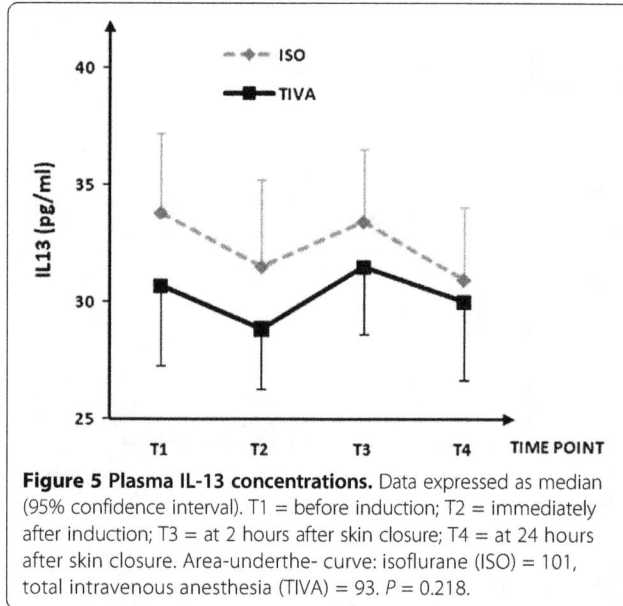

Figure 5 Plasma IL-13 concentrations. Data expressed as median (95% confidence interval). T1 = before induction; T2 = immediately after induction; T3 = at 2 hours after skin closure; T4 = at 24 hours after skin closure. Area-underthe- curve: isoflurane (ISO) = 101, total intravenous anesthesia (TIVA) = 93. P = 0.218.

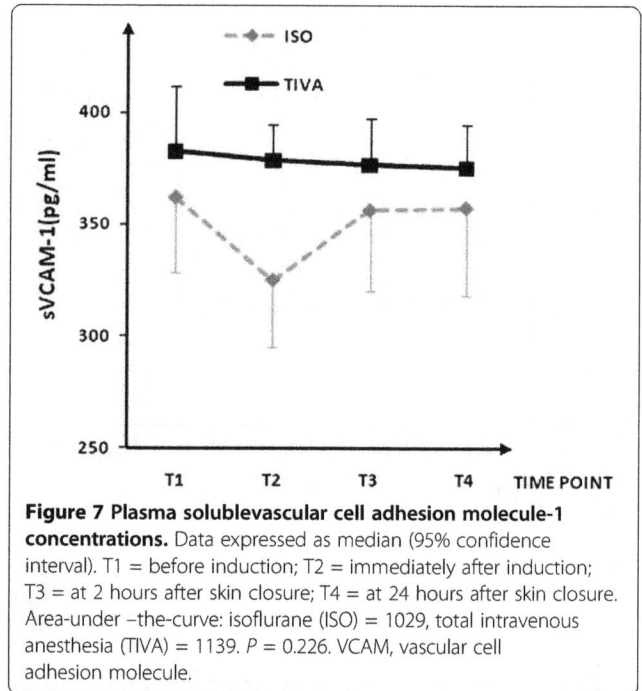

Figure 7 Plasma solublevascular cell adhesion molecule-1 concentrations. Data expressed as median (95% confidence interval). T1 = before induction; T2 = immediately after induction; T3 = at 2 hours after skin closure; T4 = at 24 hours after skin closure. Area-under –the-curve: isoflurane (ISO) = 1029, total intravenous anesthesia (TIVA) = 1139. P = 0.226. VCAM, vascular cell adhesion molecule.

effects of propofol [24,40] as compared with immune effects of inhalation agents [41]. As for adhesion molecules, our results with inhalation anesthesia are similar to other studies [42], confirming that isoflurane has an inhibitory effect on CAMs. Moreover, we have demonstrated that there are no differences between inhalation anesthesia and TIVA. The anti-inflammatory effects of propofol may thus involve mechanisms other than adhesion molecules.

Directly comparing our results with previous publications is difficult since each study evaluated different

anesthetic protocols, different surgical interventions, and used different cytokine assays. Nonetheless, our results are thus generally consistent with the previous literature and are among the largest that evaluated a single typical operation.

Our study does have some limitations. A low dose of dexamethasone (4 mg) was given to all patients for prophylaxis against postoperative nausea and vomiting, as is common in clinical practice. It is wellknown that steroids are immunosuppressive and may have ameliorated the inflammatory response to surgery. Observed differences between the randomized TIVA and volatile anesthetic groups remain valid, but it remains possible

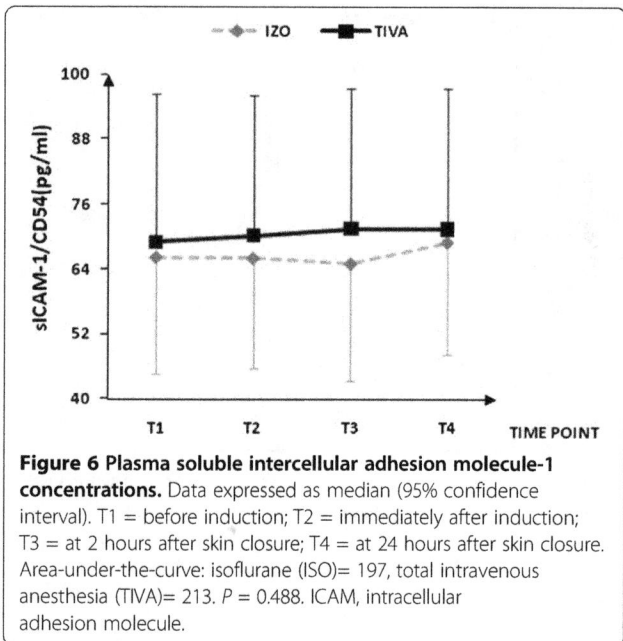

Figure 6 Plasma soluble intercellular adhesion molecule-1 concentrations. Data expressed as median (95% confidence interval). T1 = before induction; T2 = immediately after induction; T3 = at 2 hours after skin closure; T4 = at 24 hours after skin closure. Area-under-the-curve: isoflurane (ISO)= 197, total intravenous anesthesia (TIVA)= 213. P = 0.488. ICAM, intracellular adhesion molecule.

Table 3 Area under the curve between-group comparisons

	Total intravenous anesthesia (*n*= 44)	Isoflurane (*n*= 44)	*P*value
IL-1β (pg·hour/ml)	3.4 (3.0 to 4.3)	3.3 (2.9 to 4.0)	0.428
IL-6 (pg·hour/ml)	33.0 (21.6 to 44.9)	78.0 (52.2 to 109.1)	**0.006**
IL-8 (pg·hour/ml)	49.0 (39.6 to 67.0)	54.0(47.2 to 82.6)	0.285
IL-10 (pg·hour/ml)	37.0 (23.8 to 55.4)	26.0 (21.6 to 42.1)	0.151
IL-13 (pg·hour/ml)	93.0 (83.4 to 101.3)	101.0 (89.8 to 112.1)	0.218
Soluble ICAM-1 (ng·hour/ml)	213 (188.0 to 242.3)	197 (178.9 to 220.9)	0.488
Soluble VCAM-1 (ng·hour/ml)	1,139 (1,029 to 1,188)	1,029 (947 to 1,163)	0.226

Data expressed as median (95% confidence interval). Area-under-the-curve based on preoperative values. Mann–Whitney U tests were used for between-group comparisons; because multiple comparisons were made, $P<0.01$ was considered statistically significant. Bold data are significant.

that responses in both groups would be more impressive in patients not given steroids. A more serious consideration is that laparoscopic cholecystectomies produce only a moderate amount of tissue injury, and cholecystectomies presumably provoke a smaller inflammatory response than larger operations. They nonetheless well represent the types of surgery that are most commonly performed. On the contrary, having only a minor inflammatory response due to surgery, the differences may be more attributable to anesthetic technique.

Immune response is a mosaic in which interleukins and adhesion molecules are but one piece. However, it is an important piece because exaggerated or abnormally low cytokine concentrations may have a substantial effect on patient outcome. For example abnormally increased levels of IL-6 are involved in systemic inflammatory response with impact on outcome and postoperative complications, and even on prognosis and mortality in cancer patients [43,44]. However, we observed relatively small differences between isoflurane anesthesia and TIVA, and only over a short period of time; whether this difference is clinically important remains unknown — but seems somewhat unlikely.

In summary, IL-6 and IL-10 increased significantly 2 hours after incision. There were no other statistically significant or clinically important perioperative increases. The only significant difference in cytokine concentrations related to anesthetic management was a greater increase in the IL-6 AUC with isoflurane anesthesia than with TIVA. However, the increase was only a factor-of-two, which is small by cytokine standards. The AUC concentrations were greater for IL-10 ($P = 0.15$), soluble ICAM-1 ($P = 0.49$), and soluble VCAM-1 ($P = 0.23$) in patients assigned to TIVA, although not significantly.

Conclusion

TIVA significantly reduced the increase in IL-6 during the perioperative period as compared with isoflurane. IL-10 and the adhesion molecules were increased, although not significantly. This effect may be favorable in some patients (for example, increased systemic inflammatory response). Further studies on larger groups of patients and for more extensive surgical interventions are needed for a better evaluation of the extent of this effect and its clinical impact.

Abbreviations
AUC: Area under the curve; CAM: Cell adhesion molecule; CI: Confidence interval; ELISA: Enzyme-linked immunosorbent assay; IL: Interleukin; ICAM: Intercellular adhesion molecule; NK: Natural killer; TIVA: Total intravenous anesthesia; VCAM: Vascular cell adhesion molecule.

Competing interests
The authors declare that they have no competing interests.

Authors' contributions
DCI conceived the study, design study protocol, and acquisition of data, and drafted the manuscript. SCDM contributed to acquisition of data by enrolling patients and to drafting the manuscript. ANIH contributed to acquisition of data (sample preservation, storage) and the database. TNM contributed to the database and statistical analysis and interpretation of the data. NAM was responsible for immunological analysis of blood samples and interpretation. DIS revised critically the manuscript for important intellectual content and drafted parts of it. All authors read and approved the final manuscript.

Funding
This work was supported by the research grant PN 41025 funded by The National Centre for Projects Management (CNMP), Bucharest, Romania.

Author details
[1]Department of Anesthesia and Intensive Care I, 'Iuliu Hatieganu' University of Medicine and Pharmacy, Croitorilor, nr. 19-21, Cluj-Napoca 400162, Romania. [2]Outcomes Research Consortium, Cleveland, OH, USA. [3]Department of Anaesthesia and Intensive Care, Regional Institute of Gastroenterology and Hepatology'O Fodor', Croitorilor, nr. 19-21, Cluj-Napoca 400162, Romania. [4]Department of Physiology, 'Iuliu Hatieganu' University of Medicine and Pharmacy, Croitorilor, nr. 19-21, Cluj-Napoca 400162, Romania. [5]Department of Clinical Immunology, 'Iuliu Hatieganu' University of Medicine and Pharmacy, Croitorilor, nr. 19-21, Cluj-Napoca 400162, Romania. [6]Department of Outcomes Research, The Cleveland Clinic 9500 Euclid Ave -- P77, Cleveland, OH 44195, USA.

References
1. Salo M: Effects of anaesthesia and surgery on the immune response. Acta Anaesthesiol Scand 1992, 36:201–220.
2. Lin E, Calvano SE, Lowry SF: Inflammatory cytokines and cell response in surgery. Surgery 2000, 127:117–126.
3. McBride WT, Armstrong MA, Crockard AD, McMurray TJ, Rea JM: Cytokine balance and immunosuppressive changes at cardiac surgery: contrasting response between patients and isolated CPB circuits. Br J Anaesth 1995, 75:724–733.
4. Breidahl AF, Hickey MJ, Stewart AG, Hayward PG, Morrison WA: The role of cellular adhesion molecules in surgery. ANZ J Surg 1995, 5:838–847.
5. McBride WT, Armstrong MA, McBride SJ: Immunomodulation: an important concept in modern anaesthesia. Anaesthesia 1996, 51:465–473.
6. Kalawski R, Bugajski P, Smielecki J, Wysocki H, Olszewski R, More R, Sheridan DJ, Siminiak T: Soluble adhesion molecules in reperfusion during coronary bypass grafting. Eur J Cardiothorac Surg 1998, 14:290–295.
7. Yukami T, Hasegawa M, Matsushita Y, Matsushita T, Horikawa M, Komura K, Yanaba K, Hamaguchi Y, Nagaoka T, Ogawa F, Fujimoto M, Steeber DA, Tedder TF, Takehara K, Sato S: Endothelial selectins regulate skin wound healing in cooperation with L-selectin and ICAM-1. J Leukoc Biol 2007, 82:519–531.
8. Nagaoka T, Kaburagi Y, Hamaguchi Y, Hasegawa M, Takehara K, Steeber DA, Tedder TF, Sato S: Delayed wound healing in the absence of intercellular adhesion molecule-1 or L-selectin expression. Am J Pathol 2000, 157:237–247.
9. Albelda SM: Role of integrins and other cell adhesion molecules in tumor progression and metastasis. Lab Invest 1993, 68:4–17.
10. Kobayashi H, Boelte KC, Lin PC: Endothelial cell adhesion molecules and cancer progression. Curr Med Chem 2007, 14:377–386.
11. Yang L, Froio RM, Sciuto TE, Dvorak AM, Alon R, Luscinskas FW: ICAM-1 regulates neutrophil adhesion and transcellular migration of TNF-α -activated vascular endothelium under flow. Blood 2005, 106:584–592.
12. Matheny HE, Deem TL, Cook-Mills JM: Lymphocyte migration through monolayers of endothelial cell lines involves VCAM-1 signaling via endothelial cell NADPH oxidase. J Immunol 2000, 164:6550–6559.
13. Alexiou D, Karayiannakis AJ, Syrigos KN, Zbar A, Kremmyda A, Bramis I, Tsigris C: Serum levels of E-selectin, ICAM-1 and VCAM-1 in colorectal cancer patients: correlations with clinicopathological features, patient survival and tumour surgery. Eur J Cancer 2001, 37:2392–2397.
14. Maurer CA, Friess H, Kretschmann B, Wildi S, Muller C, Graber H, Schilling M, Büchler MW: Over-expression of ICAM-1, VCAM-1 and ELAM-1 might

influence tumor progression in colorectal cancer. *Int J Cancer* 1998, **79:**76–81.

15. Mantur M, Snarska J, Koper O, Dzieciol J, Płonski A, Lemancewicz D: **Serums ICAM, sVCAM and sE-selectin levels in colorectal cancer patients.** *Folia Histochem Cytobiol* 2009, **47:**621–625.

16. Alexiou D, Karayiannakis AJ, Syrigos KN, Zbar A, Sekara E, Michail P, Rosenberg T, Diamantis T: **Clinical significance of serum levels of E-selectin, intercellular adhesion molecule-1, and vascular cell adhesion molecule-1 in gastric cancer patients.** *Am J Gastroenterol* 2003, **98**(2):478–85.

17. Ding YB, Chen GY, Xia JG, Zang XW, Yang HY, Yang L: **Association of VCAM-1 overexpression with oncogenesis, tumor angiogenesis and metastasis of gastric carcinoma.** *World J Gastroenterol* 2003, **9:**1409–1414.

18. Schneemilch CE, Ittenson A, Ansorge S, Hachenberg T, Bank U: **Effect of 2 anaesthetic techniques on the postoperative proinflammatory and anti-inflammatory cytokine response and cellular immune function to minor surgery.** *J Clin Anesth* 2005, **17:**517–527.

19. Snyder GL, Greenberg S: **Effect of anaesthetic technique and other perioperative factors on cancer recurrence.** *Br J Anaesth* 2010, **105:**106–115.

20. Ke JJ, Zhan J, Feng XB, Wu Y, Rao Y, Wang Y: **A comparison of the effect of total intravenous anaesthesia with propofol and remifentanil and inhalational anaesthesia with isoflurane on the release of pro- and anti-inflammatory cytokines in patients undergoing open cholecystectomy.** *Anaesth Intensive Care* 2008, **36:**74–78.

21. Gilliland HE, Armstrong MA, Carabine U, McMurray TJ: **The choice of anaesthetic maintenance technique influences the anti-inflammatory cytokine response to abdominal surgery.** *Anesth Analg* 1997, **85:**1394–1398.

22. Crozier TA, Muller JE, Quittkat D, Sydow M, Wuttke W, Kettler D: **Effect of anaesthesia on the cytokine responses to abdominal surgery.** *Br J Anaesth* 1994, **72:**280–285.

23. Siddiqui RA, Zerouga M, Wu M, Castillo A, Harvey K, Zaloga GP, Stillwell W: **Anticancer properties of propofol–docosahexaenoate and propofol–eicosapentaenoate on breast cancer cells.** *Breast Cancer Res* 2005, **7:**R645–R654.

24. Chen RM, Chen TG, Chen T-L, Lin L-L, Chang CC, Chang HC, Wu CH: **Anti-inflammatory and antioxidative effects of propofol on lipopolysaccharide-activated macrophages.** *Ann NY Acad Sci* 2005, **1042:**262–271.

25. Marik P: **Propofol: an immunomodulating agent.** *Pharmacotherapy* 2005, **25:**28S–33S.

26. Schilling T, Kozian A, Kretzschmar M, Huth C, Welte T, Buhling F, Hedenstierna G, Hachenberg T: **Effects of propofol and desfluraneanaesthesia on the alveolar inflammatory response to one-lung ventilation.** *Br J Anaesth* 2007, **99:**368–375.

27. Weber N, Kandler J, Schlack W, Grueber Y, Frädorf J, Preckel B: **Intermitted pharmacologic pretreatment by xenon, isoflurane, nitrous oxide, and the opioid morphine prevents tumor necrosis factor α–induced adhesion molecule expression in human umbilical vein endothelial cells.** *Anesthesiology* 2008, **108:**199–207.

28. Corcoran TB, Engel A, Shorten GD: **The influence of propofol on the expression of intercellular adhesion molecule 1 (ICAM-1) and vascular cell adhesion molecule 1 (VCAM-1) in reoxygenated human umbilical vein endothelial cells.** *Eur J Anaesthesiol* 2006, **23:**942–947.

29. Apfel CC, Korttila K, Abdalla M, Kerger H, Turan A, Vedder I, Zernak C, Danner K, Jokela R, Pocock SJ, Trenkler S, Kredel M, Biedler A, Sessler DI, Roewer N, IMPACT Investigators: **A factorial trial of six interventions for the prevention of postoperative nausea and vomiting.** *N Engl J Med* 2004, **350:**2441–251.

30. Sessler DI: **Long-term consequences of anaesthetic management.** *Anesthesiology* 2009, **111:**1–4.

31. Kurz A, Sessler DI, Lenhardt RA: **Study of wound infections and temperature group: perioperative normothermia to reduce the incidence of surgical-wound infection and shorten hospitalization.** *N Engl J Med* 1996, **334:**1209–1215.

32. Greif R, Akça O, Horn E-P, Kurz A, Sessler DI, Outcomes Research™ Group: **Supplemental perioperative oxygen to reduce the incidence of surgical wound infection.** *N Engl J Med* 2000, **342:**161–167.

33. POISE Study Group, Devereaux PJ, Yang H, Yusuf S, Guyatt G, Leslie K, Villar JC, Xavier D, Chrolavicius S, Greenspan L, Pogue J, Pais P, Liu L, Xu S, Málaga G, Avezum A, Chan M, Montori VM, Jacka M, Choi P: **Effects of extended-release metoprolol succinate in patients undergoing non-cardiac surgery (POISE trial): a randomised controlled trial.** *Lancet* 2008, **371:**1839–1847.

34. Perouansky M, Hemmings HC: **Between Clotho and Lachesis: how isoflurane seals neuronal fate.** *Anesthesiology* 2009, **110:**709–711.

35. Deegan CA, Murray D, Doran P, Moriarty DC, Sessler DI, Mascha E, Kavanagh BP, Buggy DJ: **Anaesthetic technique and the cytokine and matrix metalloproteinase response to primary breast cancer surgery.** *Reg Anesth Pain Med* 2010, **35:**490–495.

36. Exadaktylos AK, Buggy DJ, Moriarty DC, Mascha E, Sessler DI: **Can anaesthetic technique for primary breast cancer surgery affect recurrence or metastasis?** *Anesthesiology* 2006, **105:**660–664.

37. Gottschalk A, Sharma S, Ford J, Durieux M, Tiouririne M: **The role of the perioperative period in recurrence after cancer surgery.** *Anesth Analg* 2010, **110:**1636–1643.

38. Monk TG, Weldon BC: **Anaesthetic depth is a predictor of mortality: it's time to take the next step.** *Anesthesiology* 2010, **112:**1070–1072.

39. Helmy SAK, Wahby MAM, El-Nawaway M: **The effect of anaesthesia and surgery on plasma cytokine production.** *Anaesthesia* 1999, **54:**733–738.

40. Corcoran TB, Engel A, Sakamoto H, O'Shea A, O'Callaghan-Enright S, Shorten GD: **The effects of propofol on neutrophil function, lipid peroxidation and inflammatory response during elective coronary artery bypass grafting in patients with impaired ventricular function.** *Br J Anaesth* 2006, **97:**825–831.

41. Inada T, Yamanouchi Y, Jomura S, Sakamoto S, Takahashi M, Kambara T, Shingu K: **Effect of propofol and isofluraneanaesthesia on the immune response to surgery.** *Anaesthesia* 2004, **59:**954–959.

42. Yuki K, Astrof NS, Bracken C, Yoo R, Silkworth W, Soriano SG, Shimaoka M: **The volatile anaestheticisoflurane perturbs conformational activation of integrin LFA-1 by binding to the allosteric regulatory cavity.** *FASEB J* 2008, **22:**4109–4116.

43. Knüpfer H, Preiss R: **Significance of interleukin-6 (IL-6) in breast cancer [review].** *Breast Cancer Res Treat* 2007, **102:**129–135.

44. Nicolini A, Carpi A, Rossi G: **Cytokines in breast cancer.** *Cytokine Growth Factor Rev* 2006, **17:**325–337.

Risk stratification by pre-operative cardiopulmonary exercise testing improves outcomes following elective abdominal aortic aneurysm surgery

Stephen J Goodyear[1*], Heng Yow[1], Mahmud Saedon[1,2], Joanna Shakespeare[1], Christopher E Hill[1], Duncan Watson[1], Colette Marshall[1], Asif Mahmood[1], Daniel Higman[1] and Christopher HE Imray[1,2]

Abstract

Background: In 2009, the NHS evidence adoption center and National Institute for Health and Care Excellence (NICE) published a review of the use of endovascular aneurysm repair (EVAR) of abdominal aortic aneurysms (AAAs). They recommended the development of a risk-assessment tool to help identify AAA patients with greater or lesser risk of operative mortality and to contribute to mortality prediction.

A low anaerobic threshold (AT), which is a reliable, objective measure of pre-operative cardiorespiratory fitness, as determined by pre-operative cardiopulmonary exercise testing (CPET) is associated with poor surgical outcomes for major abdominal surgery. We aimed to assess the impact of a CPET-based risk-stratification strategy upon perioperative mortality, length of stay and non-operative costs for elective (open and endovascular) infra-renal AAA patients.

Methods: A retrospective cohort study was undertaken. Pre-operative CPET-based selection for elective surgical intervention was introduced in 2007. An anonymized cohort of 230 consecutive infra-renal AAA patients (2007 to 2011) was studied. A historical control group of 128 consecutive infra-renal AAA patients (2003 to 2007) was identified for comparison.

Comparative analysis of demographic and outcome data for CPET-pass (AT $\geq$ 11 ml/kg/min), CPET-fail (AT < 11 ml/kg/min) and CPET-submaximal (no AT generated) subgroups with control subjects was performed. Primary outcomes included 30-day mortality, survival and length of stay (LOS); secondary outcomes were non-operative inpatient costs.

Results: Of 230 subjects, 188 underwent CPET: CPET-pass $n = 131$, CPET-fail $n = 35$ and CPET-submaximal $n = 22$. When compared to the controls, CPET-pass patients exhibited reduced median total LOS (10 vs 13 days for open surgery, $n = 74$, $P < 0.01$ and 4 vs 6 days for EVAR, $n = 29$, $P < 0.05$), intensive therapy unit requirement (3 vs 4 days for open repair only, $P < 0.001$), non-operative costs (£5,387 vs £9,634 for open repair, $P < 0.001$) and perioperative mortality (2.7% vs 12.6% (odds ratio: 0.19) for open repair only, $P < 0.05$). CPET-stratified (open/endovascular) patients exhibited a mid-term survival benefit ($P < 0.05$).

Conclusion: In this retrospective cohort study, a pre-operative AT > 11 ml/kg/min was associated with reduced perioperative mortality (open cases only), LOS, survival and inpatient costs (open and endovascular repair) for elective infra-renal AAA surgery.

Keywords: AAA, Abdominal aortic aneurysm, CPET, Cardiopulmonary exercise test, Clinical outcomes

* Correspondence: drgoodyear@hotmail.com
[1]University Hospitals Coventry and Warwickshire NHS Trust, Clifford Bridge Road, Coventry CV2 2DX, UK
Full list of author information is available at the end of the article

Background

It is more important to know what sort of person has a disease than to know what sort of disease a person has (Hippocrates, 460 to 370 BC).

Open abdominal aortic aneurysm (AAA) surgery places substantial metabolic demands upon patients during the perioperative period. These result from increased energy requirements necessary for wound healing [1], hemostasis, ventilation, significant intra-operative hemodynamic [2,3] and acid/base fluctuations in addition to the catecholamine stress response to surgery [4-6]. Failure of the cardiorespiratory system to meet these increased metabolic requirements of patients undergoing major abdominal surgery may lead to avoidable cardiorespiratory morbidity and mortality [7-10]. Aortic surgery is associated with a high (≥5%) combined incidence of cardiac death and non-fatal myocardial infarction [11]. An individual's functional status has been shown to be reliably predictive of perioperative and long-term cardiac events following non-cardiac surgery [11], which can be derived from an assessment of their ability to perform activities of daily living [12,13]. Functional capacity (a numeric measure of functional status) can be expressed in metabolic equivalent (MET) levels; the oxygen consumption (VO_2) of a 70-kg, 40-year-old man in a resting state is 3.5 ml/kg/min or 1 MET [11]. The American College of Cardiology and American Heart Association (ACC/AHA) guidelines for perioperative assessment states that patients able to demonstrate a functional capacity of 4 METS may safely proceed to surgery without further cardiac assessment [14]. This equates to the ability to climb a flight of stairs or run a short distance. However, subjective assessment of functional status by clinicians for patients undergoing AAA repair, can be easily confounded and lacks prognostic accuracy [15-17], identifying a potential role for objective testing.

Static pre-operative tests of cardiac function, such as resting left ventricular ejection fraction, correlate poorly with cardiorespiratory (physical) fitness [18,19], whilst dynamic tests such as dobutamine stress echocardiography and stress electrocardiogram (ECG) testing do not measure respiratory function and global oxygen delivery simultaneously. Cardiopulmonary exercise testing (CPET) allows the objective quantification of the level at which end-organ oxygen demand exceeds delivery [20] (the functional reserve) and may be safely performed in high-risk populations [7,15,21]. The transition point at which the production of CO_2 exceeds VO_2 is known as the anaerobic threshold (AT) and can be determined by gaseous exchange measurement during CPET [20]. More simply, the AT is the work rate at which an individual's cardiorespiratory system fails to deliver sufficient oxygen to maintain aerobic respiration, mandating usage of an anaerobic substrate. AT is recognized as a reliable measure of preoperative fitness in AAA patient populations [22].

Older *et al.* demonstrated that a critical AT ≥ 11 ml/kg/min for elderly subjects was associated with 0.8% perioperative mortality rate in major abdominal surgery, compared to 18% in individuals below this level [23]. In a further study, the same center identified a less intensive perioperative care requirement and reduced cardiovascular and all-cause mortality for elderly (major surgical) patients with AT ≥ 11, when compared to individuals below this threshold [24]. Additional work has shown anaerobic threshold >11 to be associated with fewer short-term complications and hence a shorter length of inpatient stay (LOS) following major abdominal surgery [25]. More contemporary evidence highlights other variables obtained during CPET to be at least as valuable (as AT) in predicting short- and mid-term outcomes in elective AAA surgery [7,26]. This is supported by a recent finding that AT < 10.2 ml/kg/min and peak oxygen consumption (VO_2peak) < 15 ml/kg/min were associated with increased 30- and 90-day mortality following AAA surgery [27].

The aim of elective surgery for AAA is to prolong the survival of patients. However, there is an increasing awareness that many of these individuals have significant and potentially life-threatening cardiorespiratory comorbidities [26]. Proactive screening for AAA reduces the prevalence of aneurysm-related mortality [28] and surgical intervention when the AAA ≥ 5.5 cm anterior-posterior (AP) diameter is appropriate [29] in units that have low perioperative complication rates. Large multicenter trials such as EVAR-1 have published 30-day mortality rates of 5.3% for open AAA repair [30]. However, the Vascular Society of Great Britain and Ireland's (VSGBI) quality improvement framework (QIF) target of 3.5% by 2013 suggests that this could be improved further [31].

Pre-operative CPET was introduced for elective aneurysm surgery at University Hospitals Coventry and Warwickshire (UHCW) NHS Trust in 2007 in response to a 30-day mortality rate of 12.6% for open elective surgery, determined by internal audit and following an invited review by the VSGBI. These data reflected the hospitals' all-comers policy to elective aneurysm surgery, offering operative repair to many individuals of equivocal cardiovascular health, who may have been declined intervention in vascular units with more stringent perioperative selection. The observed mortality rate for unselected patients prior to 2007 is comparable with the findings of Carlisle and Swart (30-day mortality rate: 9%) [26], who studied infra-renal AAA outcomes during a similar era. Whilst 12.6% 30-day mortality for unstratified (pre-CPET era) open AAA surgery appears unacceptably high at first glance, there is a significant moral dilemma to be addressed when consideration is given to the overall mortality rate for ruptured AAA, generally accepted as 90% [32]. Nevertheless, these mortality data fell beyond the established range quoted in the literature [33] and a trust-wide guideline of pre-operative CPET-stratification-based selection (for all elective AAA patients) was introduced, to facilitate ongoing AAA intervention at the established diameter of 5.5 cm, on a risk-benefit basis. Conservative management was offered to individuals considered to be at high risk of perioperative mortality following stratification, based upon an extrapolation of the 2007 Carlisle and Swart data [26].

This study aimed to assess the outcomes of pre-operative CPET-stratification on the duration of postoperative inpatient stay, intensive therapy unit (ITU) usage, end-organ support, 30-day mortality rates and longer-term survival following elective open and endovascular infra-renal AAA repair.

Methods

This study is a retrospective, anonymized, single-center, cohort study performed at UHCW NHS Trust, a centralized vascular unit serving a population of 950,000. A review of the study proposal was undertaken by the trust's Research and Development department; ethical approval was deemed unnecessary, based upon National Research Ethics Service guidance [34].

From November 2007, all patients considered for elective AAA repair (AAA ≥ 5.5 cm) surgery were recommended pre-operative CPET. An evidence-based minimum anaerobic threshold of 11.0 ml/kg/min was selected to identify individuals with adequate cardiopulmonary reserves who would be able to tolerate general anesthesia and open abdominal surgery, with acceptable perioperative mortality rates (the CPET-pass subgroup). These individuals were offered the option of endovascular aneurysm repair (EVAR), if anatomically applicable, or open AAA repair. Individuals attaining an AT < 11 ml/kg/min (the CPET-fail subgroup) were counseled regarding conservative management if EVAR (a less cardiovascularly challenging procedure) was not anatomically feasible. CPET-fail patients with unfavorable anatomy for infra-renal EVAR who requested open repair (rather than expectant management), were permitted to proceed following careful discussion and documentation of the perceived increased mortality risk. Individuals who were unable to demonstrate AT during CPET due to mechanical co-morbidities, suboptimal effort, suboptimal compliance with the investigation or ECG changes at minimal exertion (the CPET-submaximal subgroup) were managed as per the CPET-fail subgroup.

Data collection and analysis

The data for 230 consecutive infra-renal AAA (≥5.5 cm AP diameter) patients considered for elective surgery between November 2007 and July 2011 (the CPET era) were studied. A control group of 128 consecutive individuals who underwent open or endovascular (infra-renal) AAA repair between January 2003 and October 2007 (the pre-CPET era) were identified for comparison. Patients diagnosed with thoracoabdominal or suprarenal aneurysms were excluded from the data collection, in addition to individuals who had undergone repairs of ruptured or urgent (symptomatic, non-ruptured) AAA.

Individuals were identified (with permission) by the Department of Clinical Coding using KMR1 diagnoses and procedures. To ensure completeness of data, results were cross-referenced with (computerized and written) operating theatre registries, the Dr Foster national outcomes database and the results of an internal audit of mortality/morbidity for elective AAA patients. Cardiopulmonary exercise testing data for CPET-era patients were collected (with full permission of the Department of Respiratory Physiology) from the UHCW CPET database.

Demographic and outcome data were identified by a systematic review of the hospitals' Clinical Results Reporting System (CRRS) and the patient case notes. Data loss was minimized by cross-referencing, using anonymized patient identification (PID) numbers, with the ITU patient digital registry and the CPET database. Information relating to length of ITU stay and the number of end organs supported was obtained from the ITU patient digital registry. Mortality data were sourced (with permission) from CRRS, the hospitals' Bereavement Services Department and by liaison with primary care providers. Survival was calculated from the date of intervention until death or censorship, in days. For individuals managed conservatively (CPET era), survival was calculated from the date of CPET until death or censorship. Survival could be observed for up to eight years in the control cohort and a maximum of four years for the CPET-era cohort, within the constraints of this study and this is regarded as mid-term survival. Tariffs for ITU and ward stays were obtained from the Department of Health Report 2010/2011 for UHCW via the Finance Section of the Information Services department. ITU cost data were calculated on an individual basis. A variable tariff applied, based upon the total number of end organs postoperatively supported (Table 1) multiplied by the duration of ITU stay. Ward costs were calculated by multiplication of a standard tariff (Table 1) by duration of ward stay. Financial analysis did not consider the costs of staff, equipment and consumables, which are essentially constant throughout NHS organizations offering similar interventions.

Surgical technique

All elective infra-renal AAA repairs were discussed and planned within a multidisciplinary team. Open aneurysm

Table 1 Ward-based and critical care unit costs per 24 h stay

Location	Discriminator	Cost per day (£)
CPET	One-off tariff	150
Surgical ward	Influenceable costs	110
	Fully absorbed costs	250
ITU	0 organs supported	260
	1 organ supported	769
	2 organs supported	1106
	3 organs supported	1386
	4 organs supported	1511
	5 organs supported	1568
	6 organs supported	1638

repairs were performed by a consultant vascular surgeon, or a consultant-supervised higher surgical trainee, using a transperitoneal inlay repair with knitted Dacron graft prostheses. Endovascular aneurysm repairs were planned and performed by a consultant vascular surgeon and consultant interventional radiologist. The EVAR devices used were the Cook Zenith® (Cook, Brisbane, Australia) endovascular system, Medtronic Endurant® (Medtronic, Minneapolis, MN, USA) and Lombard Aorfix™ (Lombard Medical, Oxfordshire, UK).

Cardiopulmonary exercise testing

Prior to testing, the patient's body mass index (BMI) was determined by measurement of height and weight. Resting spirometry was performed to measure forced expiratory volume per second (FEV_1) and forced vital capacity (FVC), from which FEV_1/FVC ratios were calculated. Predicted FEV_1 and FVC values were derived as a function of age, height, ethnicity and gender (calculated by the CPET software – see below). FEV_1 data were used to assess an individual's maximum predicted ventilation. The patient's weight and predicted maximum oxygen uptake (VO_2max) were used to calculate the individually required work rate on the cycle ergometer. Patients were subsequently attached to a 12-lead ECG and a form-fitting face-mask connected to a metabolic cart with protocol specific software (Viasprint Ergometer and MasterScreen CPX software v5.21.0.60, CareFusion Corporation, CA, USA). Patients were initially made to pedal for an unloaded phase (work rate 0 W at 50 rpm for 3 min) followed by a ramped phase requiring a constant 70 rpm against increasing resistance until they reached their peak oxygen uptake (VO_2peak). The test could be stopped at any point during the test protocol due to patient fatigue, presence of ischemic ECG changes, chest pain or if the maximum heart rate was achieved. The AT was derived using the V-slope method as described by Beaver et al. [35].

Statistical analysis

All data were tabulated using a Microsoft Excel® spreadsheet (Microsoft, CA, USA) and statistical analyses performed using Graphpad Prism4® (Graphpad, La Jolla, CA, USA). The normality of data was assessed with the D'Agostino and Pearson omnibus normality test. Nonparametric unpaired data were analyzed using the Mann–Whitney U test or Kruskal–Wallace analysis of variance (ANOVA), whilst categorical variables were analyzed using the chi-squared test or Fisher's exact test. Parametric data were assessed with a Student's t-test or one-way ANOVA. Survival data were evaluated by Kaplan–Meier curves. A P value of less than 0.05 was considered significant.

Results

Of 128 control subjects in the pre-CPET era, there were 103 (80.5%) open AAA repairs and 25 (19.5%) EVARs. Following introduction of CPET, 230 consecutive subjects with elective infra-renal AAA were studied. Operated cases included open repair in 100 (59.2%) patients and EVAR in 69 (40.8%), representing a significant increase in the proportion of endovascular cases ($P < 0.001$). A further 61 individuals did not have intervention.

Composition of the CPET-era open surgery, EVAR and no intervention groups, with respect to CPET outcomes, are demonstrated in Figure 1.

CPET subgroups

Of the 230 subjects identified in the CPET era, 188 underwent CPET. Tested individuals were stratified by their anaerobic threshold into three cohorts: CPET-pass ($n = 131$, AT ≥ 11.0 ml/kg/min), CPET-fail ($n = 35$, AT < 11.0) and CPET-submaximal ($n = 22$, unable to generate an AT). Of the patients, 42 were not referred for CPET (Figure 1).

Table 2 shows demographic data for pre-CPET era controls and CPET-era subgroups. Control subjects were of comparable age (median age: 74.0 years, 95% CI: 71.9 to 74.4) and equivalent aneurysm size (median aneurysm diameter: 6.3 cm, 95% CI: 6.5 to 6.9) to those in the CPET-stratified subgroups. BMI was infrequently recorded during the pre-CPET era rendering these data unsuitable for comparison. However, the median age was significantly higher in the CPET-submaximal group compared to CPET-pass patients ($P < 0.01$), the untested cohort ($P < 0.01$) and the pre-CPET cohort ($P < 0.01$). In addition, BMI was significantly lower in the CPET-pass cohort than the CPET-fail group ($P < 0.05$).

Length of inpatient stay

The median length of inpatient stay was significantly longer for open AAA surgery than EVAR in both the

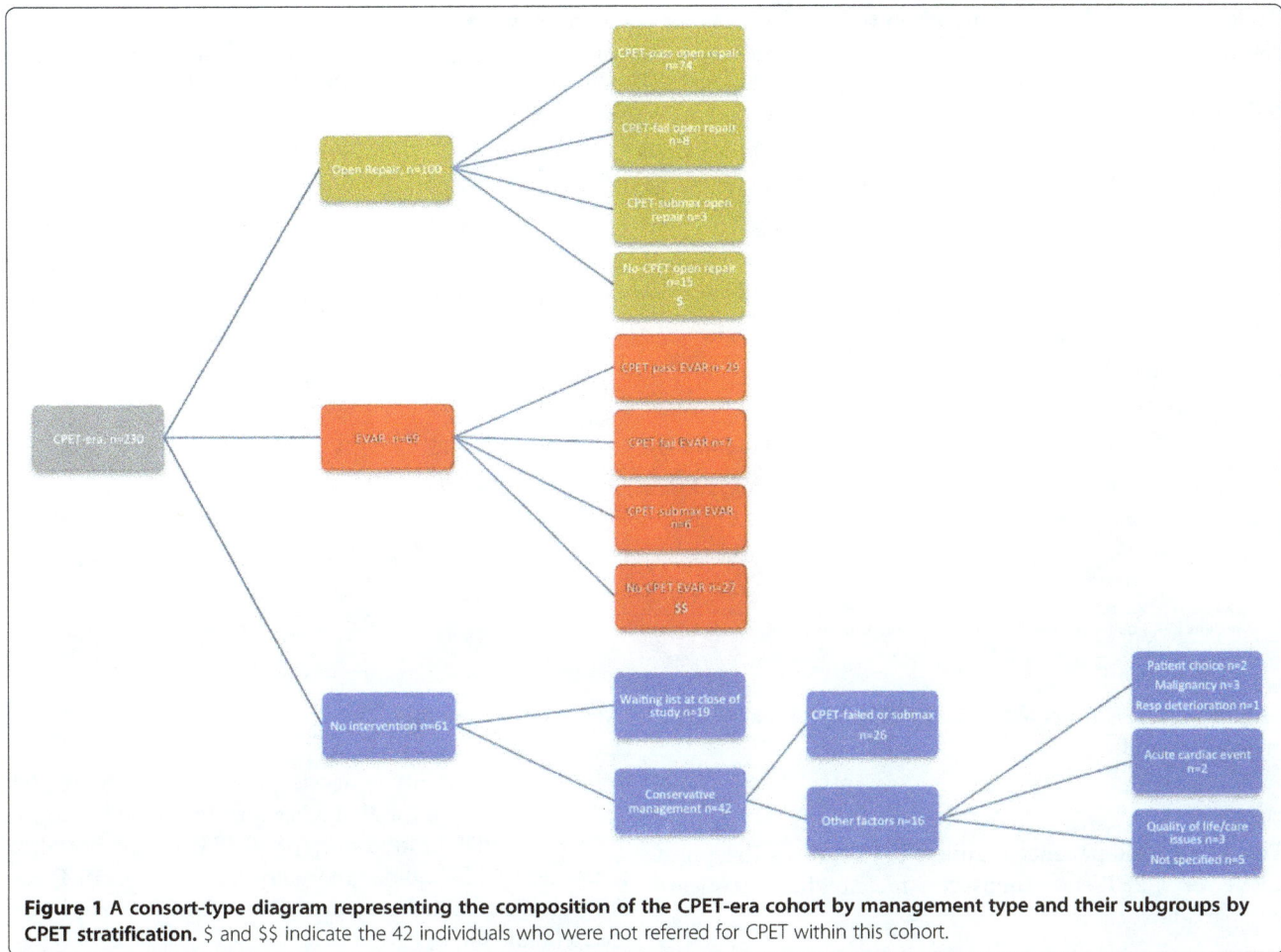

Figure 1 A consort-type diagram representing the composition of the CPET-era cohort by management type and their subgroups by CPET stratification. $ and $$ indicate the 42 individuals who were not referred for CPET within this cohort.

pre-CPET (open surgery: 13 days, 95% CI: 13.9 to 19.0; EVAR: 6 days, 95% CI: 4.3 to 8.3 days; *P* < 0.001) and post-CPET (open surgery: 10 days, 95% CI: 10.3 to 13.5; EVAR: 4 days, 95% CI: 4.6 to 6.7 days; *P* < 0.001) cohorts.

Open surgery

The length of inpatient stay following open AAA surgery in the CPET era (median: 10 days, 95% CI: 10.3 to 13.5) was shorter than that in the pre-CPET era (median: 13 days, 95% CI: 13.9 to 19.0; *P* < 0.001) principally due to the reduced duration of stay seen in the CPET-pass subgroup (Table 3, Figure 2a).

EVAR

The length of inpatient stay following EVAR in the CPET era (median: 4.0 days, 95% CI: 4.6 to 6.7) was shorter than that in the pre-CPET era (median: 6.0 days, 95% CI: 5.3 to 8.6; *P* < 0.05), due to the reduced duration of stay seen in the CPET-pass subgroup (Table 3, Figure 2b).

Duration of ITU stay
Open surgery

The length of ITU stay was reduced in the CPET era compared to pre-CPET controls (CPET era: 3 days, 95% CI: 3.2 to 4.4, pre-CPET: 4 days, 95% CI: 5.5 to

Table 2 Demographic data for CPET-era elective infra-renal AAA patients compared to pre-CPET era controls

	Pre-CPET era (n = 128)		Elective AAA patients – CPET performed (n = 188)						No CPET (n = 42)	
			CPET-pass (n = 131)		CPET-fail (n = 35)		CPET-submaximal (n = 22)			
	Median	95% CI	Median	95% CI	Median	95% CI	Median	95% CI	Median	95% CI
Age (years)	74.0 (**)	71.9 to 74.4	74.0 (**)	72.1 to 74.7	75	73.1 to 78.3	**80.5**	76.7 to 81.4	72.5 (**)	70.1 to 74.8
BMI (kg/m^2)	N/A	N/A	27.3 (*)	26.8 to 28.2	**30.0**	27.6 to 31.4	27.6	25.7 to 31.3	N/A	N/A
Aneurysm size (cm)	6.3	6.5 to 6.9	6.1	6.2 to 6.6	6.1	6.0 to 6.7	6.3	6.0 to 6.9	5.9	5.9 to 6.5

*P < 0.05, **P < 0.01; significance when compared to the figure highlighted in bold for the given row.

Table 3 Mann–Whitney *U* comparison of length of stay for open and endovascular AAA repairs

Cohort		Median total length of stay (days) (95% CI)	P value	Median length of ITU stay (days) (95% CI)	P value
Open surgery					
Pre-CPET (*n* = 103)		13 (13.9 to 19.0)		4 (5.5 to 11.2)	
CPET era (*n* = 100)	**CPET-era open (100/100)**	**10 (10.3 to 13.5)**	**P < 0.001**	**3 (3.2 to 4.4)**	**P < 0.01**
	CPET-pass (74/100)	10 (10.6 to 14.9)	*P < 0.01*	3 (2.9 to 4.3)	*P < 0.001*
	CPET-fail (8/100)	11.5 (8.6 to 3.9)	*P = 0.25*	4.95 (2.1 to 8.4)	*P = 0.88*
	CPET-submaximal (3/100)	11 (−5.4 to 22.0)	*P = 0.18*	11 (−5.3 to 22.0)	*P = 0.59*
	No-CPET (15/100)	8 (6.6 to 11.1)	*P < 0.001*	5 (3.1 to 6.1)	*P = 0.82*
EVAR[a]					
Pre-CPET (*n* = 25)		6 (5.3 to 8.6)		N/A	N/A
CPET era (*n* = 69)	**CPET-era EVAR (69/69)**	**4 (4.6 to 6.7)**	**P < 0.05**	**N/A**	**N/A**
	CPET-pass (29/69)	4 (3.6 to 5.7)	*P < 0.05*	N/A	N/A
	CPET-fail (7/69)	4 (2.5 to 8.1)	*P = 0.23*	N/A	N/A
	CPET-submaximal (6/69)	4 (0 to 14.3)	*P = 0.56*	N/A	N/A
	No-CPET (27/69)	4 (4.4 to 8.8)	*P = 0.14*	N/A	N/A

[a] Insufficient EVAR patients required ITU management for reasonable comparison.

11.2; *P* < 0.01), reflected only by the CPET-pass subgroup (Table 3).

EVAR

Too few EVAR patients required ITU care in the pre-CPET or CPET-era groups for meaningful statistical comparison.

Total non-operative inpatient costs
Open surgery

Total non-operative (fully absorbed) costs of inpatient stay was significantly lower for the CPET-era cohort (mean: £5,229, 95% CI: 4,452 to 6,006; *P* < 0.001) compared with pre-CPET controls (mean: £9,637, 95% CI: 7,768 to 11,510). This trend is reflected only by the CPET-pass subgroup (mean: £5,387, 95% CI: 4,382 to 6,392; *P* < 0.001) (Figure 3). This is principally due to the reduced duration of ITU requirement (Table 3) and median number of end organs requiring support (pre-CPET: 2 organs, 95% CI 1.9 to 2.4; CPET-pass: 1 organ 95% CI 1.0 to 1.5; *P* < 0.001) in the CPET-pass subgroup.

The cost benefit is maintained when calculations are repeated using influenceable ward costs (pre-CPET: £8,203 c.f. CPET-era: £4,071; *P* < 0.001, CPET-pass subgroup: £4,068; *P* < 0.001).

EVAR

Non-operative costs are considered a function of total length of stay due to the minimal requirement for ITU in both the pre-CPET and CPET-era cohorts (Table 3).

Total 30-day mortality
Open surgery

Total 30-day mortality for elective open surgery in the pre-CPET era was significantly higher than following the introduction of CPET stratification (pre-CPET 30-day mortality: 12.6%, post-CPET 30-day mortality: 4.0%; *P* < 0.05). These findings are reflected only by those in the CPET-pass subgroup (Table 4).

EVAR

No significant difference was demonstrated in 30-day mortality following endovascular repair between the pre-CPET and CPET-era cohorts (pre-CPET 30-day mortality: 0%, CPET-era 30-day mortality: 1.4%; *P* = 1.00).

Survival

Kaplan–Meier survival analysis demonstrated reduced mid-term survival (from surgery, or from CPET for conservatively managed patients, to censorship at closure of the study) for pre-CPET EVAR and open AAA repair patients (logrank test: *P* < 0.05; Figure 4a) compared to the respective operated cohorts following CPET stratification. Median survival for pre-CPET era open AAA repairs was 2,640 days (7.23 years); however, median survival of the other subgroups could not be calculated for the period studied. The mortality-rate trends were confirmed by linear regression and remained significant (*P* < 0.001).

Survival analysis comparison between pre-CPET EVAR patients and CPET-stratified conservatively managed individuals showed no significant difference (Figure 4b) at 45 months (logrank test: *P* = 0.96).

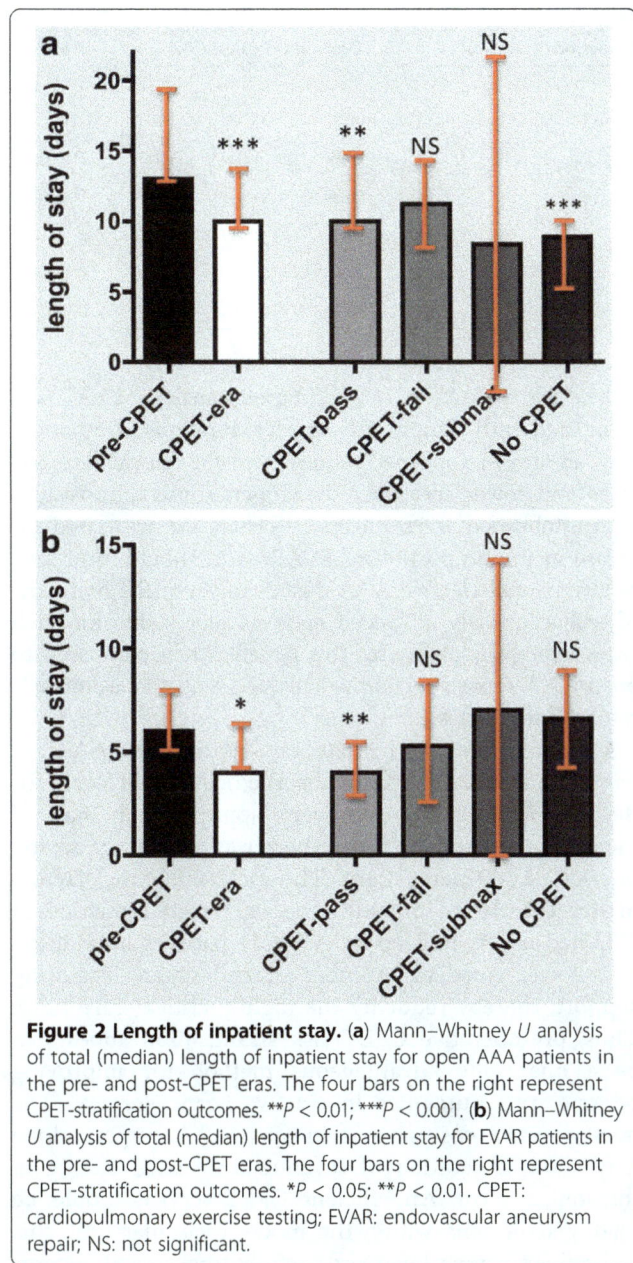

Figure 2 Length of inpatient stay. (a) Mann–Whitney U analysis of total (median) length of inpatient stay for open AAA patients in the pre- and post-CPET eras. The four bars on the right represent CPET-stratification outcomes. **$P < 0.01$; ***$P < 0.001$. (b) Mann–Whitney U analysis of total (median) length of inpatient stay for EVAR patients in the pre- and post-CPET eras. The four bars on the right represent CPET-stratification outcomes. *$P < 0.05$; **$P < 0.01$. CPET: cardiopulmonary exercise testing; EVAR: endovascular aneurysm repair; NS: not significant.

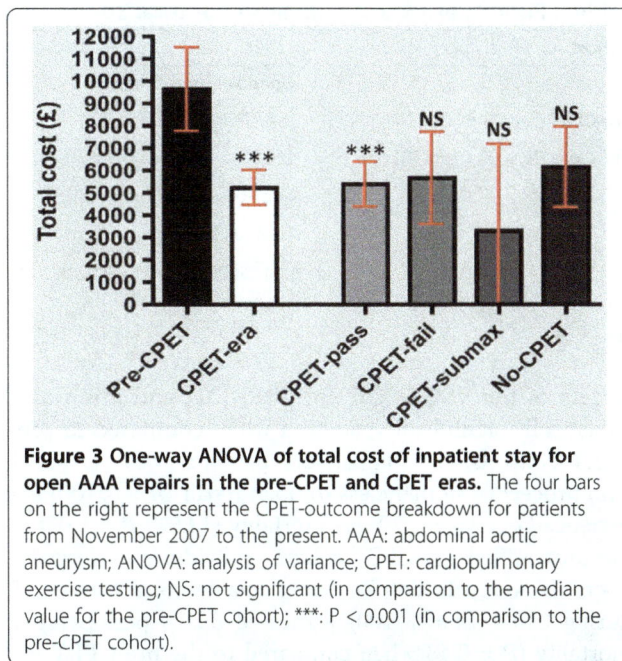

Figure 3 One-way ANOVA of total cost of inpatient stay for open AAA repairs in the pre-CPET and CPET eras. The four bars on the right represent the CPET-outcome breakdown for patients from November 2007 to the present. AAA: abdominal aortic aneurysm; ANOVA: analysis of variance; CPET: cardiopulmonary exercise testing; NS: not significant (in comparison to the median value for the pre-CPET cohort); ***: $P < 0.001$ (in comparison to the pre-CPET cohort).

Similarly, survival analysis comparison between pre-CPET open AAA repair patients and CPET-stratified conservatively managed individuals did not show significance (Figure 4c) at 45 months (logrank test: $P = 0.62$).

Non-operated patients (CPET era)

Of the 230 patients identified with elective infra-renal AAA following the introduction of CPET at UHCW NHS Trust, 61 (26.5%) had not undergone surgery prior to closure of the study. Within this group, 19 subjects were pending open or endovascular intervention (that is, on the waiting list) and 42 (18.3%) were managed conservatively. Conservative management was principally in

respect of failed or submaximal CPET, reflected by the significantly lower mean AT for this cohort (Figure 5a) despite the normal distribution of AT for the entire 2007 to 2011 cohort (Figure 5b). However, in some cases, alternate non-cardiorespiratory co-morbidities (e.g. ongoing malignancy), poor quality of life or loss of independence were quoted as indications for non-operative treatment. Two individuals chose to be managed conservatively despite an adequate AT for open intervention (Figure 1).

Conservatively managed individuals from the CPET era exhibited comparable all-cause mortality (28.6%) to the unstratified pre-CPET control group (41.4%; $P = 0.15$). However, all-cause mortality for operated patients in the CPET era was significantly lower than those treated conservatively. These findings hold true for open and endovascular repair and were reflected only in CPET-pass patients on subgroup analysis (Table 5). A summary of all-cause mortality for conservatively managed patients is shown in Table 6. This reduction in all-cause mortality translates into a significant survival advantage for CPET-stratified operated patients compared to conservatively managed individuals over the studied period (Figure 6; logrank test (curve comparison): $P < 0.05$).

Discussion

Since the advent of CPET stratification for elective AAA patients at UHCW, a significant reduction in 30-day perioperative mortality rate (4%; Table 4) for all open repairs ($n = 100$) has been noted. Individuals achieving AT ≥ 11 ml/kg/min upon CPET who subsequently underwent open AAA repair ($n = 74/100$ open repairs) exhibited 2.7% perioperative mortality, exceeding the

Table 4 Fisher's exact test comparison of total 30-day mortality

Cohort		30-day mortality (%)	Odds ratio (95% CI)	P value
	Open surgery			
Pre-CPET (Jan 03 to Oct 07)	Pre-CPET (n = 103)	12.6		
CPET era (Nov 07 to Jul 11)	CPET era (total) (n = 100)	4.0	**0.29** (0.09 to 0.92)	**$P < 0.05$**
	CPET-pass (74/100)	2.7	**0.19** (0.04 to 0.88)	**$P < 0.05$**
	CPET-fail (8/100)	12.5	0.989 (0.11 to 8.70)	$P = 1.00$
	CPET-submaximal (3/100)	33.3	2.31 (0.22 to 23.90)	$P = 0.43$
	No-CPET (15/100)	0	0.18 (0.01 to 3.20)	$P = 0.21$

targets of the VSGBI QIF for 2013 [31] and this was a statistically significant reduction when compared to pre-CPET controls. By comparison, patients with AT < 11 who proceeded nonetheless to open repair (n = 8/100) experienced equivalent 30-day mortality (12.5%; P = 1.00) to the unstratified pre-CPET cohort. Individuals undergoing open AAA repair despite being unable to generate AT during CPET (n = 3/100) witnessed 33.3% perioperative mortality (P = 0.43 when compared to the pre-CPET era cohort). No perioperative deaths were reported following open AAA repair among the 15 individuals who were submitted for surgery without CPET; however this did not achieve statistical significance (P = 0.21) when compared to pre-CPET era controls.

A pre-operative AT ≥ 11 ml/kg/min was also associated with reduced total LOS following open repair (P < 0.01) and EVAR (P < 0.05). Of interest, the 15 individuals submitted for open surgery without CPET also demonstrated a significant reduction in total LOS (P < 0.001) when compared to pre-CPET controls. Conversely, the 27 individuals who underwent EVAR without CPET risk stratification did not show such a reduction in LOS (P = 0.14).

Following open surgery, the CPET-pass subgroup also benefited from reduced ITU LOS (P < 0.001) and median number of end organs supported (P < 0.001), which were not observed among individuals with AT < 11, no AT, or those who were not referred for CPET.

The reduction in length of inpatient stay demonstrated for both open and endovascular AAA repair may have considerable beneficial financial implications for trusts offering pre-operative CPET stratification.

EVAR patients exhibited a reduction in median length of stay from 6 to 4 days following the introduction of testing; hence there was a proportionate reduction in non-operative costs attributable to fewer bed-nights on general surgical wards. Confounding factors in this analysis include a shift from pre-discharge (inpatient) computed tomography assessment of stent-graft position prior to 2007, to 30-day surveillance as an outpatient in more recent times. This may contribute to the reduction in inpatient stay witnessed within this cohort, although of note, the reduction in bed-nights required was only significant for

individuals with AT ≥ 11 on subgroup analysis. EVAR was associated with significantly shorter durations of inpatient stay, an almost abolished requirement for critical care services and lower mortality than open surgery, consistent with established work [30,36,37]. Thus, the witnessed increase in the proportion of EVAR cases should intuitively reduce overall elective AAA costs. However, the high cost of technologically advanced endovascular stents for such cases effectively abrogates this benefit when compared to open AAA repairs for individuals of adequate cardiorespiratory fitness [30,38].

A marked financial benefit was seen in open AAA repairs. Non-operative (fully absorbed) inpatient costs for the CPET-pass subgroup were approximately half of those for the pre-CPET era; there was an average saving of over £4,000 per patient. The most influential factors in this calculation included the significant reduction in ITU bed-nights utilized by AT ≥ 11 patients in addition to a lower (median) number of end organs requiring support, thereby reducing the nightly critical care tariff. Thus, pre-operative CPET risk stratification appears to be a financially advantageous method for improving perioperative outcomes in elective aortic surgery. The non-operative cost savings in open AAA surgery alone may allow generation of revenue from such testing in the longer term. An efficient CPET service should be readily achievable within the modern vascular unit; this technology having been successfully transported, assembled and utilized in a field laboratory on the South Col of Mt. Everest [39], 8,000 m above sea level.

All-cause mortality for the CPET-era cohort (2007 to 2011) was shown to be greater among individuals managed conservatively (28.6%; Tables 5 and 6) following CPET risk stratification, when compared to individuals concurrently submitted for open or endovascular surgery (6.5%; P < 0.001). A significant survival advantage was confirmed for surgically managed patients compared with those treated conservatively (for the period studied) according to Kaplan–Meier analysis (Figure 6). Individuals within this subgroup were shown to have poorer cardiorespiratory fitness than those within the operative subgroups (Figure 5a, mean AT 9.2 ml/kg/min c.f. 13.3 ml/kg/min;

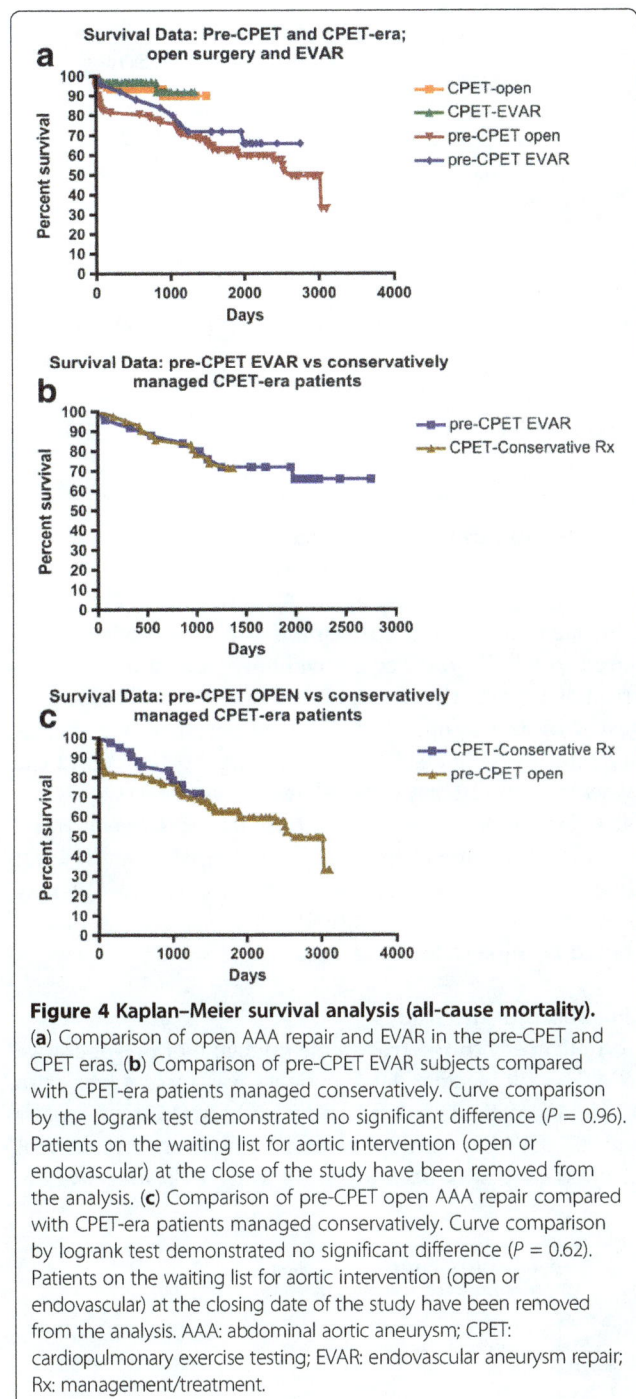

Survival Data: Pre-CPET and CPET-era;
open surgery and EVAR

a

Survival Data: pre-CPET EVAR vs conservatively
managed CPET-era patients

b

Survival Data: pre-CPET OPEN vs conservatively
managed CPET-era patients

c

Figure 4 Kaplan–Meier survival analysis (all-cause mortality).
(**a**) Comparison of open AAA repair and EVAR in the pre-CPET and
CPET eras. (**b**) Comparison of pre-CPET EVAR subjects compared
with CPET-era patients managed conservatively. Curve comparison
by the logrank test demonstrated no significant difference (*P* = 0.96).
Patients on the waiting list for aortic intervention (open or
endovascular) at the close of the study have been removed from
the analysis. (**c**) Comparison of pre-CPET open AAA repair compared
with CPET-era patients managed conservatively. Curve comparison
by logrank test demonstrated no significant difference (*P* = 0.62).
Patients on the waiting list for aortic intervention (open or
endovascular) at the closing date of the study have been removed
from the analysis. AAA: abdominal aortic aneurysm; CPET:
cardiopulmonary exercise testing; EVAR: endovascular aneurysm repair;
Rx: management/treatment.

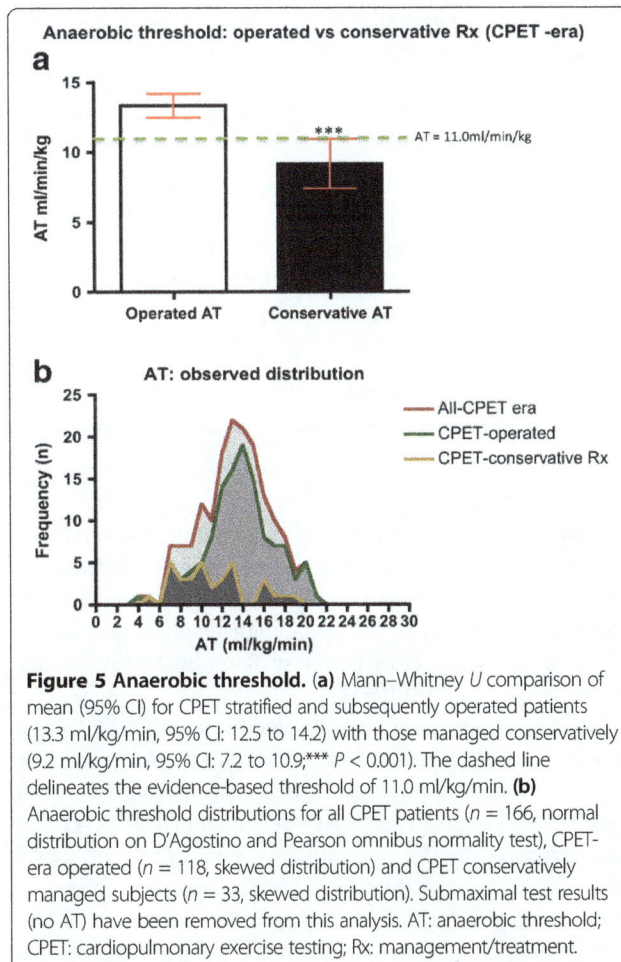

Anaerobic threshold: operated vs conservative Rx (CPET -era)

a

b   AT: observed distribution

Figure 5 Anaerobic threshold. (**a**) Mann–Whitney *U* comparison of
mean (95% CI) for CPET stratified and subsequently operated patients
(13.3 ml/kg/min, 95% CI: 12.5 to 14.2) with those managed conservatively
(9.2 ml/kg/min, 95% CI: 7.2 to 10.9;*** *P* < 0.001). The dashed line
delineates the evidence-based threshold of 11.0 ml/kg/min. (**b**)
Anaerobic threshold distributions for all CPET patients (*n* = 166, normal
distribution on D'Agostino and Pearson omnibus normality test), CPET-
era operated (*n* = 118, skewed distribution) and CPET conservatively
managed subjects (*n* = 33, skewed distribution). Submaximal test results
(no AT) have been removed from this analysis. AT: anaerobic threshold;
CPET: cardiopulmonary exercise testing; Rx: management/treatment.

P < 0.001). Data for the conservatively treated subgroup (Table 6) suggest mortality predominantly resulted from significant underlying co-morbidities and supports a non-operative approach, consistent with the findings of previous studies [40]. Known mortality from ruptured AAA for the conservatively managed subgroup was 2.4%, within the limitations of this retrospective study. By implication, therefore, only a minority of deaths within this subgroup could have been prevented by intervention (open or en-

dovascular AAA repair). However, for an individual of poor cardiorespiratory status, such an intervention would have been associated with a high risk of perioperative complications and mortality [36,40]; that is, death or serious morbidity may have been hastened by surgery. Longer-term follow-up would be required, ideally within the confines of a prospective study, to ascertain the natural progression of CPET-stratified conservatively managed patients. Assessment of the frequency of AAA-related and other deaths, morbidity and survival may develop a clearer evidence base for the optimum management of unfit individuals.

A remaining equivocation relates to the degree of stringency with which pre-operative CPET stratification is applied as a gateway to open surgery. The findings of this study show that a dramatic reduction in 30-day mortality (12.6% to 2.7%) is achievable if an AT ≥ 11.0 is considered an absolute requirement. By contrast CPET-guided pre-operative decision-making (allowing for clinical discretion) resulted in 4% 30-day mortality and permitted surgical management of a further 26 individuals. Ultimately, individual vascular units offering this service

Table 5 Fisher's exact test comparison of all-cause mortality

Cohort	Group	All-cause deaths	P value	Odds ratio
CPET era	Conservative Rx (n = 42)	12 (28.6%)		
Pre-CPET	All (n = 128)	53	0.15	N/A
	Open (n = 103)	45	0.10	N/A
	EVAR (n = 25)	8	0.79	N/A
CPET era	All operated (n = 169)	11 (6.5%)	<0.001	0.17 (0.07 to 0.43)
	All open (n = 100)	8 (8%)	<0.01	0.22 (0.08 to 0.58)
	CPET-pass OPEN (n = 74)	6 (8.1%)	<0.01	0.22 (0.08 to 0.64)
	All EVAR (n = 69)	3 (4.3%)	<0.001	0.11 (0.03 to 0.43)
	CPET-pass EVAR (n = 25)	0 (0%)	<0.01	0.05 (0.005 to 0.85)

CPET: cardiopulmonary exercise testing; EVAR: endovascular aneurysm repair; Rx: management/treatment.

will have to choose between optimizing perioperative mortality, or allowing patients of borderline cardiorespiratory fitness the chance of an elective AAA repair. This controversy, perhaps, warrants high-level debate as we move towards the 2013 target of 3.5% 30-day mortality, as set by the VSGBI QIF [31].

Patients undergoing open or endovascular AAA repair in the pre-CPET era exhibited reduced mid-term survival when compared to the CPET-era operated cohorts. Indeed, at 45 months no significant survival advantage was conferred to the unstratified open surgery or EVAR patients, when compared to CPET-stratified conservatively managed individuals (Figure 4b,c). For pre-CPET EVAR patients, who demonstrated negligible perioperative mortality rates, a prevalence of significant underlying co-morbidities in subjects selected for this intervention may contribute to these data, consistent with the findings of Goodney et al. [41]. The less metabolically demanding EVAR is routinely offered to carefully selected patients who fail to achieve a satisfactory AT on exercise testing. Equivalent survival between these patients and conservatively managed individuals, again, suggests a requirement for further study; conservative management may be more appropriate for such

patients [40], based upon specific morbidities, quality-of-life outcomes and mode of death.

For pre-CPET-era open AAA repairs, the finding of equivalent survival at 45 months (Figure 4c) when compared to CPET-stratified individuals rejected for surgery, strongly reflects the perioperative death rate. This is suggested by the significantly reduced perioperative mortality rates for CPET-stratified open AAA patients and the concurrent mid-term survival advantage seen for this cohort (Figure 4a). Moreover, the improved survival trend for CPET-stratified open AAA patients suggests that their superior cardiorespiratory fitness (Figure 5a) may preserve the survival advantage in the longer term and should be subject to further study.

Limitations of the study

Compliance with the trust-wide guideline of pre-operative CPET for all elective AAA patients was incomplete, with 42 (18.3%) patients submitted for surgery (15 open repairs and 27 EVAR) without testing. Moreover, an element of cross-over was permitted following risk stratification;

Table 6 A summary of all-cause mortality in non-operated patients following CPET stratification

Cohort	Group	Deaths	Frequency
CPET era (n = 230)	Conservatively managed (n = 42)	Total	12 (28.6%)
		Community deaths (unknown cause)	6 (14.3%)
		Ruptured AAA	1 (2.4%)
		Cardiorespiratory disease	1 (2.4%)
		Malignancy	2 (4.8%)
		Sepsis	2 (4.8%)

AAA: abdominal aortic aneurysm; CPET: cardiopulmonary exercise testing.

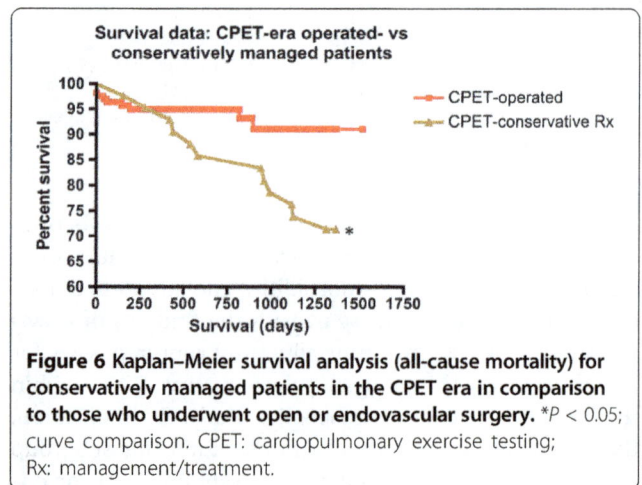

Figure 6 Kaplan–Meier survival analysis (all-cause mortality) for conservatively managed patients in the CPET era in comparison to those who underwent open or endovascular surgery. *P < 0.05; curve comparison. CPET: cardiopulmonary exercise testing; Rx: management/treatment.

individuals within the CPET-fail (AT < 11) or CPET-submaximal (no AT) subgroups were not prevented from proceeding to open surgery upon request. A number of patients were disinclined to manage their AAA expectantly (when consideration was given to the accepted 90% mortality following rupture [32]), instead they accepted the increased risk of perioperative mortality and proceeded to intervention. Morally, this was a difficult view to oppose. Such limitations of this retrospective study dictated a need for subgroup analysis of the open repair and EVAR patient groups within the CPET-era cohort (see Figure 1) to avoid confounding results.

Furthermore, despite exhaustive efforts to identify all patients with elective infra-renal AAA within both cohorts, no conservatively managed individuals could be detected in the pre-CPET era. Notwithstanding the trust's all-comers policy to aneurysm repair prior to 2007, the authors are reluctant to accept that there were no such patients. By implication, a degree of misclassification and data loss has to be assumed (leading to information bias). Such bias is compensated in part, by the subgroup analyses performed. However, potentially valuable comparisons between subjectively determined conservatively managed individuals of the pre-CPET era and those objectively identified by CPET, were not possible.

Conclusion

The introduction of pre-operative CPET risk stratification for elective AAA repair patients (as a quality improvement strategy) has shown improved perioperative outcomes.

In this retrospective study, an anaerobic threshold of ≥ 11.0 ml/kg/min has been positively associated with reduced perioperative (30-day) mortality, total LOS, length of ITU stay and support requirements for open surgical patients. As a consequence, non-operative costs were significantly reduced for these individuals. For EVAR patients, AT ≥ 11.0 was similarly associated with a reduced total LOS and thus, non-operative costs.

A significant mid-term survival advantage is also seen for CPET-stratified open repair and EVAR cohorts over controls, consistent with previous findings [26]. A consequence of CPET stratification (and clinical discretion) was the generation of a conservatively managed, unfit patient cohort. These individuals demonstrated greater all-cause mortality than surgically managed patients, principally of non-aneurysmal etiology, justifying the non-operative approach.

Recommendations for further study

A prospective randomized controlled trial (RCT) would be scientifically most appropriate to confirm the findings of this study, potentially implicating CPET as an appropriate risk assessment tool contributing to mortality prediction in AAA surgery, as per NICE recommendations for further research [42]. A recently published study suggests that the paucity of robust data should preclude routine adoption of CPET in risk-stratifying patients undergoing major vascular surgery [15]. However, to the authors' knowledge, this manuscript describes the largest current single-center UK series of patients risk-stratified in this manner for elective AAA repair, with numerous potentially advantageous outcomes. Thus, there is precedent for a RCT to clarify this ongoing and controversial issue.

Abbreviations
AAA: Abdominal aortic aneurysm; ANOVA: Analysis of variance; AT: Anaerobic threshold; BMI: Body mass index; CPET: Cardiopulmonary exercise testing; CRRS: Clinical results reporting system; ECG: Electrocardiogram; EVAR: Endovascular aneurysm repair; FEV$_1$: Forced expiratory volume in 1 second; FVC: Forced vital capacity; ITU: Intensive therapy unit; MET: Metabolic equivalent; NHS: National Health Service; NICE: National Institute for Health and Care Excellence; NS: Not significant; QIF: Quality improvement framework; RCT: Randomized controlled trial; Rx: Management/treatment; UHCW: University Hospitals Coventry and Warwickshire; VSGBI: Vascular Society of Great Britain and Ireland.

Competing interests
The authors declare that they have no competing interests.

Authors' contributions
SJG: data collection, interpretation, analysis, drafting and revision of manuscript, intellectual content of study. HY: concept and design, data collection. MS: data collection and analysis. JS: data collection, drafting of manuscript, critical revisions. CH: data collection. DW: data analysis, interpretation, critical revisions for intellectual content. CM: revision of manuscript, intellectual content. AM: revision of manuscript, intellectual content. DH: concept, intellectual content. CHEI: concept and design, data interpretation, drafting and revision of manuscript, intellectual content of study. All authors read and approved the final manuscript.

Authors' information
SJG: MBChB MD MRCS. SpR in Vascular/General Surgery, West Midlands Deanery. HY: MBChB FRCS. SpR in Vascular/General Surgery, West Midlands Deanery. MS: MBChB MRCS. Research Registrar in Vascular Surgery, UHCW NHS Trust. JS: MSc BSc. Clinical Service Manager, Department of Respiratory Physiology, University Hospitals Coventry and Warwickshire NHS Trust. CEH: MBChB MRCS. SpR in Trauma and Orthopedics. West Midlands Deanery. DW: FRCA. Consultant in Critical Care and Anesthetics. Medical Lead Central England Critical Care Network and Chair of the National Forum of Medical Leads for Critical Care Networks. CM: MBBS FRCS. Consultant Vascular Surgeon. UHCW NHS Trust. AM: MD FRCS. Consultant Vascular and Endovascular Surgeon, UHCW NHS Trust. DH: MS MMedEd FRCS. Consultant Vascular Surgeon and Clinical Lead, UHCW NHS Trust. CHEI: (Professor) PhD FRCS FRCP. Director of Research and Development, Associate Medical Director. Consultant Vascular, Endovascular and Renal Transplant Surgeon
Warwick Medical School and University Hospitals Coventry and Warwickshire NHS Trust.

Collaborators
Andrew Taylor (Finance Manager, Surgical Directorate, UHCW NHS Trust), Andrew Roberts (Information Systems Manager Department of Critical Care, UHCW NHS Trust), Julie Aughton (Specialist Respiratory Physiologist), Mr P Blacklay and Mr K Zayyan (Consultant Vascular Surgeons), Dr A Scase, Dr A Thacker, Dr E Borman, Dr B Dudkovsky, Dr S Sreevathsa and Dr A Kelly (Consultant Anesthetists).

Funding
This research received no specific grant from any funding agency in the public, commercial or not-for-profit sectors.

Author details
[1]University Hospitals Coventry and Warwickshire NHS Trust, Clifford Bridge Road, Coventry CV2 2DX, UK. [2]Warwick Medical School, University of Warwick, Coventry CV4 7AL, UK.

References
1. Waxman K: Hemodynamic and metabolic changes during and following operation. *Crit Care Clin* 1987, **3**(2):241–250.
2. Silverstein PR, Caldera DL, Cullen DJ, Davison JK, Darling RC, Emerson CW: Avoiding the hemodynamic consequences of aortic cross-clamping and unclamping. *Anesthesiology* 1979, **50**(5):462–466.
3. Attia RR, Murphy JD, Snider M, Lappas DG, Darling RC, Lowenstein E: Myocardial ischemia due to infrarenal aortic cross-clamping during aortic surgery in patients with severe coronary artery disease. *Circulation* 1976, **53**(6):961–965.
4. Pearson S, Hassen T, Spark JI, Cabot J, Cowled P, Fitridge R: Endovascular repair of abdominal aortic aneurysm reduces intraoperative cortisol and perioperative morbidity. *J Vasc Surg* 2005, **41**(6):919–925.
5. Salatash K, Sternbergh WC, York JM, Money SR: Comparison of open transabdominal AAA repair with endovascular AAA repair in reduction of the postoperative stress response. *Ann Vasc Surg* 2001, **15**:53–59.
6. Baxendale BR, Baker DM, Hutchinson A, Chuter TA, Wenham PW, Hopkinson BR: Haemodynamic and metabolic response to endovascular repair of infra-renal aortic aneurysms. *Br J Anaesth* 1996, **77**(5):581–585.
7. Struthers R, Erasmus P, Holmes K, Warman P, Collingwood A, Sneyd JR: Assessing fitness for surgery: a comparison of questionnaire, incremental shuttle walk, and cardiopulmonary exercise testing in general surgical patients. *Br J Anaesth* 2008, **101**(6):774–780.
8. Shoemaker WC, Appel PL, Kram HB, Waxman K, Lee TS: Prospective trial of supranormal values of survivors as therapeutic goals in high-risk surgical patients. *Chest* 1988, **94**(6):1176–1186.
9. Older P, Smith R: Experience with the preoperative invasive measurement of haemodynamic, respiratory and renal function in 100 elderly patients scheduled for major abdominal surgery. *Anaesth Intensive Care* 1988, **16**(4):389–395.
10. Buck N, Devlin HB, Lunn JN: *The Report of a Confidential Enquiry into Perioperative Deaths.* London: The Nuffield Provincial Hospital Trust and the Kings Fund; 1987.
11. Eagle KA, Berger PB, Calkins H, Chaitman BR, Ewy GA, Fleischmann KE, Fleisher LA, Froehlich JB, Gusberg RJ, Leppo JA, Ryan T, Schlant RC, Winters WL Jr, Gibbons RJ, Antman EM, Alpert JS, Faxon DP, Fuster V, Gregoratos G, Jacobs AK, Hiratzka LF, Russell RO, Smith SC Jr: ACC/AHA guideline update for perioperative cardiovascular evaluation for noncardiac surgery – executive summary: a report of the American College of Cardiology/American Heart Association Task Force on Practice Guidelines (Committee to Update the 1996 Guidelines on Perioperative Cardiovascular Evaluation for Noncardiac Surgery). *J Am Coll Cardiol* 2002, **39**(3):542–553.
12. Aronow WS, Ahn C: Incidence of heart failure in 2,737 older persons with and without diabetes mellitus. *Chest* 1999, **115**(3):867–868.
13. Reilly DF, McNeely MJ, Doerner D, Greenberg DL, Staiger TO, Geist MJ, Vedovatti PA, Coffey JE, Mora MW, Johnson TR, Guray ED, Van Norman GA, Fihn SD: Self-reported exercise tolerance and the risk of serious perioperative complications. *Arch Intern Med* 1999, **159**(18):2185–2192.
14. Fleisher LA, Beckman JA, Brown KA, Calkins H, Chaikof EL, Fleischmann KE, Freeman WK, Froehlich JB, Kasper EK, Kersten JR, Riegel B, Robb JF, Smith SC Jr, Jacobs AK, Adams CD, Anderson JL, Antman EM, Buller CE, Creager MA, Ettinger SM, Faxon DP, Fuster V, Halperin JL, Hiratzka LF, Hunt SA, Lytle BW, Nishimura R, Ornato JP, Page RL, Riegel B, *et al*: ACC/AHA 2007 Guidelines on Perioperative Cardiovascular Evaluation and Care for Noncardiac Surgery: Executive Summary: A Report of the American College of Cardiology/American Heart Association Task Force on Practice Guidelines (Writing Committee to Revise the 2002 Guidelines on Perioperative Cardiovascular Evaluation for Noncardiac Surgery)

Developed in Collaboration With the American Society of Echocardiography, American Society of Nuclear Cardiology, Heart Rhythm Society, Society of Cardiovascular Anesthesiologists, Society for Cardiovascular Angiography and Interventions, Society for Vascular Medicine and Biology, and Society for Vascular Surgery. *J Am Coll Cardiol* 2007, **50**(17):1707–1732.
15. Young EL, Karthikesalingam A, Huddart S, Pearse RM, Hinchliffe RJ, Loftus IM, Thompson MM, Holt PJ: A systematic review of the role of cardiopulmonary exercise testing in vascular surgery. *Eur J Vasc Endovasc Surg* 2012, **44**:64–71.
16. Bauer SM, Cayne NS, Veith FJ: New developments in the preoperative evaluation and perioperative management of coronary artery disease in patients undergoing vascular surgery. *J Vasc Surg* 2010, **51**(1):242–251.
17. Thompson AR, Peters N, Lovegrove RE, Ledwidge S, Kitching A, Magee TR, Galland RB: Cardiopulmonary exercise testing provides a predictive tool for early and late outcomes in abdominal aortic aneurysm patients. *Ann R Coll Surg Engl* 2011, **93**(6):474–481.
18. Franciosa JA, Park M, Levine TB: Lack of correlation between exercise capacity and indices of resting left ventricular ejection performance in heart failure. *Am J Cardiol* 1981, **47**:33–39.
19. Lipkin DP: The role of exercise testing in chronic heart failure. *Br Heart J* 1987, **58**:559–566.
20. Smith TB, Stonell C, Purkayastha S, Paraskevas P: Cardiopulmonary exercise testing as a risk assessment in non cardio-pulmonary surgery: a systematic review. *Anaesthesia* 2009, **64**:883–893.
21. Henry K, Gilliland C, Sharkey R, Daly JG, Kelly MG, Mc Cune K, *et al*: The use of cardiopulmonary exercise testing in the pre-operative assessment of patients awaiting abdominal aortic aneurysm repair in a District General Hospital. *Irish J Med Sci* 2010, **179**:S496.
22. Kothmann E, Danjoux G, Owen SJ, Parry A, Turley AJ, Batterham AM: Reliability of the anaerobic threshold in cardiopulmonary exercise testing of patients with abdominal aortic aneurysms. *Anaesthesia* 2009, **64**(1):9–13.
23. Older P, Smith R, Courtney P, Hone R: Preoperative evaluation of cardiac failure and ischaemia in elderly patients by cardiopulmonary exercise testing. *Chest* 1993, **104**:701–704.
24. Older P, Hall A, Hader R: Cardiopulmonary exercise testing as a screening test for perioperative management of major surgery in the elderly. *Chest* 1999, **116**:355–362.
25. Snowden CP, Prentis JM, Anderson HL, Roberts DR, Randles D, Renton M, Manas DM: Submaximal cardiopulmonary exercise testing predicts complications and hospital length of stay in patients undergoing major elective surgery. *Ann Surg* 2010, **251**(3):535–541.
26. Carlisle J, Swart M: Mid-term survival after abdominal aortic aneurysm surgery predicted by cardiopulmonary exercise testing. *Br J Surg* 2007, **94**:966–969.
27. Hartley RA, Pichel AC, Grant SW, Hickey GL, Lancaster PS, Wisely NA, McCollum CN, Atkinson D: Preoperative cardiopulmonary exercise testing and risk of early mortality following abdominal aortic aneurysm repair. *Br J Surg* 2012, **99**(11):1539–1546.
28. Scott RAP, Ashton HA, Buxton MJ, Day NE, Day NE, Marteau TM, *et al*: The Multicentre Aneurysm Screening Study (MASS) into the effect of abdominal aortic aneurysm screening on mortality in men: a randomised controlled trial. *Lancet* 2002, **360**:1531–1539.
29. The UK Small Aneurysm Trial Participants: Mortality results for randomised controlled trial of early elective surgery or ultrasonographic surveillance for small abdominal aortic aneurysms. *Lancet* 1998, **352**:1649–1655.
30. EVAR trial participants: Comparison of endovascular aneurysm repair with open repair in patients with abdominal aortic aneurysm (EVAR trial 1), 30-day operative mortality results: randomised controlled trial. *Lancet* 2004, **364**:844–848.
31. Vascular Society of Great Britain and Ireland: UK National AAA Quality Improvement Framework document, 2009 - Updated 2011. [http://www.vascularsociety.org.uk/vascular/wp-content/uploads/2012/11/VSGBI-AAA-QIF-2011-v4.pdf] (last accessed 24/05/2013).
32. Bengtsson H, Bergqvist D: Ruptured abdominal aortic aneurysm: a population-based study. *J Vasc Surg* 1993, **18**:74–80.
33. Blankensteijn JD, Lindenburg FP, Van der Graaf Y, Eikelboom BC: Influence of study design on reported mortality and morbidity rates after abdominal aortic aneurysm repair. *Br J Surg* 1998, **85**:1624–1630.

34. National Research Ethics Service: *Changes to the Remit of Research Ethics Committees*; 2011. Available at www.nres.nhs.uk/EasySiteWeb/GatewayLink. aspx?alld=134047. Last accessed 05/05/2013.

35. Beaver WL, Wasserman K, Whipp BJ: **A new method of detecting anaerobic threshold by gas exchange.** *J Appl Physiol* 1986, **60**:2020–2027.

36. Prentis JM, Trenell MI, Jones DJ, Lees T, Clarke M, Snowden CP: **Submaximal exercise testing predicts perioperative hospitalization after aortic aneurysm repair.** *J Vasc Surg* 2012, **56**(6):1564–1570.

37. Shiels H, Desmond AN, Parimkayala R, Cahill J: **The impact of abdominal aortic aneurysm surgery on intensive care unit resources in an Irish tertiary centre.** *Ir J Med Sci* 2012.

38. Finlayson SR, Birkmeyer JD, Fillinger MF, Cronenwett JL: **Should endovascular surgery lower the threshold for repair of abdominal aortic aneurysms?** *J Vasc Surg* 1999, **29**:973–985.

39. Levett DZH, Martin DS, Wilson MH, Mitchell K, Dhillon S, Rigat F, *et al*: **Design and conduct of Caudwell Xtreme Everest: an observational cohort study of variation in human adaptation to progressive environmental hypoxia.** *BMC Med Res Methodol* 2010, **10**:98.

40. EVAR Trial Participants: **Endovascular aneurysm repair and outcome in patients unfit for open repair of abdominal aortic aneurysm (EVAR trial 2): randomised controlled trial.** *Lancet* 2005, **365**:2187–2192.

41. Goodney PP, Travis L, Lucas FL, Fillinger MF, Goodman DC, Cronenwett JL, Stone DH: **Survival after open versus endovascular thoracic aortic aneurysm repair in an observational study of the Medicare population.** *Circulation* 2011, **358**:464–474.

42. National Institute for Health and Care Excellence (NICE): *technology appraisal guidance 167. Endovascular Stent Grafts for the Treatment of Abdominal Aortic Aneurysms.* http://www.nice.org.uk/nicemedia/live/12129/43289/43289.pdf (last accessed 05/05/2013).

Coagulation during elective neurosurgery with hydroxyethyl starch fluid therapy: an observational study with thromboelastometry, fibrinogen and factor XIII

Caroline Ulfsdotter Nilsson[1*], Karin Strandberg[2], Martin Engström[3] and Peter Reinstrup[1]

Abstract

Background: Several studies have described hypercoagulability in neurosurgery with craniotomy for brain tumor resection. In this study, hydroxyethyl starch (HES) 130/0.42 was used for hemodynamic stabilization and initial blood loss replacement. HES can induce coagulopathy with thromboelastographic signs of decreased clot strength. The aim of this study was to prospectively describe perioperative changes in coagulation during elective craniotomy for brain tumor resection with the present fluid regimen.

Methods: Forty patients were included. Perioperative whole-blood samples were collected for EXTEM and FIBTEM assays on rotational thromboelastometry (ROTEM) and plasma fibrinogen analysis immediately before surgery, after 1 L of HES infusion, at the end of surgery and in the morning after surgery. Factor (F)XIII activity, thrombin-antithrombin complex (TAT) and plasmin-α2-antiplasmin complex (PAP) were analysed in the 25 patients receiving ≥1 L of HES.

Results: Most patients (37 of 40) received HES infusion (0.5–2 L) during surgery. Preoperative ROTEM clot formation/structure, plasma fibrinogen and FXIII levels were generally within normal range but approached a hypocoagulant state during and at end of surgery. ROTEM variables and fibrinogen levels, but not FXIII, returned to baseline levels in the morning after surgery. Low perioperative fibrinogen levels were common. TAT levels were increased during and after surgery. PAP levels mostly remained within the reference ranges, not indicating excessive fibrinolysis. There were no differences in ROTEM results and fibrinogen levels in patients receiving <1 L HES and ≥1 L HES.

Conclusions: Only the increased TAT levels indicated an intra- and postoperative activation of coagulation. On the contrary, all other variables deteriorated towards hypocoagulation but were mainly normalized in the morning after surgery. Although this might be an effect of colloid-induced coagulopathy, we found no dose-dependent effect of HES. The unactivated fibrinolysis indicates that prophylactic use of tranexamic acid does not seem warranted under normal circumstances in elective neurosurgery. Individualized fluid therapy and coagulation factor substitution is of interest for future studies.

Keywords: Factor XIII, Fibrinogen, Hydroxyethyl starch derivatives, Neurosurgery, Thromboelastography

---

* Correspondence: caroline.nilsson@med.lu.se
[1]Department of Anaesthesia and Intensive Care, Skåne University Hospital, Lund University, Lund, Sweden
Full list of author information is available at the end of the article

Background

In neurosurgery, it is imperative to avoid intracranial bleeding. Perioperative bleeding can be associated with a number of factors including antihemostatic drugs and coagulation status but is also linked to the tumor's vascularity, type, size and localization and the use of local hemostatics (Gerlach et al. 2004; Nittby et al. 2016). On the other hand, there is an increased risk of venous thromboembolism after elective neurosurgery (Collen et al. 2008). Hypercoagulation has been described in patients undergoing brain tumor surgery (Iberti et al. 1994; Nielsen et al. 2014).

In order to balance thrombosis and bleeding, we need to know the perioperative changes in coagulation. Among routine coagulation analyses are activated partial thromboplastin time (aPTT), prothrombin time (PT), platelet count and fibrinogen levels (Kozek-Langenecker 2010). Additional parameters that can be used are measurements of activated coagulation and fibrinolysis (e.g. thrombin-antithrombin complex (TAT) and plasmin-α2-antiplasmin complex (PAP)). Measurement of coagulation factor XIII (FXIII) levels or activity is becoming increasingly recognized as important during surgery (Levy and Greenberg 2013). Viscoelastic instruments such as thromboelastography (TEG) and rotational thromboelastometry (ROTEM) are point-of-care instruments that are helpful for quickly assessing global hemostatic function in whole blood and for guiding treatment of bleeding (Afshari et al. 2011).

Hydroxyethyl starch (HES) is a colloid solution that can be used to replace initial blood loss and to treat hypovolemia during elective surgery. However, HES can induce a hypocoagulable state by diluting fibrinogen and FXIII, as well as it affects fibrin polymerization and clot structure (Fenger-Eriksen et al. 2009). After the publication of several large randomized controlled trials indicating a risk of kidney injury in critically ill patients receiving HES, its use has been diminished over the last few years. However, there is still controversy as to whether HES should be avoided in all clinical situations, and evidence of HES-induced kidney injury in the perioperative setting is lacking (Greenberg and Tung 2015; European Medicines Agency 2014). The European Medicines Agency currently states that HES may be used to treat acute hypovolemia, but not in patients with sepsis, critical illness, severe coagulopathy and renal injury (European Medicines Agency 2014).

The local routine at our hospital was to use HES (130/0.42) for hemodynamic stabilization and initial blood loss replacement during elective brain tumor resection. The aim of this prospective observational study was to describe perioperative coagulation changes with ROTEM, TAT, PAP, FXIII activity and fibrinogen levels in these patients.

Methods

Ethical approval and patients

The study was approved by the regional ethics committee (Lund, Protocol DNR 2012/43) and was performed at Skåne University Hospital in Lund, Sweden. The study included 40 patients undergoing elective craniotomy and tumor resection.

All patients were >18 years old and gave written consent to participate. Patients with a known congenital hemophilic or thrombophilic coagulation disorder and/or who were treated with anticoagulants/antiplatelet agents within 5 days before surgery were not enrolled. Preoperative coagulation tests PT, aPTT and platelet count were not routinely analysed in patients with no history of bleeding disorders (according to previous findings (Seicean et al. 2012)). Patients with abnormal aPTT and/or PT and a platelet count below the reference range were excluded. Patients with abnormal serum-creatinine (>90 µmol/L for women and >105 µmol/L for men) were also excluded. For logistical reasons, only patients scheduled for surgery in the morning were chosen to participate. Patients meeting the inclusion criteria were enrolled consecutively from February through May 2012.

The majority of patients had dexamethasone treatment prior to surgery in order to reduce tumor edema. All patients received a preoperative prophylactic dose of peroral rifampicin. Standard anaesthesia with fentanyl, propofol, isoflourane and rocuronium was used.

All patients received mechanical calf compression thromboprophylaxis during surgery and 24 h postoperatively. The fluid protocol included isotonic saline infusion as maintenance fluid (1.5–2.0 mL/kg/h). Bleeding (200–300 mL) was initially substituted with saline (1:2 bleeding to saline). Additional bleeding was substituted with HES (Venofundin® 60 mg/mL [6% hydroxyethyl, molecular weight (MW) 130 kDa, substitution 0.42, in saline solution, Braun, Melsungen Germany], 1:1 bleeding to HES), with a maximum dose of 30 mL/kg. HES was also used to keep mean arterial blood pressure (MAP) at >65 mmHg. Red blood cell transfusion was given when hemoglobin levels declined below 95–100 g/L. Blood loss of more than 30 % of calculated blood volume was substituted with red blood cells, fresh frozen plasma and platelet concentrates.

Local hemostatics (SurgiSeal®, Adhezion Biomedica, PA, USA, and TachoSil®, Takeda, High Wycomb, UK) were applied at the discretion of the surgeon. The coagulation assays TAT, PAP, fibrinogen and FXIII were performed in a batch after the completion of the study enrolment. TAT, PAP and FXIII were analysed in a subset of patients (those receiving ≥1 L HES) due to the initial plan to focus in depth coagulation studies on these patients (more homogenous with respect to HES volumes administered). Perioperative ROTEM analyses, especially abnormal EXTEM-MCF and FIBTEM-MCF, were shown to the anaesthetist in charge, who evaluated the hemostatic status together with the surgeon to decide whether plasma, platelet transfusion or fibrinogen concentrate were to be administered. Apart from this safety measure of informing the anaesthetist in charge, there was no intervention in the management of patients.

Blood sampling

Arterial blood samples were drawn from an indwelling radial arterial catheter with continuous flushing and a sampling membrane which eliminates the need for disposing blood samples.

Blood sampling for the study was performed before surgery (after the induction of anaesthesia, baseline), after 1 L of HES infusion (only analysed in patients receiving ≥1 L HES), at the end of surgery and in the morning after surgery (the first postoperative day).

Blood was collected in citrated tubes (BD Vacutainer® 4.5 mL 0.129 M for laboratory plasma analysis and 2.7 mL 0.109 M for ROTEM analysis). The blood samples intended for laboratory plasma analysis were immediately centrifuged for 20 min at 2000 rpm at a temperature of 20 °C to obtain the plasma fractions. Plasma vials for the separate tests (TAT, PAP, fibrinogen and FXIII) were frozen and stored in a −85 °C freezer until analysis.

Surgical blood loss

The amount of bleeding during surgery was assessed by weighing sponges and measuring losses in the suction device.

ROTEM

ROTEM analysis (TEM International GmbH, Munich, Germany) was performed according to the manufacturer's instructions with EXTEM (tissue factor activation) and FIBTEM (tissue factor activation and platelet inhibition) reagents. The parameters obtained with EXTEM were clotting time (CT), clot formation time (CFT), α-angle and maximum clot firmness (MCF), whereas MCF was obtained with FIBTEM. Reference intervals provided by the ROTEM manufacturer were used: EXTEM: CT 38–79 s, CFT 34–159 s, α-angle 63–83°, MCF 50–72 mm, and FIBTEM: MCF 9–25 mm. A ROTEM variable within the reference interval indicated normal coagulability, whereas a variable outside the reference interval indicated increased or decreased coagulability.

Laboratory plasma analyses

Fibrinogen was measured with a photometric assay (Multifibren U, Siemens, AG, Gerlangen, Germany). Thrombin (50 U/mL) was added in excess to plasma

samples. Clotting time was recorded with an automated coagulometer (Symex CA 7000, Siemens AG, Gerlangen, Germany) and compared to clotting times with known fibrinogen concentrations. The reference interval for fibrinogen is 2–4 g/L, according to the manufacturer.

FXIII activity was determined with the automated Berichrom FXIII (Siemens Healthcare Diagnostics, Marburg, Germany) method, on the BCS-XP Coagulation analyser (Siemens Healthcare Diagnostics, Marburg, Germany). FXIII in the plasma sample is converted to FXIIIa after the addition of thrombin. FXIIIa is detected in an enzymatic reaction in which ammonia is released. The absorbance at 340 mm is proportional to the FXIIIa activity in the sample. The reference interval in healthy adults is 0.70–1.40 kIU/L according to the manufacturer.

TAT was measured using Enzygnost TAT micro (Siemens Healthcare Diagnostics, Marburg, Germany), a solid-phase enzyme-linked immunoassay (ELISA). The reference interval in healthy adults is 1.0–4.1 µg/L (2.5–97.5 percentile, $n = 196$) according to the manufacturer.

PAP was determined using DRG PAP micro ELISA (DRG Instruments GmbH, Marburg, Germany), a solidphase ELISA based on a sandwich principle. The reference interval in healthy adults is 120–700 µg/L (2.5–97.5 percentile, $n = 466$) according to the manufacturer.

Statistical analysis

Data was processed using Microsoft Excel® and Graph-Pad Prism. Results are presented as median and range. The Wilcoxon matched-pairs signed rank test was performed to find changes in the variables from baseline compared to after 1 L HES, at the end of surgery and in the morning after surgery.

Statistics were also performed with patients divided into groups receiving a low dose (<1 L) or higher dose (≥1 L) of HES in order to investigate a possible dose-response. The Mann-Whitney U test for unpaired data was used to detect differences between the groups at baseline, at the end of surgery and in the morning after surgery.

After Bonferroni correction for the number of significance tests per each variable ($n = 6$), a P value of <0.0083 (0.05/6) was considered statistically significant at a $P < 0.05$ level.

For five measured FXIII activity levels, the activity was > 1.299 kIU/L. This right-truncated data (>1.299) was treated as =1.299 in statistical calculations and in graphs.

Fibrinogen and FXIII levels were correlated with FIBTEM-MCF levels using the Spearman rank correlation.

Results

Study population and clinical data

The study included 40 patients (16 males and 24 females), aged 35–81 years (median 56 years), with median BMI 25 (range 17.5–39). Meningioma was the most common diagnosis (18 patients); other tumor types included metastasis, astrocytoma, schwannoma, glioblastoma, ependymoma, craniopharyngioma and chordoma. Operation times ranged from 2 to 10 h, with a median time of 5 h.

Preoperative hemoglobin levels were 128 g/L (range 96–169 g/L). Median bleeding during surgery was 450 mL, ranging from 50 to 2500 mL. Nine patients had bleeding of ≥1 L during surgery. Of the six patients with bleeding of >1 L, all but one had surgery for meningioma. Fifteen patients received <1 L HES (between 500 and 800 mL), including three patients who did not receive any HES at all. Twenty-five patients received ≥1 L HES, with only one patient receiving a large volume of 2 L. Twelve patients were transfused with blood components during surgery (red blood cells, plasma and/or platelets). One patient was given one dose of tranexamic acid during surgery. Seven patients were also given 5 % albumin in waiting for plasma. No patient needed reoperation because of postoperative hematoma. Characteristics of the patients divided into groups (<1 L HES and ≥1 L HES) are seen in Table 1.

ROTEM

Preoperative hypercoagulation as seen with ROTEM variables was only found in one patient with a shortened CT (36 s). Signs of preoperative decreased coagulability were seen in eight patients with ROTEM. Five patients had low alpha angle and/or low FIBTEM-MCF. Three patients had impaired CFT, alpha angle, MCF and FIBTEM-MCF, and two of these had prolonged CT.

Statistical analysis for all patients ($n = 40$) showed that all ROTEM variables (CFT, alpha angle, MCF and FIBTEM-MCF) except for CT were changed towards impaired coagulation at the end of surgery compared to baseline ($P < 0.0001$, Table 2, Fig. 1). All ROTEM variables were also impaired after administration of 1 L HES compared to baseline ($P < 0.0001$). ROTEM variables returned to baseline values in the morning of the first postoperative day.

Table 1 Group characteristics

	<1 L HES	≥1 L HES
Number of patients	15	25
Age (years)	57 (31–79)	55 (35–81)
Operation duration (h)	3.5 (2–7)	6 (2–10)
Bleeding during surgery (mL)	200 (50–2000)	700 (70–2500)
Number of patients receiving blood component therapy (red blood cells, plasma and/or platelets) during surgery	2	10
Reoperation due to hematoma	0	0

Group characteristics for patients receiving <1 L HES and ≥1 L HES. Median (range)

There were no statistically significant differences between the groups (patients receiving <1 L HES and ≥1 L HES) at baseline, at the end of surgery and in the morning after surgery for any of the ROTEM variables ($P > 0.0083$).

Laboratory plasma analyses

Twenty patients had low fibrinogen (<2.0 g/L) before surgery. At the end of surgery, 21 of 40 patients had a fibrinogen level of ≤1.5 g/L. Fibrinogen decreased from the baseline median of 1.9 to 1.5 g/L by the end of surgery ($P < 0.0001$, Table 2, Fig. 2) but increased again until the first morning after surgery (median 2.4 g/L). Fibrinogen was decreased compared to baseline after the administration of 1 L HES ($P < 0.0001$). All patients with low preoperative FIBTEM-MCF (<9 mm, $n = 5$) had low fibrinogen levels (0.9–1.4 g/L). There were no differences in fibrinogen levels between the groups (patients receiving <1 L HES or ≥1 L HES) at baseline, at the end of surgery and in the morning after surgery ($P > 0.0083$).

In the 25 patients who received ≥1 L HES ($n = 25$), six patients had low preoperative FXIII which remained below the reference range during the observation period. FXIII activity was decreased compared to baseline after 1 L HES and at the end of surgery, and it remained decreased in the morning after surgery ($P < 0.0001$, Table 2, Fig. 2).

TAT levels (>4.1 µg/L) were significantly elevated at the end of surgery and remained elevated the morning after surgery (Table 2, Fig. 2). TAT levels were borderline significantly elevated after 1 L HES (Table 2). PAP was decreased after 1 L HES and at the end of surgery but returned to preoperative levels in the morning after surgery (Table 2, Fig. 2). However, PAP mainly remained within the normal reference range.

Variable correlation

FXIII activity correlated poorly with FIBTEM-MCF with a correlation coefficient of 0.54 ($P < 0.01$). Fibrinogen correlated better with FIBTEM-MCF with a correlation coefficient of 0.70 ($P < 0.01$).

Discussion

Increased ("hyper") or decreased ("hypo") coagulability was defined as variables outside the reference intervals (Görlinger et al. 2013). Based on this definition, the preoperative coagulation state in our neurosurgical patients mostly appeared normal on ROTEM but approached a hypocoagulable state during surgery and at the end of surgery, only to return to baseline levels in the first postoperative morning (or, for CT, at end of surgery). Signs of perioperative hypercoagulability were uncommon.

Like our results, previous viscoelastic studies of elective neurosurgical patients describe both a mainly normal

Table 2 Descriptive data and statistics

	Reference interval	Baseline	After 1 L HES (patients receiving ≥1 L HES)	P value Baseline vs after 1 L HES (patients receiving ≥1 L HES)	End of surgery	P value Baseline vs end of surgery	Morning after surgery	P value Baseline vs morning after surgery
Analysed in all patients (n = 40)								
CT (s)	38–79	50.5 (36–121)	63 (37–125)	<0.0001	57 (38–101) [3]	0.027	54 (36–97) [5]	0.41
CFT (s)	34–159	110.5 (64–286)	170 (97–325)	<0.0001	135 (74–311) [3]	<0.0001	116 (57–276) [5]	0.13
Alpha angle (°)	63–83	68 (51–80)	58 (48–70)	<0.0001	64 (46–75) [3]	<0.0001	68 (45–79) [5]	0.034
MCF (mm)	50–72	59 (39–69)	50 (38–74)	<0.0001	55 (38–65) [3]	<0.0001	58 (46–69) [6]	0.24
FIBTEM-MCF (mm)	9–25	12 (4–24)	7 (0–12)	<0.0001	9 (2–18) [5]	<0.0001	14 (5–26) [5]	0.051
Fibrinogen (g/L)	2–4	1.9 (0.9–3.3)	1.4 (0.6–2.8)	<0.0001	1.5 (0.6–2.8)	<0.0001	2.4 (0.6–3.4) [5]	0.012
Analysed in patients receiving ≥1000 mL HES (n = 25)								
FXIII (kIU/L)	0.7–1.4	0.9 (0.43–>1.30)	0.62 (0.32–1.16)	<0.0001	0.68 (0.39–1.19) [3]	<0.0001	0.84 (0.44–>1.30) [3]	<0.0001
TAT (µg/L)	1.0–4.1	4.4 (2–68) [1]	7.2 (2–98)	0.0087	23.4 (2–142) [3]	0.0004	8.1 (3–449) [2]	0.0032
PAP (µg/L)	120–700	541.3 (275–1997)	419.5 (218–1478)	<0.0001	392.4 (276–1339) [3]	<0.0001	481.0 (288–2297) [2]	0.80

Data is presented as median values (range) [missing]. Italicized P values are statistically significant (P < 0.0083)
HES hydroxyethyl starch, CT clotting time, CFT clot formation time, MCF maximum clot firmness, TAT thrombin-antithrombin complex, PAP plasmin-α2-antiplasmin complex, FXIII factor XIII

preoperative coagulation status in accordance with our findings (Goobie et al. 2001; El Kady et al. 2009; Lindroos et al. 2014) but, unlike our findings, an increased coagulability (varying definitions) during and after surgery (Nielsen et al. 2014; Goobie et al. 2001; El Kady et al. 2009; Abrahams et al. 2002; Goh et al. 1997). Two studies found that patients who developed a postoperative hematoma had impaired coagulation as compared to patients who did not develop a hematoma (El Kady et al. 2009; Goh et al. 1997). Thus, the impaired coagulation we identified during surgery might increase the risk for postoperative intracranial hematomas. Explanations for this impaired coagulation could be blood loss, coagulation factor consumption or dilution by fluids including HES-induced coagulopathy. A possible HES effect needs to be validated in a randomized trial comparing HES to another fluid regime including its implications for bleeding and thrombotic events in neurosurgery.

Although modern starches (such as 130/0.4) seem to have little effect on perioperative bleeding in major surgery (Kozek-Langenecker 2015), a dose-response of the negative impact on clot strength by HES 130/0.4 has previously been described, primarily by in vitro studies (Hartog et al. 2011). In the present study, we did not see a dose-response of HES on coagulation (ROTEM and fibrinogen levels), as we compared patients who received either <1 L HES or ≥1 L HES; however, this is a small study in which almost all patients received HES, making conclusions about a dose-response difficult. Although

our study is underpowered to detect a correlation between the different variables and clinical bleeding/postoperative complications, no patient needed reoperation due to hematoma. Median bleeding volume was higher in patients who received the higher doses of HES, but probably reflects that more bleeding prompted more volume replacement. Of the six patients who bled >1 L, all but one had meningioma surgery. Meningiomas are known to be highly vascular and bleeding can be a problem during resection and postoperatively (Gerlach et al. 2004).

Other studies have looked at HES in neurosurgery. A study by Lindroos et al. that included 30 patients detected signs of impaired ROTEM FIBTEM clot formation and strength during neurosurgery with HES infusion (130/0.4), but not with Ringer's acetate (Lindroos et al. 2014). ROTEM EXTEM was unaffected. The mean HES volume was 440 mL, which is less than the HES volumes that was used for our patients and could explain why we saw a more pronounced impaired coagulation. Two retrospective studies of more than 4000 patients (Feix et al. 2015) and more than 40,000 patients (Jian et al. 2014) did not find an association between the use of HES 130/0.4 (average volume 700 mL and median volume 500 mL, respectively) and a risk of reoperation for intracranial hematoma after craniotomy. As mentioned, evidence so far do not suggest that modern day HES increases bleeding in other types of major surgery. However, this fluid still impairs fibrin polymerization and clot strength (Kozek-Langenecker 2015) and this

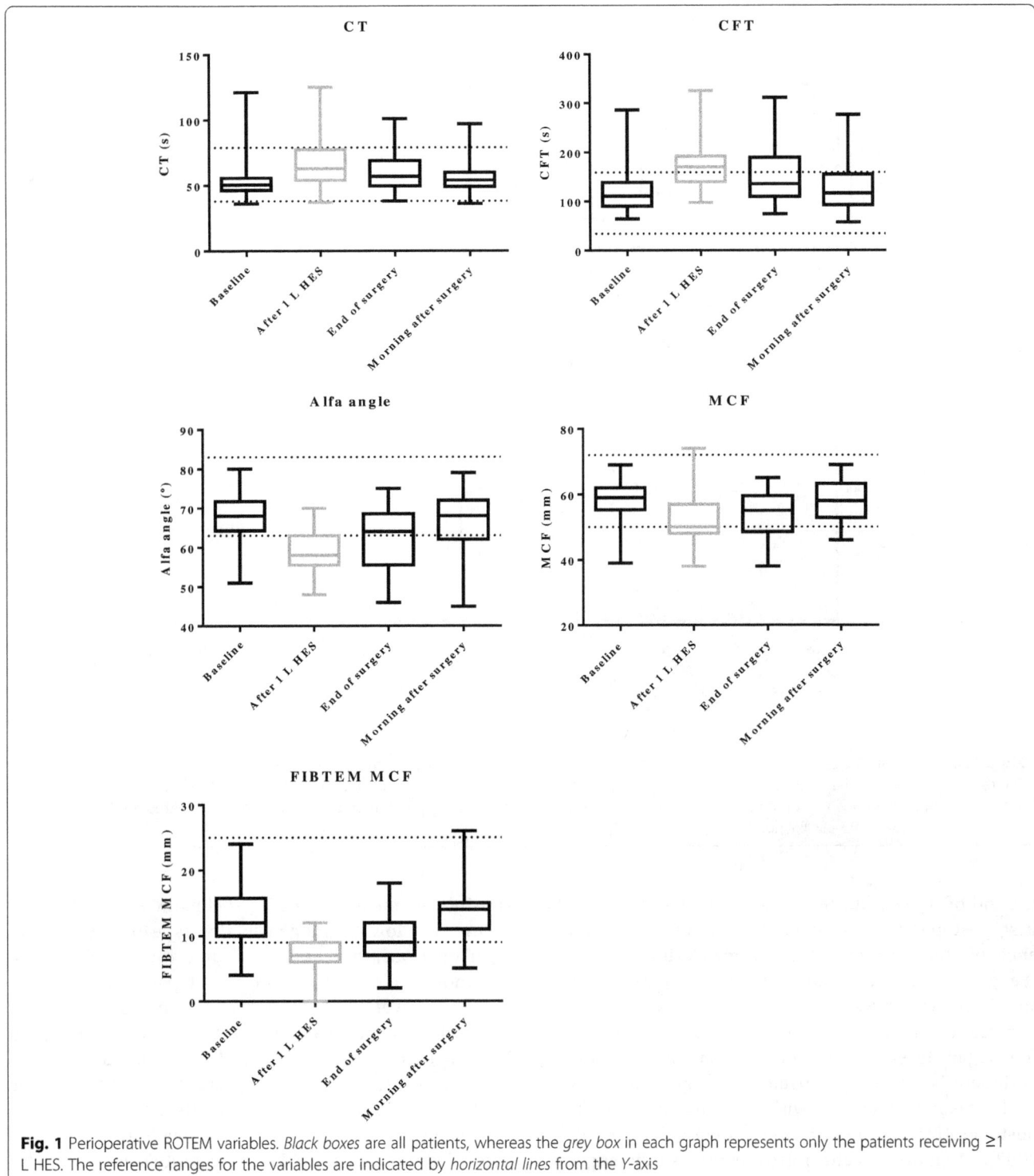

Fig. 1 Perioperative ROTEM variables. *Black boxes* are all patients, whereas the *grey box* in each graph represents only the patients receiving ≥1 L HES. The reference ranges for the variables are indicated by *horizontal lines* from the *Y*-axis

effect in neurosurgery has not been properly evaluated. Currently, the role of HES in the perioperative setting is still largely unknown, and further studies regarding the safety, timing and choice of colloids are necessary (Coriat et al. 2014). Furthermore, preoperative coagulation testing could possibly indicate which patients can tolerate larger volumes of HES and which patients should be given HES or other colloids with care, but this "dilutive capacity strategy" in patients needs to be tested in prospective studies.

Preoperative low fibrinogen (<2 g/L) was common in the present study and decreased further during and at

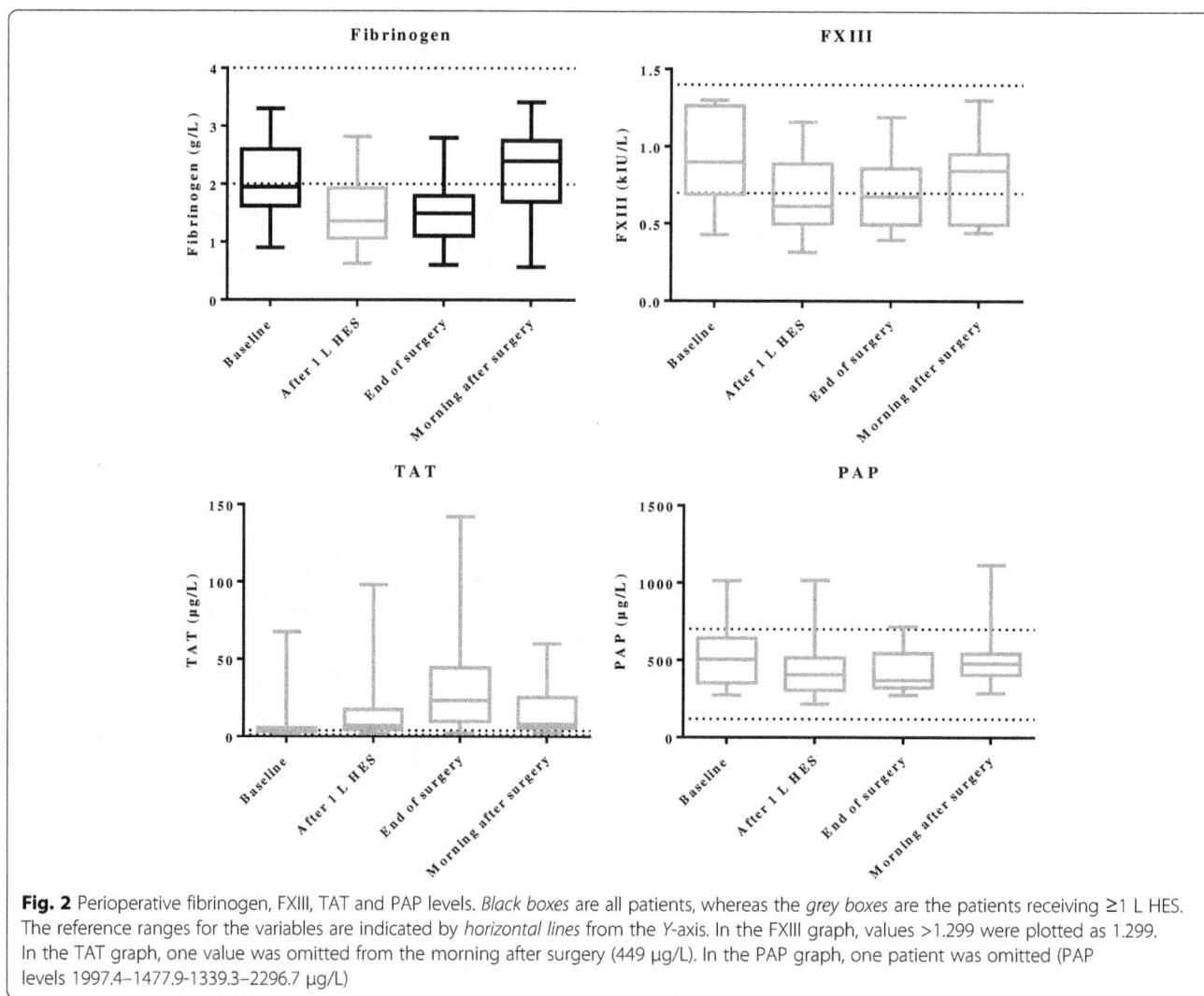

Fig. 2 Perioperative fibrinogen, FXIII, TAT and PAP levels. *Black boxes* are all patients, whereas the *grey boxes* are the patients receiving ≥1 L HES. The reference ranges for the variables are indicated by *horizontal lines* from the Y-axis. In the FXIII graph, values >1.299 were plotted as 1.299. In the TAT graph, one value was omitted from the morning after surgery (449 µg/L). In the PAP graph, one patient was omitted (PAP levels 1997.4–1477.9-1339.3–2296.7 µg/L)

the end of surgery but returned to baseline levels on the first postoperative morning. HES is known to influence photometric methods for measuring fibrinogen (Fenger-Eriksen et al. 2010) with falsely high values, so fibrinogen levels could have been even lower in our study. There is no specific recommendation for fibrinogen levels during intracranial surgery, but a perioperative low fibrinogen (<1.5 g/L) has previously been associated with an increased risk of postoperative intracranial hematoma (Gerlach et al. 2002). A more recent retrospective study suggests targeting a perioperative fibrinogen level >2 g/L to avoid postoperative hematomas (Wei et al. 2015). The importance of fibrinogen has also been shown by Adelmann et al., who studied 290 patients undergoing elective neurosurgery and found lower fibrinogen levels (mean 1.7 g/L) at the end of surgery in patients who developed postoperative hematoma compared to patients who had no hematoma

(fibrinogen mean 2.4 g/L) (Adelmann et al. 2014). It seems that low fibrinogen in this type of surgery can be dangerous, and as we found low levels to be common (in our study, 21 of 40 patients had a fibrinogen level of ≤1.5 at the end of surgery), how and when to prophylactically treat a low fibrinogen level in neurosurgery remains to be studied.

FIBTEM-MCF can be an indicator of low fibrinogen; we found a correlation between FIBTEM-MCF and fibrinogen ($R = 0.7$), which is comparable to previous findings (Solomon et al. 2011). This test is however also affected by other proteins such as FXIII (Schöchl et al. 2011), even though we found the correlation between FXIII and FIBTEM-MCF to be poor.

Acquired FXIII deficiency and substitution of FXIII is increasingly studied during surgical procedures (Levy and Greenberg 2013; Gerlach et al. 2009), much due to better FXIII assays. A large observational study of more than 1200 neurosurgical intracranial procedures found an increased risk of postoperative hematoma in patients who had low postoperative FXIII activity (Gerlach et al. 2000). A subsequent prospective study of more than 800 patients has found an association between decreased perioperative FXIII (FXIII activity of <60 %, which corresponds to <0.6 kIU/L) and an increased risk of postoperative intracranial hematoma (Gerlach et al. 2002). Of the 25 patients receiving ≥1 L HES in our study, 11 patients had FXIII activity of <0.6 kIU/L after HES infusion and FXIII activity was still low on the first postoperative morning. However, in the study by Adelmann et al. (mentioned above), FXIII activity was not lower in elective neurosurgical patients who developed postoperative hematoma compared to patients who did not (Adelmann et al. 2014). Many questions still remain to be answered on how and when to treat surgical patients with FXIII concentrates. Although FXIII supplementation was not beneficial in cardiac surgery (Karkouti et al. 2013), this does not necessarily translate to neurosurgery.

TAT is a marker for the generation of thrombin and thus for coagulation activation (Amiral and Fareed 1996), but unlike ROTEM variables, it does not provide information on clot structure. Elevated TAT levels indicate procoagulant plasma reactions during surgery as seen in our study, probably as a response to the surgical trauma. This is supported by two previous studies who also found elevated TAT levels during neurosurgery (Fujii et al. 1994; Heesen et al. 1997).

PAP is a marker for plasmin generation and an indicator of fibrinolytic activation (Montes et al. 1996). Unlike in a previous neurosurgical study that found increased PAP during surgery (Fujii et al. 1994), the present study found perioperative levels within the reference range. Our results therefore do not advocate the prophylactic use of tranexamic acid for fibrinolysis inhibition, as has been suggested for many types of surgery (Ker et al. 2012).

The strengths of this study are the meticulous repeated blood sampling and the inclusion of both ROTEM and advanced plasma analysis of hemostasis. Limitations are primarily the small study population and the lack of a control group (no HES or another colloid).

Conclusions

In conclusion, perioperative signs of increased coagulability were extremely uncommon in this prospective observational study. Only TAT levels indicated activation of coagulation. PAP levels showed no fibrinolytic activa-

tion, thus not advocating routine prophylactic use of tranexamic acid. There was an overall impaired coagulation during and at the end of surgery compared to the pre-surgery coagulation status, which was mainly normalized the day after surgery. The impaired coagulation could possibly be an effect of HES but needs to be further studied in randomized controlled studies. A more advanced perioperative coagulation testing method with thromboelastometry, fibrinogen levels and FXIII activity could help to reduce bleeding by an individualized regimen of fluids, transfusion and coagulation factor substitution, but this requires further studies.

Abbreviations
APTT, activated thromboplastin time; CFT, clot formation time; CT, clotting time; FXIII, factor XIII; HES, hydroxyethyl starch; MCF, maximum clot firmness; PAP, plasmin-antiplasmin complex; PT, prothrombin time; ROTEM, rotational thromboelastometry; TAT, thrombin-antithrombin complex; TEG, thromboelastography

Acknowledgements
Not applicable.

Funding
The study was financed through an external Project 829 *Project Intensiv- o periop* vård, Skåne University Hospital, with a research grant from CSL Behring Sweden.

Authors' contributions
CUN contributed to study planning, data collection and analysis, and manuscript preparation. KS, ME and PR contributed with data analysis and manuscript preparation. All authors read and approved the final manuscript.

Competing interests
The authors declare that they have no competing interests.

Author details
₁Department of Anaesthesia and Intensive Care, Skåne University Hospital, Lund University, Lund, Sweden. ²Department of Laboratory Medicine, Skåne University Hospital Malmö, Lund University, Malmö, Sweden. ³Department of Anaesthesia and Intensive Care, Lund University, Lund, Sweden.

References
Abrahams JM, Torchia MB, McGarvey M, Putt M, Baranov D, Sinson GP. Perioperative assessment of coagulability in neurosurgical patients using thrombelastography. Surg Neurol. 2002;58:5–11.
Adelmann D, Klaus DA, Illievich UM, Krenn CG, Krall C, Kozek-Langenecker S, et al. Fibrinogen but not factor XIII deficiency is associated with bleeding after craniotomy. Br J Anaesth. 2014;113:628–33.
Afshari A, Wikkelsø A, Brok J, Møller AM, Wetterslev J. Thrombelastography (TEG) or thromboelastometry (ROTEM) to monitor haemotherapy versus usual care in patients with massive transfusion. Cochrane Database Syst Rev. 2011; 16:CD007871.
Amiral J, Fareed J. Thromboembolic diseases: biochemical mechanisms and new possibilities of biological diagnosis. Semin Thromb Hemost. 1996;22 Suppl 1: 41–8.
Collen JF, Jackson JL, Shorr AF, Moores LK. Prevention of venous thromboembolism in neurosurgery: a metaanalysis. Chest. 2008;134:237–49.
Coriat P, Guidet B, de Hert S, Kochs E, Kozek S, Van Aken H, et al. Counter statement to open letter to the Executive Director of the European

Medicines Agency concerning the licensing of hydroxyethyl starch solutions for fluid resuscitation. Br J Anaesth. 2014;113:194–5.

El Kady N, Khedr H, Yosry M, El Mekavy S. Perioperative assessment of coagulation in paediatric neurosurgical patients using thromboelastography. Eur J Anaesthesiol. 2009;26:293–7.

European Medicines Agency. Hydroxyethyl starch solutions for infusion. 2014. http://www.ema.europa.eu/ema/index.jsp?curl=pages/medicines/human/referrals/Hydroxyethyl_starchcontaining_medicines/human_referral_prac_000029.jsp&mid=WC0b01ac05805c516f. Accessed 12 July 2016.

Feix JA, Peery CA, Gan TJ, Warner DS, James ML, Zomorodi A, et al. Intra-operative hydroxyethyl starch is not associated with post-craniotomy hemorrhage. Springerplus. 2015;4:350.

Fenger-Eriksen C, Tønnesen E, Ingerslev J, Sørensen B. Mechanisms of hydroxyethyl-starch-induced dilutional coagulopathy. J Thromb Haemost. 2009;7:1099–105.

Fenger-Eriksen C, Moore GW, Rangarajan S, Ingerslev J, Sørensen B. Fibrinogen estimates are influenced by methods of measurement and hemodilution with colloid plasma expanders. Transfusion. 2010;50:2571–6.

Fujii Y, Tanaka R, Takeuchi S, Koike T, Minakawa T, Sasaki O. Serial changes in hemostasis after intracranial surgery. Neurosurgery. 1994;35:26–33.

Gerlach R, Raabe A, Zimmermann M, Siegemund A, Seifert V. Factor XIII deficiency and postoperative hemorrhage after neurosurgical procedures. Surg Neurol. 2000;54:260–4.

Gerlach R, Tölle F, Raabe A, Zimmermann M, Siegemund A, Seifert V. Increased risk for postoperative hemorrhage after intracranial surgery in patients with decreased factor XIII activity: implications of a prospective study. Stroke. 2002;33:1618–23.

Gerlach R, Raabe A, Scharrer I, Meixensberger J, Seifert V. Post-operative hematoma after surgery for intracranial meningiomas: causes, avoidable risk factors and clinical outcome. Neurol Res. 2004;26:61–6.

Gerlach R, Krause M, Seifert V, Goerlinger K. Hemostatic and hemorrhagic problems in neurosurgical patients. Acta Neurochir (Wien). 2009;151:873–900.

Goh KY, Tsoi WC, Feng CS, Wickham N, Poon WS. Haemostatic changes during surgery for primary brain tumours. J Neurol Neurosurg Psychiatry. 1997;63:334–8.

Goobie SM, Soriano SG, Zurakowski D, McGowan FX, Rockoff MA. Hemostatic changes in pediatric neurosurgical patients as evaluated by thrombelastograph. Anesth Analg. 2001;93:887–92.

Görlinger K, Dirkmann D, Solomon C, Hanke AA. Fast interpretation of thromboelastometry in non-cardiac surgery: reliability in patients with hypo-, normo-, and hypercoagulability. Br J Anaesth. 2013;110:220–30.

Greenberg S, Tung A. But is it safe? Hydroxyethyl starch in perioperative care. Anesth Analg. 2015;120:519–21.

Hartog CS, Reuter D, Loesche W, Hofmann M, Reinhart K. Influence of hydroxyethyl starch (HES) 130/0.4 on hemostasis as measured by viscoelastic device analysis: asystematic review. Intensive Care Med. 2011;37:1725–37.

Heesen M, Kemkes-Matthes B, Deinsberger W, Boldt J, Matthes KJ. Coagulation alterations in patients undergoing elective craniotomy. Surg Neurol. 1997;47:35–8.

Iberti TJ, Miller M, Abalos A, Fischer EP, Post KD, Benjamin E, et al. Abnormal coagulation profile in brain tumor patients during surgery. Neurosurgery. 1994;34:389–94.

Jian M, Li X, Wang A, Zhang L, Han R, Gelb AW. Flurbiprofen and hypertension but not hydroxyethyl starch are associated with post-craniotomy intracranial haematoma requiring surgery. Br J Anaesth. 2014;113:832–9.

Karkouti K, von Heymann C, Jespersen CM, Korte W, Levy JH, Ranucci M, et al. Efficacy and safety of recombinant factor XIII on reducing blood transfusions in cardiac surgery: a randomized, placebo-controlled, multicenter clinical trial. J Thorac Cardiovasc Surg. 2013;146:927–39.

Ker K, Edwards P, Perel P, Shakur H, Roberts I. Effect of tranexamic acid on surgical bleeding: systematic review and cumulative meta-analysis. BMJ. 2012;17(344):e3054.

Kozek-Langenecker SA. Perioperative coagulation monitoring. Best Pract Res Clin Anaesthesiol. 2010;24:27–40.

Kozek-Langenecker SA. Fluids and coagulation. Curr Opin Crit Care. 2015;21:285–91.

Levy JH, Greenberg C. Biology of factor XIII and clinical manifestations of factor XIII deficiency. Transfusion. 2013;53:1120–31.

Lindroos AC, Niiya T, Randell T, Niemi TT. Stroke volume-directed administration of hydroxyethyl starch (HES 130/0.4) and Ringer's acetate in prone position during neurosurgery: a randomized controlled trial. J Anesth. 2014;28:189–97.

Montes R, Páramo JA, Anglès-Cano E, Rocha E. Development and clinical application of a new ELISA assay to determine plasmin-alpha2-antiplasmin complexes in plasma. Br J Haematol. 1996;92:979–85.

Nielsen VG, Lemole Jr GM, Matika RW, Weinand ME, Hussaini S, Baaj AA, et al. Brain tumors enhance plasmatic coagulation: the role of hemeoxygenase-1. Anesth Analg. 2014;118:919–24.

Nittby HR, Maltese A, Ståhl N. Early postoperative haematomas in neurosurgery. Acta Neurochir (Wien). 2016;158:837–46.

Schöchl H, Cotton B, Inaba K, Nienaber U, Fischer H, Voelckel W, et al. FIBTEM provides early prediction of massive transfusion in trauma. Crit Care. 2011;15:R265.

Seicean A, Schiltz NK, Seicean S, Alan N, Neuhauser D, Weil RJ. Use and utility of preoperative hemostatic screening and patient history in adult neurosurgical patients. J Neurosurg. 2012;116:1097–105.

Solomon C, Cadamuro J, Ziegler B, Schöchl H, Varvenne M, Sørensen B, et al. A comparison of fibrinogen measurement methods with fibrin clot elasticity assessed by thromboelastometry, before and after administration of fibrinogen concentrate in cardiac surgery patients. Transfusion. 2011;51:1695–706.

Wei N, Jia Y, Wang X, Zhang Y, Yuan G, Zhao B, Wang Y, Zhang K, Zhang X, Pan Y, Zhang J. Risk factors for postoperative fibrinogen deficiency after surgical removal of intracranial tumors. PLoS One. 2015;10:e0144551.

A case management report: a collaborative perioperative surgical home paradigm and the reduction of total joint arthroplasty readmissions

Navid Alem[1][*] (iD), Joseph Rinehart[1], Brian Lee[1], Doug Merrill[1], Safa Sobhanie[1], Kyle Ahn[1], Ran Schwarzkopf[2], Maxime Cannesson[3] and Zeev Kain[4]

Abstract

Background: Efforts to mitigate costs while improving surgical care quality have received much scrutiny. This includes the challenging issue of readmission subsequent to hospital discharge. Initiatives attempting to preclude readmission after surgery require planned and unified efforts extending throughout the perioperative continuum. Patient optimization prior to discharge, enhanced disease monitoring, and seamless coordination of care between hospitals and community providers is integral to this process. The perioperative surgical home (PSH) has been proposed as a model to improve the delivery of perioperative healthcare via patient-centered risk stratification strategies that emphasize value and evidence-based processes.

Results: This case report seeks to specifically describe implementation of readmission reduction strategies via a PSH paradigm during total joint arthroplasty (TJA) procedures at the University of California Irvine (UCI) Health. An orthopedic surgeon open to collaborate within a PSH paradigm for TJA procedures was recruited to UCI Health in October of 2012. Institution specific data was then prospectively collected for 2 years post implementation of the novel program. A total of 328 unilateral, elective primary TJA (120 hip, 208 knee) procedures were collectively performed. Demographic analysis reveals the following: mean age of 64 ± 12; BMI of 28.5 ± 6.2; ASA Score distribution of 0.3 % class 1, 23 % class 2, 72 % class 3, and 4.3 % class 4; and 62.5 % female patients. In all, a 30-day unplanned readmission rate of 2.1 % (95 % CI 0.4–3.8) was observed during the study period. As a limitation of this case report, this reported rate does not reflect readmissions that may have occurred at facilities outside UCI Health.

Conclusions: As healthcare evolves to emphasize value over volume, it is integral to invest efforts in longitudinal patient outcomes including patient disposition subsequent to hospital discharge. As outlined by this case management report, the PSH provides an institution-led means to implement a series of care initiatives that optimize the important metric of readmission following TJA, potentially adding further value to patients, surgical colleagues, and health systems.

Keywords: Anesthesia, Perioperative surgical home (PSH), Surgical readmissions, Perioperative medicine, Readmission reduction, Hospital discharge, Total joint arthroplasty (TJA)

* Correspondence: alemn@uci.edu
[1]Department of Anesthesiology & Perioperative Care, School of Medicine, University of California, Irvine, 333 City Boulevard West Side, Orange, CA 92868-3301, USA
Full list of author information is available at the end of the article

Background

Repeat admission after hospital discharge remains a significant and complex problem (Joynt and Jha 2012; Lucas and Pawlik 2014; Allaudeen et al. 2011; Merkow et al. 2015; Garrison et al. 2013; Zmistowski et al. 2013; Saucedo et al. 2014). Nearly one in every five patients is readmitted within 30 days of hospital discharge, accounting for an estimated $15 billion in healthcare spending annually (Allaudeen et al. 2011). This alarmingly high rate of unplanned readmission and the associated costs are both unsustainable and unacceptable. As the Affordable Care Act and other efforts to reduce the cost of healthcare are assimilated into payer policies, there is urgency for the healthcare industry to implement collaborative care models that emphasize value over volume (Ho and Sandy 2014; Szokol and Stead 2014; Schroeder and Frist 2013; Hertzberg 2013). Accountable care organizations (ACOs) are rapidly proliferating and can be defined as an integrated group motivated to provide enhanced patient care at a reduced cost for a defined population of patients (Barnes et al. 2014; Decamp et al. 2014; Epstein et al. 2014).

The Centers for Medicare & Medicaid Services (CMS) established the Hospital Readmissions Reduction Program in 2013.[1] Under this program, payments are now reduced for hospitals with 30-day readmission rates higher than a national benchmark for patients with the diagnoses of heart attack, heart failure, or pneumonia. Payment reduction is expanding and now includes readmission after surgical procedures (specifically elective total hip or total knee arthroplasty and coronary artery bypass graft surgery). CMS has also begun to associate 30-day readmission rates after elective total joint arthroplasty (TJA) procedures as an overall surrogate measure of hospital quality (Grosso et al. 2012). Payers, providers, and policymakers have much impetus to enhance the quality of patient care during TJA procedures while reducing expenditures (Bozic et al. 2014).

The perioperative surgical home (PSH) has been proposed as a model to improve the delivery of perioperative healthcare via patient-centered optimization strategies that involve risk stratification and standardization of care (Kash et al. 2014; Cyriac et al. 2016; Raphael et al. 2014; Garson et al. 2014; Cannesson et al. 2014; Schweitzer et al. 2013; Mackey and Schweitzer 2014; Vetter et al. 2013, 2014; Desebbe et al. 2016). The PSH also introduces clinical opportunities for varied providers to collectively enhance care of the surgical patient (Kash et al. 2014). A prime example is the reduction of surgical readmissions, as in theory this would yield improved longitudinal care at reduced costs (Joynt and Jha 2012). As such, this case report will outline one model of a collaborative perioperative team operating within a PSH practice-model to reduce surgical readmissions after TJA procedures.

Methods

Implementation of a perioperative surgical home for total joint arthroplasty (TJA) procedures

With unique and cumulative insights, a multitude of disciplines including anesthesiology, orthopedic surgery, nursing, pharmacy, case management, social work, nutrition, physical therapy, and information technology closely collaborated to institute a PSH for primary TJA (hip and knee) procedures at UCI Health in October of 2012 (Cyriac et al. 2016; Raphael et al. 2014; Garson et al. 2014). Weekly meetings were coordinated and LEAN Six Sigma methodology (De Koning et al. 2006) was used to ultimately manifest clinical pathways that paralleled "patient-centered, multidisciplinary, and integrated care (Grocott and Mythen 2015)" as opposed to fragmented, variable, and inefficient care (Mackey 2012; Berwick and Hackbarth 2012). As an integral component of the implemented TJA PSH paradigm, concerted strategies designed to avert post-surgical readmissions were employed at all phases encountered during the perioperative continuum.

Preoperative measures to optimize readmission risk

The Center for Perioperative Care (CPC) at UCI Health took the role of closely working with the Case Management team before surgery to ensure that longitudinal patient disposition was planned as early as possible, long before admission. Factors that contribute to an unplanned readmission were proactively confronted. For example, transportation needs were assessed and durable medical equipment arrangements were made at the time that a surgery date was scheduled. Moreover, "preferred" pharmacies, rehabilitation services, and skilled nursing facilities were identified with the patient and family. Financial arrangements were not made, and patients maintained selection autonomy. However, the term "preferred" denoted that the case management, surgery, and anesthesiology teams met with these providers and outlined post-hospital (discharge) protocols, goals and expectations as outlined by the tailored PSH clinical care pathways (Kash et al. 2014; Cyriac et al. 2016; Raphael et al. 2014; Garson et al. 2014; Vetter et al. 2013; Desebbe et al. 2016). Another important role for the CPC included the accurate identification of the patient's primary care provider (PCP) and specialists such as chronic pain providers. This allowed for the PSH team (Fig. 1) to play a role as the liaison that manages care transitions between the community and hospital period, aspiring to achieve a seamless "handshake" between the two (Fig. 2). Transitions or "handoffs" are particularly vulnerable exchange points that expose patients to lapses in quality and safety (Naylor et al. 2011; Auerbach et al. 2016). Lastly, the CPC clinic provided educational classes that both managed patient expectations and elucidated

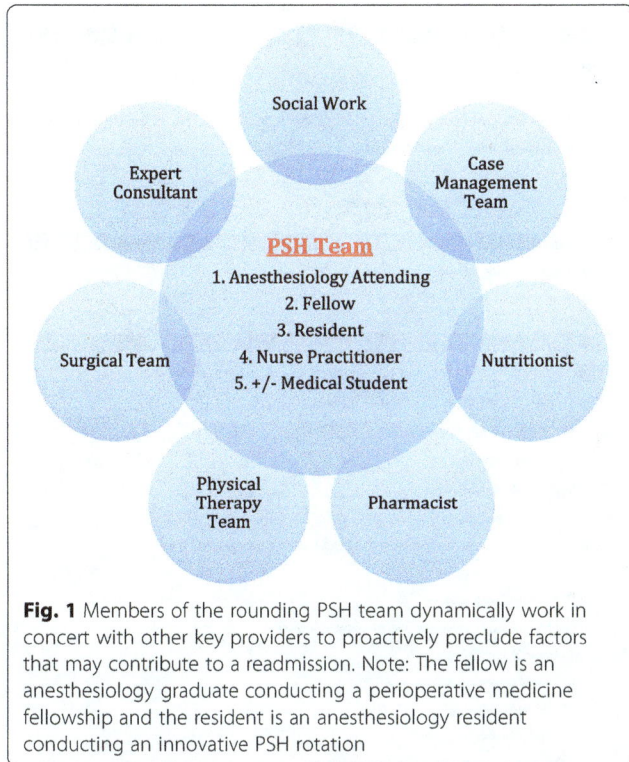

Fig. 1 Members of the rounding PSH team dynamically work in concert with other key providers to proactively preclude factors that may contribute to a readmission. Note: The fellow is an anesthesiology graduate conducting a perioperative medicine fellowship and the resident is an anesthesiology resident conducting an innovative PSH rotation

important safety initiatives. An important point is that the specific nature of the patient formed the center of the care model, rather than the diagnosis or planned procedure, a shift in focus that was significant in improving the quality and value of care (Brummett and Clauw 2015).

Postoperative measures to optimize readmission risk

Postoperatively, a collaborative PSH team longitudinally followed all enrolled PSH patients until the day of discharge. Leveraging evidence-based medicine and technology, care that transpired after the surgical intervention was managed for discharge optimization. This included providing fulltime coverage for a diverse array of post-surgical patients, often with multiple medical comorbidities. Goals included enhancement of discharge processes

by continually working with other key disciplines (Fig. 1) and the proactive identification and confrontation of factors known to contribute to a readmission after surgery (Table 1). As a final step, a discharge readiness checklist was created as a tool for review by the PSH team with the patient before a discharge ensues (Fig. 3).

Post-discharge measures to optimize readmission risk

The post-discharge period was a critical time to continue guiding a patient to enhanced recovery. A phone call was made by designated inpatient orthopedic nursing staff to all patients within 72 h of discharge to assure that discharge milestones were being met appropriately. The simple standardized list of questions was scripted in advance as a component of the PSH clinical pathway and integrated into the electronic medical record (Fig. 4). While the majority of calls were uneventful, triage occurred when answers indicated that an intervention may be required. Further measures taken to ensure that post-discharge care was not fragmented included sending a PSH note replete with information regarding the patient's perioperative medical care to the patient's PCP at the time of discharge (Fig. 5). To further bolster the transition in care, the PSH team supplemented with planned phone calls to the PCP and/or specialist provider for all high-risk patients with perioperative complications.

In addition, when emergency care was needed, all program enrolled patients were instructed to return to our own institution when feasible. When a PSH patient presented to the emergency room within 30 days of discharge, an automated page was immediately sent to the PSH team for the opportunity to contribute a value-added (Hertzberg 2013) assessment and care plan. Simultaneous with the patient's presenting signs and symptoms, assessment was made, and appropriate steps were taken to intervene and help manage the patient as deemed appropriate. Efforts were made to collaborate with other specialists as indicated, and Table 2 specifically outlines some of the point of care opportunities at the patient's

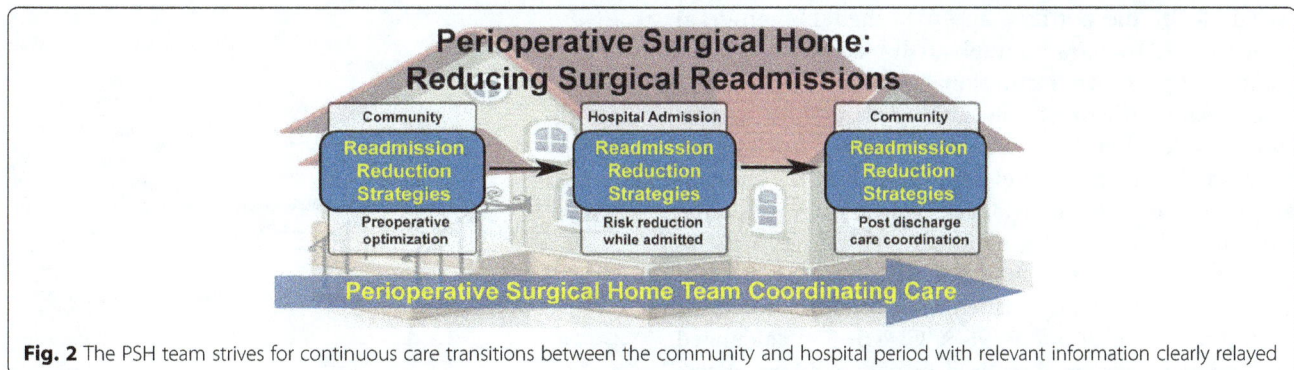

Fig. 2 The PSH team strives for continuous care transitions between the community and hospital period with relevant information clearly relayed

Table 1 Most common risk factors and causes that contribute to readmission risk after a surgical intervention

Risk factors (Lucas and Pawlik 2014)	Causes (Merkow et al. 2015)
Multiple comorbidities	Surgical site infection
Long length of hospital stay	Ileus
Postoperative complications	Postoperative bleeding

bedside for an anesthesiologist to potentially avert an unnecessary readmission.

Results and Discussion

This report describes our findings for unplanned 30-day readmissions in the first 2 years of the novel PSH program (October 1 2012 until September 30 2014). Institutional Review Board (IRB) approval was obtained for prospective data collection, analysis, and reporting (IRB HS # 2012-9273). Data was corroborated using hospital-based decision support, electronic medical record (Allscripts, Chicago, IL), and AIMS (SIS, Alpharetta, GA). A total of 328 unilateral, primary, and elective TJA (120 hip, 208 knee) procedures were collectively performed in year 1 and year 2. Demographic analysis reveals the following: mean age of 64 ± 12; BMI of 28.5 ± 6.2; ASA Score distribution of 0.3 % class 1, 23 % class 2, 72 % class 3, and 4.3 % class 4; and 62.5 % female patients.

In all, a 30-day unplanned readmission rate of 2.1 % (95 % CI 0.4–3.8) was observed during the study period (Table 3) (Cyriac et al. 2016). During the 2-year study period, unplanned 30-day readmissions were noted to be due to variable etiologies, but surgically related complications such as dislocation or fracture of the prosthetic joint predominated (Table 3). The increased readmission rate observed in year 2 of the program (Table 3) is not attributable to dissimilar patient demographics or comorbidities (Cyriac et al. 2016) and is likely an incidental finding reflective of the small sample size. While the program protocol included approaches to send patients to our own institution for emergency care when possible, it should be emphasized that the reported readmission rates do not incorporate readmissions that potentially occurred beyond UCI Health.

UCI Health did not have an established TJA program prior to 2012 to allow an unplanned readmission evaluation relative to an institutional baseline. As such, a comparison with previously published national results was considered to be useful. A systematic review and meta-analysis by Bernatz et al. (2015) listed the individual results of nine individual studies on readmission rates for TKA or THA nationally. A de novo meta-analysis of these nine studies reveals a total of 6076 readmissions in 78,505 patients—a 30-day unplanned readmission rate of 5.5 % (95 % CI 4.5–6.7) calculated by the inverse variance method using a random effects

Patient Information

Patient Name: ______

Surgeon: ______

The patient will be going to (select one): ☐ Home ☐ Skilled Nursing Facility

The patient's primary helper/ "coach" will be: ______

Primary language spoken: ______

Interpreter Needed? ☐ Yes ☐ No

Pain Management

Does patient have history of chronic pain? ☐ Yes ☐ No

Was acute pain service involved in care? ☐ Yes ☐ No

Telephone Follow-up

☐ I informed patient to expect an important telephone call in the next 72 hours.

Best time to call patient in the next 48 – 72 hours: ______

Best number to call 1: ______

Best number to call 2: ______

Best Email contact: ______

Does patient have an iPhone with face-time ability? ☐ Yes ☐ No

Specific follow-up reviewed with patient (please check all that were performed):

☐ Surgeon follow-up
☐ Primary Care Follow-up
☐ Physical therapy/Occupational Therapy follow-up
☐ Home Health follow-up
☐ Pain Management follow-up
☐ Specialist follow-up
☐ Other follow-up or pending labs/tests: ______
☐ Pharmacy patient will obtain medications from

Patient Questionnaire

Do you have assistance at home or plans to go to a nursing home or rehab facility?
☐ Home with assistance ☐ Nursing home

Do you have any transportation needs, including directions, to follow-up on appointments made for you? If yes, please explain:
☐ Yes ☐ No

Have you made arrangements for your medical record during this hospitalization to be made available to all your doctors and care members? How can we get this report out to your doctors so we can smoothly transition your post-hospital care?
☐ Yes ☐ No

Have you had all of your questions regarding medications answered including expected side effects and dosing intervals?
☐ Yes ☐ No

Have all your questions regarding diet/nutrition been answered? Will you need to take oral supplements, such as iron, or other drinks?
☐ Yes ☐ No

Have all your questions regarding surgical wound care been answered?
☐ Yes ☐ No

Has a physical therapist (PT) provided you with education related to techniques for mobility, walking, transfer training, and special positioning precautions?
☐ Yes ☐ No

Has an occupational therapist (OT) provided you with proper techniques in dressing, grooming, toilet/tub transfers and activities of daily living (ADL) modifications?
☐ Yes ☐ No

Have all your arrangements for equipment, such as a walker, crutches, cane, bedside commode, been made if needed?
☐ Yes ☐ No

In your own words, the following are barriers/challenges expected when I go home:
______
______
______

Fig. 3 Discharge readiness checklist to be reviewed with the patient by the PSH team prior to discharge

Discharge Information

Discharge Date: _____

Discharge RN: _____

Discharged to: _____

Type of Surgery: _____

PATIENT LABEL HERE

Time of Interview

Date of Telephone Interview: _____ Telephone number used: _____

> *First telephone call within 3 days of discharge.*
> *If no response, second call within next 3 days.*

If no response to two telephone calls, please note dates of 1st and 2nd telephone calls below:

Date of 1st Phone Call Attempt: _____ RN Signature _____

Date of 2nd Phone Call Attempt: _____ RN Signature _____

Patient Questionnaire

"Good (morning, afternoon, evening). My name is _____ and I'm calling from UC Irvine Health to see how you are doing since you have been discharged. May I have a few minutes of your time for follow-up questions?"

How well has your pain been managed at home?

1 (worst)   2   3   4   5 (best)

Comments:

Do you have any concerns about your surgical site or dressing?

☐ Yes   ☐ No

Comments:

Can you tell me when your follow-up appointment with your surgeon is?

☐ Yes   ☐ No

Comments:

Do you have any concerns about your homecare or medical equipment?

☐ Yes   ☐ No

Comments:

Are you taking all of your discharge prescription medications?

☐ Yes   ☐ No

Comments:

If appropriate for patient, when is your next appointment with the Coumadin Clinic?

Comments:

Are there any staff or physicians that you really liked that we may recognize?

☐ Yes   ☐ No

Comments:

I want to thank you for coming to UCI and for taking the time to speak with me. You may also receive an email or paper survey from the hospital. Thank you in advance for filling it out and sending it back!

Fig. 4 Standardized list of post-discharge questions during nurse follow-up calls

Perioperative Surgical Home Discharge Note

Date of Surgery: _____

Surgery performed: _____

Surgeon: _____

Brief Hospital Course: [<<PATIENT_NAME>>] had an uneventful hospital course and followed the expected pathways and protocols related to surgery. [<<HE_SHE>>] was discharged on [[[date]]] to [[[home or SNF name]]] and will follow up with their surgeon on [<<date>>].

$$\left\{ \text{ OR } \right\}$$

Brief Hospital Course: [<<PATIENT_NAME>>] had an eventful hospital course that included [[[list issues]]]. [<<HE_SHE>>] was discharged on [[[date]]] to [[[home or SNF name]]] and will follow up with their surgeon as scheduled.

Acute problems and interventions during hospitalization:

1)_____
2)_____
3)_____

Medications

Allergies: _____

Inpatient Medications	Home Medications

Discharge Recommendations

Medications (*list specific medication adjustments/taper schedule for medications below*):
1)_____
2)_____
3)_____

Follow-up visits (*list follow-up appointments for patient in items below*):
1)_____
2)_____
3)_____

Anticipated barriers/case management (*list barriers to adequate post-discharge care in items below*):
1)_____
2)_____
3)_____

If you should have any questions about [<<PATIENT_NAME>>]'s hospital course, please call the Perioperative Surgical Home team at 714-456-xxxx. Thank you.

Perioperative Surgical Home:
☐PSH – followed pathway
☐ PSH – deviated from pathway

Fig. 5 This standardized discharge note prepared by the PSH team is replete with information regarding the patient's perioperative medical care. It is integrated into the electronic medical record and sent to the patient's community primary care provider on the day of discharge

Table 2 Point of care (POC) assessment and intervention prospects to avert hospital readmissions

Opportunities to avert a readmission in the emergency room
1. Point of care (POC) ultrasonography (Ramsingh et al. 2015) for bedside assessment of cardiopulmonary function, volume status, vascular access, gastric volume, bladder volume
2. Advanced pain management intervention including multimodal therapy with regional techniques ± indwelling catheters
3. Liaisons to surgical services that may be confined to the operating room and delayed in patient assessment
4. Patient education, medication reconciliation, expectation management, multimodal anxiolysis
5. Postoperative nausea and emesis management
6. Assessment and management of perioperative medical complications
7. Assistance with transitions in care with community primary care providers (PCPs) or other specialists to provide rapid and appropriate disposition planning

model, with significant heterogeneity between studies ($Q = 145.5$, $p < 0.0001$). For the meta-analysis, we used the statistical methodology of Bernatz et al. (2015) to analyze the same final data sample they used in their study, with the addition of our own data as a new group. When comparing these nine pooled results to our own results using the same meta-analytical method, we find the difference is significant at the 0.05 level ($Q = 6.07$; $p = 0.014$ for difference) (Fig. 6). Further comparison of our readmission data to a national benchmark rate of 4.6 % after TJA should also be noted.[2] This reported national estimate is specific to Medicare beneficiaries and is again inclusive of unplanned readmission to an any acute care hospital within 30 days after discharge from a hospital.

Conclusions

Preventable readmissions remain a common target for the improvement of healthcare (Joynt and Jha 2012; Lucas and Pawlik 2014; Allaudeen et al. 2011; Merkow et al. 2015; Garrison et al. 2013; Zmistowski et al. 2013;

Saucedo et al. 2014; Jencks et al. 2009; Tsai et al. 2013; Joynt et al. 2011). Although surgical readmissions account for less than a quarter of all hospital readmissions (Jencks et al. 2009), analysis has revealed significant disparities in re-hospitalization rates after surgery between institutions (Lucas and Pawlik 2014; Tsai et al. 2013). It can be debated as to whether this appropriately parallels the quality of care rendered by a particular hospital or rather is a reflection of greater readmission risk for hospitals providing care to patient populations with greater disease burden or lower socioeconomic status and support (Tsai et al. 2013; Joynt et al. 2011). Regardless, a large review demonstrated that the majority of surgical readmissions are attributable to new complications that can be predicted and are characteristic of a particular procedure (Merkow et al. 2015). These findings suggest that appropriate risk stratification and thoroughly preparing patients for post-hospital care present significant potential for healthcare systems endeavoring to reduce surgical readmissions.

In this case management report, we outline the use of the PSH as a model to reduce the incidence of readmission after TJA surgery. Our model resulted in lower readmission rates than those reported nationally in a statistically significant manner. There are several limitations that should be noted, including a limited sample size and duration, lack of control group of patients not enrolled in the program, and the ability to only capture institution-specific readmissions. Nevertheless, we submit that understanding general risk factors and causes (Table 1) for readmission in surgical patient populations will facilitate the development of evidence-based models aimed at both optimizing patients for early discharge as well as decreasing preventable readmission. While there are certainly recurring factors that must be accounted for, efforts aimed at decreasing unplanned readmissions are ultimately much more complex and dynamic. Corrective efforts must be holistic and tailored to the patient, surgery, and the facility, as each readmission ultimately reflects multifactorial underpinnings. For instance, we learned that at our institution post-

Table 3 Post PSH implementation TJA and readmission data year 1 and year 2

	Year 1 post PSH implementation	Year 2 post PSH implementation	2-year cumulative
Total number of total joint arthroplasty	144	184	328
Total number of unplanned 30-day readmissions	1	6	7
Readmission diagnosis	• Disruption of external wound	• Dislocation of prosthetic joint • Malaise • Stress fracture of femoral neck • Peri-prosthetic fracture • Contracture of tendon • Acute renal failure	
30-day readmission rate[a]	0.7 %	3.3 %	2.1 %

[a]Institution specific

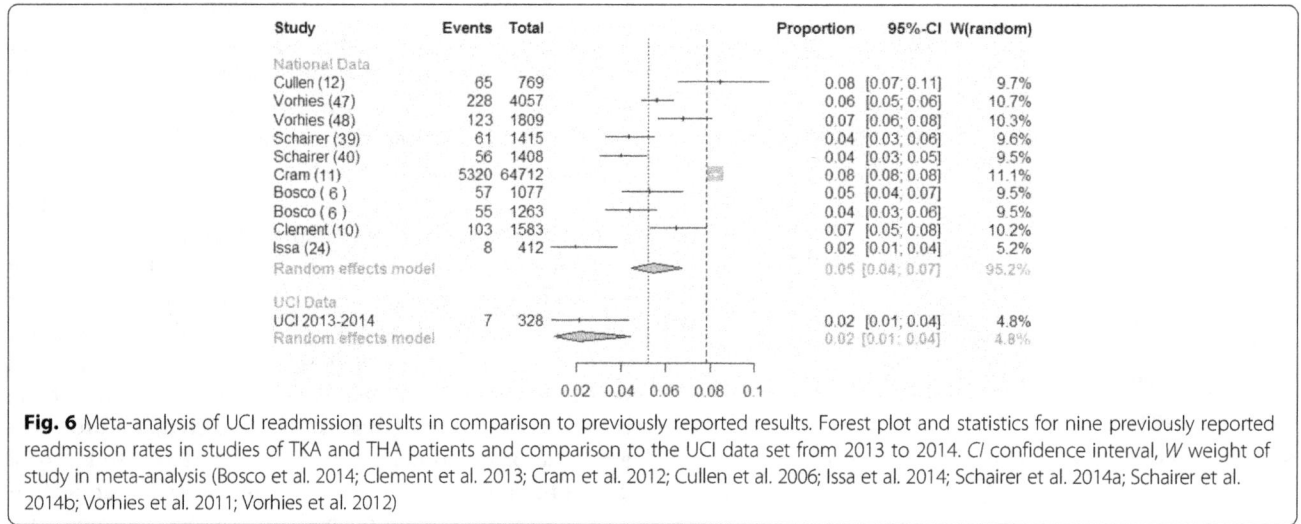

Fig. 6 Meta-analysis of UCI readmission results in comparison to previously reported results. Forest plot and statistics for nine previously reported readmission rates in studies of TKA and THA patients and comparison to the UCI data set from 2013 to 2014. *CI* confidence interval, *W* weight of study in meta-analysis (Bosco et al. 2014; Clement et al. 2013; Cram et al. 2012; Cullen et al. 2006; Issa et al. 2014; Schairer et al. 2014a; Schairer et al. 2014b; Vorhies et al. 2011; Vorhies et al. 2012)

surgical joint dislocations and fractures were the primary culprits for unplanned readmissions (Table 3), and future pathway revisions will evolve to optimize patient education and physical therapy for fall prevention. A delicate balance must also be achieved for proper "discharge optimization," as the inherent investment of time and resources required may be significant. Frank divergence exists between reducing readmission and other important hospital goals, such as a fast-track discharge (Kehlet and Wilmore 2005) and decreased length of stay (Pearson et al. 2001).

Pathways and systems that are integrated into discharge processes need thorough vetting and contribution from practitioners with diversified perspectives. The PSH provides an institution-led means to optimize patient care by unifying resources available throughout the perioperative continuum (Kash et al. 2014; Cyriac et al. 2016; Raphael et al. 2014; Garson et al. 2014; Cannesson et al. 2014; Schweitzer et al. 2013; Mackey and Schweitzer 2014; Vetter et al. 2013, 2014). Beginning with an indication for surgery and extending to the post-discharge transfer of care back to a PCP, there are an abundance of opportunities to incorporate the evidence-based initiatives of the PSH. By means of interdisciplinary discharge planning and oversight of process outcomes that re-compose variable practices into uniformly implemented evidence-based models, potential gaps in care that expose patients to harm or potential readmission can be minimized. As outlined by the Institute for Healthcare Improvement's "Triple Aim," much of healthcare reform has revolved around the multifaceted goals of improving patient satisfaction, while decreasing morbidity and costs of care (Vetter et al. 2014). With this in mind, it is important to continually search for ways to improve longitudinal patient outcomes as illustrated by this case report describing the potential impact of the PSH care model on the important metric of readmission following elective TJA surgery.

Endnotes

[1]Centers for Medicare & Medicaid Services. Readmission Reductions Program, 2014. Available from URL: https://www.cms.gov/medicare/medicare-fee-for-service-payment/acuteinpatientpps/readmissions-reduction-program.html, (Last Viewed June 2016)

[2]Medicare.gov. 30-day unplanned readmission and death measures: complication rate for hip/knee replacement patients. 2016. Available from URL: https://www.medicare.gov/hospitalcompare/Data/30-day-measures.html, (Last Viewed August 2016)

Abbreviations

CMS: Centers for Medicare & Medicaid Services; CPC: Center for Perioperative Care; IRB: Institutional Review Board; PCP: Primary care provider; POC: Point of care; PSH: Perioperative surgical home; TJA: Total joint arthroplasty; UCI: University of California, Irvine

Acknowledgements

We thank Dr. Patrick Hu for his assistance with figure preparation. This work was received from the School of Medicine and Department of Anesthesiology & Perioperative Care, University of California Irvine

Funding

Not applicable.

Authors' contributions

NA participated in the case-study design, figure design, contributed to the statistical analysis, and authored the manuscript; JR performed statistical analysis and co-authored the manuscript; BL participated in case-study design and figure design and co-authored the manuscript; DM participated in case-study design and co-authored the manuscript; SS participated in figure design and co-authored the manuscript; KA participated in case-study design and co-authored the manuscript; RS participated in case-study design and co-authored the manuscript; MC participated in case-study design and co-authored the manuscript; ZK participated in case-study design, contributed to figure design, contributed to statistical analysis, and co-authored the manuscript. All authors read and approved the final manuscript.

Competing interests
The authors declare that they have no competing interests.

Author details
[1]Department of Anesthesiology & Perioperative Care, School of Medicine, University of California, Irvine, 333 City Boulevard West Side, Orange, CA 92868-3301, USA. [2]Division of Adult Reconstruction, Department of Orthopedic Surgery, NYU Langone Medical Center, Hospital For Joint Diseases, New York, USA. [3]Department of Anesthesiology & Perioperative Care, School of Medicine, University of California, Los Angeles, Los Angeles, USA. [4]Center for Stress & Health & Department of Anesthesiology & Perioperative Care, School of Medicine, University of California, Irvine, Orange, USA.

References
Allaudeen N, Vidyarthi A, Maselli J, Auerbach A. Redefining readmission risk factors for general medicine patients. J Hosp Med. 2011;2:54–60.

Auerbach AD, Kripalani S, Vasilevskis EE, Sehgal N, Lindenauer PK, Metlay J, Fletcher G, Ruhnke GW, Flanders SA, Kim C, Williams MV, Thomas L, Giang V, Herzig SJ, Patel K, Boscardin J, Robinson EJ, Schnipper JL. Preventability and causes of readmissions in a national cohort of general medicine patients. JAMA. 2016;176(4):484–93.

Barnes AJ, Unruh L, Chukmaitov A, Ginneken EV. Accountable care organizations in the USA: types, developments and challenges. Healthy Policy. 2014;118:1–7.

Bernatz, JT, Tueting JL, Anderson PA. Thirty-day readmission rates in orthopedics: a systematic review and meta-analysis. PLoS One 2015;10(4):1–20.

Berwick DM, Hackbarth AD. Eliminating waste in US health care. JAMA. 2012; 307(14):1513–6.

Bosco 3rd JA, Karkenny AJ, Hutzler LH, Slover JD, Iorio R. Cost burden of 30-day readmissions following Medicare total hip and knee arthroplasty. J Arthroplasty. 2014;29(5):903–5.

Bozic JK, Ward L, Vail TP, Maze M. Bundled payments in total joint arthroplasty: targeting opportunities for quality improvement and cost reduction. Clin Orthop Relat Res. 2014;472:188–93.

Brummett C, Clauw D. Flipping the paradigm: from surgery-specific to patient-driven perioperative analgesic algorithms. Anesthesiology. 2015;122:731–3.

Cannesson M, Ani F, Mythen M, Kain Z. Anesthesiology and perioperative medicine around the world: different names, same goals. BJA. 2014;231:1–2.

Clement RC, Derman PB, Graham DS, Speck RM, Flynn DN, Levin LS, et al. Risk factors, causes, and the economic implications of unplanned readmissions following total hip arthroplasty. J Arthroplasty. 2013;28(8 Suppl):7–10.

Cram P, Cai X, Lu X, Vaughan-Sarrazin MS, Miller BJ. Total knee arthroplasty outcomes in top-ranked and non-top-ranked orthopedic hospitals: an analysis of Medicare administrative data. Mayo Clin Proc. 2012;87(4):341–8.

Cullen C, Johnson DS, Cook G. Re-admission rates within 28 days of total hip replacement. Ann R Coll Surg Engl. 2006;88(5):475–8.

Cyriac J, Garson L, Schwarzkopf R, Ahn K, Rinehart J, Vakharia S, Cannesson M, Kain Z. Total Joint Replacement Perioperative Surgical Home Program: 2 year follow-up. Anesth Analg. 2016;123(1):51–62.

De Koning H, Verver JP, Van Den Heuvel J, Bisgaard S, Does RJ. Lean six sigma in healthcare. J Healthc Qual. 2006;28:4–11.

Decamp M, Sugarman J, Berkowitz S. Shared savings in accountable care organizations. How to determine fair distributions. JAMA. 2014;311(10):1011–2.

Desebbe O, Lanz T, Kain Z, Cannesson M. The perioperative surgical home: an innovative, patient-centered and cost-effective perioperative care model. Anaesthe Crit Care Pain Med. 2016;35:59–66.

Epstein AM, Jha AK, Orah J, Liebman DL, Audet AM, Zezza MA, Guterman S. Analysis of early accountable care organizations defines patient, structural, cost, and quality-of-care characteristics. Health Aff. 2014;33(1):95–102.

Garrison G, Mansukhani M, Bohn B. Predictors of thirty-day readmission among hospitalized family medicine patients. J Am Board Fam Med. 2013;26(1):71–7.

Garson L, Schwartzkopf R, Vakharia S, Alexander B, Stead S, Cannesson M, Kain Z. Implementation of a total joint replacement-focused perioperative surgical home: a management case report. Anesth Analg. 2014;118:1081–9.

Grocott MP, Mythen MG. Perioperative medicine: the value proposition for anesthesia? Anesthesiology Clin. 2015;33:617–28.

Grosso LM, Curtis JP, Lin Z, et al. Hospital-level 30 day all-cause risk-standardized readmission rate following elective primary total hip arthroplasty (THA) and/ or total knee arthroplasty. Review prepared for Medicare and Medicaid Services (CMS). 2012.

Hertzberg LB. Evolution of value-added services. American Society of Anesthesiologists Newsletter. 2013;77(5):30–1.

Ho S, Sandy LG. Getting value from health spending: going beyond payment reform. J Gen Intern Med. 2014;29(5):796–7.

Issa K, Cherian JJ, Kapadia BH, Robinson K, Bhowmik-Stoker M, Harwin SF, et al. Readmission rates for cruciate-retaining total knee arthroplasty. J Knee Surg. 2014;28(3): 239-42.

Jencks S, Williams M, Coleman E. Rehospitalizations among patients in the Medicare fee-for-service program. N Engl J Med. 2009;360(14):1418–28.

Joynt KE, Jha AK. Thirty-day readmissions—truth and consequences. N Engl J Med. 2012;366(15):1366–9.

Joynt K, Orav EJ, Jha A. Thirty-day readmission rates for Medicare beneficiaries by race and site of care. JAMA. 2011;305:675–81.

Kash B, Zhang Y, Cline K, Menser T, Miller T. The perioperative surgical home (PSH): a comprehensive review of US and non-US studies shows predominantly positive quality and cost outcomes. The Millbank Quarterly. 2014;92(4):796–821.

Kehlet H, Wilmore D. Fast-track surgery. Br J Surg. 2005;92(1):3–4.

Lucas D, Pawlik T. Readmission after surgery. Adv Surg. 2014;48:185–99.

Mackey DC. Can we finally conquer the problem of medical quality? The systems-based opportunities of data registries and medical teamwork. Anesthesiology. 2012;117(2):225–6.

Mackey DC, Schweitzer MP. The future of surgical care in the U.S.: state surgical quality collaborative, optimized perioperative care, and the perioperative surgical home. American Society of Anesthesiologists Newsletter. 2014;78(12):10–3.

Merkow RP, Ju MH, Chung JW, Hall BL, Cohen ME, Williams MV, Tsai TC, Ko CY, Bilimoria KY. Underlying reasons associated with hospital readmission following surgery in the United States. JAMA. 2015;313(5):483–95.

Naylor M, Aiken L, Kurtzman E, Olds D, Hirschman K. The importance of transitional care in achieving health reform. Health Aff. 2011;30(4):746–54.

Pearson S, Kleefield S, Soukop J, Cook F, Lee T. Critical pathways intervention to reduce length of hospital stay. Am J Med. 2001;110(3):175–80.

Ramsingh D, Rinehart J, Kain Z, Strom S, Canales C, Alexander B, Capatina A, Ma M, Le K, Cannesson M. Impact assessment of perioperative point-of-care ultrasound training on anesthesiology residents. Anesthesiology. 2015;123(3):670–82.

Raphael D, Cannesson M, Schwarzkopf R, Garson L, Vakharia S, Gupta R, Kain Z. Total joint perioperative surgical home: an observational financial review. Perioperative Medicine Journal. 2014;3(6):1–7.

Saucedo JM, Marecek GS, Wanke TR, Lee J, Stulberg SD, Puri L. Understanding readmission after primary total hip and knee arthroplasty: who's at risk? J Arthroplasty. 2014;29(2):256–60.

Schairer WW, Sing DC, Vail TP, Bozic KJ. Causes and frequency of unplanned hospital readmission after total hip arthroplasty. Clin Orthop Relat Res. 2014a; 472(2):464–70.

Schairer WW, Vail TP, Bozic KJ. What are the rates and causes of hospital readmission after total knee arthroplasty? Clin Orthop Relat Res. 2014b;472(1):181–7.

Schroeder SA, Frist W. Phasing out fee-for-service payment. National commission on physician payment reform. N Engl J Med. 2013;368(21):2029–32.

Schweitzer MP, Fahy B, Leib M, Rosenquist R. The perioperative surgical home model. American Society of Anesthesiologists Newsletter. 2013;77(6):58–9.

Szokol J, Stead S. The changing anesthesia economic landscape: emergence of large multispecialty practices and accountable care organizations. Curr Opin Anesthesiology. 2014;27(2):183–9.

Tsai T, Joynt K, Orav E, Gawande A, Jha A. Variation in surgical readmission rates and quality of hospital care. N Engl J Med. 2013;369(12):1134–42.

Vetter T, Goeddel L, Boudreaux A, Hunt T, Jones K, Pittet J. The perioperative surgical home: how can it make the case so everyone wins? BMC Anesthesiol. 2013;13(6):1–11.

Vetter T, Boudreaux A, Jones K, Hunter J, Pittet J. The perioperative surgical home: how anesthesiology can collaboratively achieve and leverage the triple aim in health care. Anesth Analg. 2014;118(5):1131–8.

Vorhies JS, Wang Y, Herndon J, Maloney WJ, Huddleston JI. Readmission and length of stay after total hip arthroplasty in a national Medicare sample. J Arthroplasty. 2011;9:26 (6 Suppl):119–23

Implementation of goal-directed fluid therapy during hip revision arthroplasty: a matched cohort study

Marit Habicher[1*], Felix Balzer[1], Viktor Mezger[1], Jennifer Niclas[1], Michael Müller[2], Carsten Perka[2], Michael Krämer[1] and Michael Sander[1,3]

Abstract

Background: Several randomized controlled trials (RCTs) have demonstrated that intraoperative goal-directed fluid therapy (GDFT) can decrease postsurgical complications in patients undergoing major abdominal surgery. However, very few studies have demonstrated the value of goal-directed therapy (GDT) in patients undergoing orthopaedic surgery and confirmed it is as useful in real-life conditions. Therefore, we initiated a GDFT implementation programme in patients undergoing hip revision arthroplasty in order to assess its effects on postoperative complications (e.g. infection, cardiac, neurological, renal) (primary outcome) and hospital and intensive care unit (ICU) length of stay (secondary outcomes).

Methods: We developed a GDFT protocol for the haemodynamic management of patients undergoing hip revision arthroplasty. The GDFT protocol was based on continuous monitoring and optimization of stroke volume during the surgical procedure. From December 2012 and for a period of 17 months, 130 patients were treated according to the GDFT protocol (GDFT group). The pre-, intra-, and postoperative characteristics of patients from the GDFT group were compared to those of 130 historical matched patients (control group) who had the same surgery between January 2011 and August 2012.

Results: Patients from the GDFT and from the control group were comparable in terms of age, comorbidities, and P-POSSUM score. Duration of anaesthesia and surgery were also comparable. The GDFT group had a significantly lower morbidity rate (49.2 vs. 66.9%; $p = 0.006$) and a shorter median hospital length of stay (11 days (9–15) vs. 9 days (8–12); $p = 0.003$) than the control group. Patients from the control group post-anaesthesia care unit (PACU)/ICU stayed significantly longer at PACU/ICU than patients from the GDFT group (control group vs. GDFT group, 960 min (360–1210) vs. 400 min (207–825); $p < 0.001$) Patients from the GDFT group received less crystalloids but more colloids during surgery. They also received more often inotropic therapy.

Conclusions: In patients undergoing hip revision arthroplasty, the implementation of GDT as a new standard operating procedure was successful and associated with reduced postsurgical complications, most importantly a reduction in postoperative bleeding as well as hospital and ICU stay.

Trial registration: ClinicalTrials.gov, NCT01753050

Keywords: Goal-directed fluid therapy, Hip surgery, Postoperative outcome, Haemodynamic monitoring, Hip revision arthroplasty

* Correspondence: marit.habicher@charite.de
[1]Department of Anaesthesiology and Intensive Care Medicine, Charité University Hospital Berlin, Campus Charité Mitte and Campus Virchow-Klinikum, Berlin, Germany
Full list of author information is available at the end of the article

Background

More than 230 million major surgical procedures are undertaken every year worldwide (Weiser et al. 2008). The most operations were performed under general anaesthesia. A survey in 2013 in the UK showed over 2,766,600 general anaesthesia during 1 year (Sury et al. 2014). Morbidity rates >25% have repeatedly been reported after major surgery (Ghaferi et al. 2009). Therefore, strategies to improve outcome and prevent postoperative complications are required in surgical patients.

Many randomized controlled trials (RCTs) and meta-analysis suggest that perioperative goal-directed fluid therapy (GDFT) decreases postsurgical complications and length of hospital stay in patients undergoing major abdominal procedures (Benes et al. 2010; Gan et al. 2002; Grocott et al. 2012; Hamilton et al. 2011; Lopes et al. 2007). However, (1) larger and multicentre studies have yielded conflicting results (Pearse et al. 2014; Pestaña et al. 2014; Scheeren et al. 2013). Pearse et al. demonstrated in their randomized trial of high-risk patients undergoing major gastrointestinal surgery that the use of a cardiac output-guided haemodynamic therapy algorithm when compared did not significantly reduce postoperative complications and 30-day mortality (Pearse et al. 2014); (2) RCTs are done in highly selected patients with extra human and financial resources, such that the extrapolation of their results to the real world may be questioned (Vincent 2009); and (3) only a few studies have been done in orthopaedic patients and none in patients undergoing hip revision arthroplasty. Patients undergoing revision hip surgery are usually old and often have comorbidities, increasing their risk of complications after surgery.

Therefore, we made the decision to implement GDFT in patients undergoing hip revision arthroplasty and to assess its effects on postoperative outcome as an enhanced recovery project for these patients.

Methods
Study outline

We enrolled prospectively 130 patients over a period of 17 months (from December 1, 2012, to April 30, 2014) who were managed according to our GDFT protocol (GDFT group). All consecutive patients admitted for revision hip surgery were screened for inclusion. Inclusion criteria were age ≥18 years and one of the following surgical procedures (hip revision arthroplasty): hip revision with change of the prosthesis, explantation of existing hip arthroplasty, or patients after Girdlestone resection arthroplasty, who underwent new implantation of hip prosthesis. Patients from the GDFT group were compared to 130 historical matched control patients (control group) who underwent the same surgical procedure from January 1, 2011, to August 30, 2012, before we developed the

algorithm for the prospective group. During this time frame, no patients were treated with additional monitoring that could measure intraoperative stroke volume.

The study protocol was registered at ClinicalTrials.gov (NCT01753050) and approved by the ethics committee at Charité – Universitätsmedizin Berlin (EA1/315/12). Informed written consent was obtained from all prospective GDFT patients. Retrospective patients (control group) provided their consent to use their data in anonymized fashion for scientific purposes by signing the treatment contract with our university hospital. The study was performed at the Charité – University hospital Berlin, Campus Charité Mitte. Stroke volume monitors were loaned by Edwards Lifesciences, which had no role in the development of the study protocol and the data analysis.

Patient management

All patients underwent general anaesthesia during surgery. Anaesthesia was induced according to our written SOP with fentanyl (1–2 $\mu g\ kg^{-1}$), propofol (1–2 $mg\ kg^{-1}$), and cisatracurium (0.15 $mg\ kg^{-1}$). After endotracheal intubation, the maintenance of anaesthesia was performed at the discretion of the attending anaesthesiologist with either sevoflurane or propofol continuously. Fentanyl and cisatracurium boli were given as needed.

Standard monitoring in both groups included electrocardiogram, pulse oximetry, temperature, and inspiratory and expiratory gas concentrations as well as monitoring of depth of anaesthesia. In the retrospective group, the choice between non-invasive or invasive blood pressure measurement was at the discretion of the attending anaesthesiologist. None of the patients from the retrospective group was monitored with a device that was able to measure stroke volume (SV) or any other flow-related parameter. In all patients of the GDFT group, invasive blood pressure was monitored via right or left radial artery. Haemodynamic optimization in this group was done as follows: SV was monitored using a pulse contour method (Vigileo 03.06, Edwards Lifesciences, Irvine, CA, USA) and a special pressure transducer (FloTrac system, Edwards Lifesciences). Baseline SV was measured after induction of anaesthesia and patient positioning. An intravenous colloid bolus of 250 mL (Volulyte® 6%, Fresenius Kabi Deutschland GmbH, Bad Homburg, Germany, or Gelafundin ISO 40 $mg\ mL^{-1}$, B. Braun Melsungen AG, Melsungen, Germany) was given within 5 min and repeated until reaching a SV plateau value (increase in SV < 10%). The optimum stroke volume (SV_{opt}) was defined as the last successful fluid challenge, e.g. the last SV value just before reaching the plateau value, and $SV_{trigger}$ as SV_{opt} minus 10%. Our GDT protocol is shown in Fig. 1. During surgery, our goal was to maintain SV above $SV_{trigger}$ using fluid boluses, or inotropes (dobutamine or enoximone at 3 $\mu g\ kg^{-1}\ h^{-1}$),

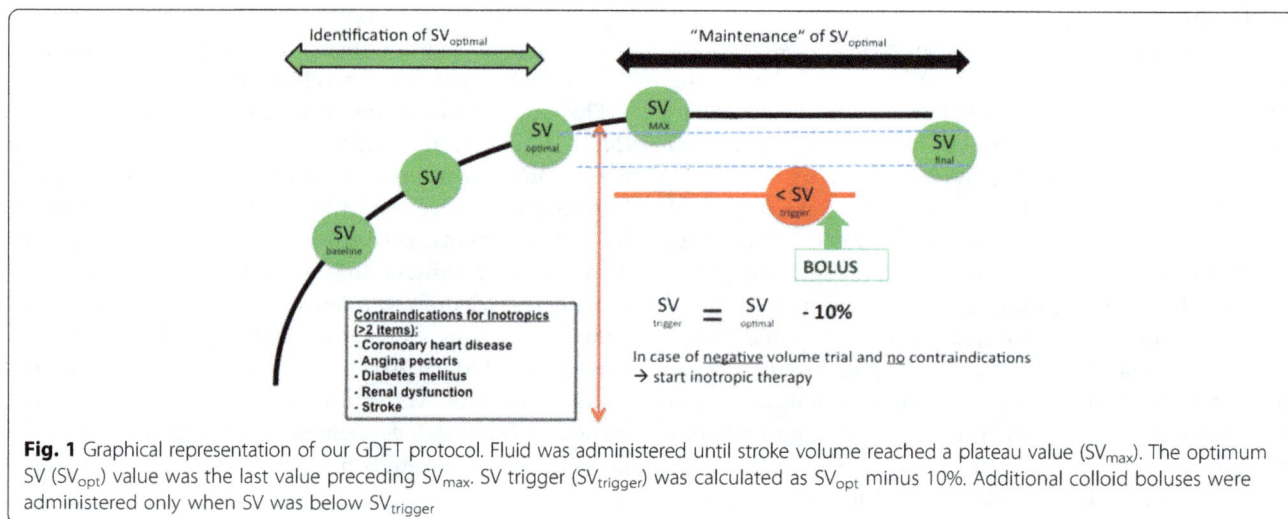

Fig. 1 Graphical representation of our GDFT protocol. Fluid was administered until stroke volume reached a plateau value (SV_{max}). The optimum SV (SV_{opt}) value was the last value preceding SV_{max}. SV trigger ($SV_{trigger}$) was calculated as SV_{opt} minus 10%. Additional colloid boluses were administered only when SV was below $SV_{trigger}$

when fluid loading was unable to restore SV values above $SV_{trigger}$. Inotropes were not used in patients with two or more of the following conditions: existing coronary heart disease or angina pectoris, presence of diabetes mellitus, impaired renal function, or stroke in the patient's history (Kristensen et al. 2014). Compliance to the haemodynamic treatment protocol was monitored using case report forms (CRFs) and evaluated postoperatively by two independent anaesthesiologists. Disagreement, if any, was solved by discussion with a third anaesthesiologist. The compliance rate was calculated as the number of protocol deviations divided by the total number of interventions during surgery and expressed as a percentage.

In the control group, haemodynamic management was left at the discretion of the attending anaesthesiologist.

Outcome variables

The *primary outcome* measurement was the proportion of patients developing one or more postoperative complications during the hospital stay. All complications were extracted retrospectively from the electronic patient database management system by an independent medical documentation assistant, both for the GDFT and the control group using ICD-10-coded diagnoses in the medical records. The following postoperative complications were considered for analysis: infectious complications (wound infections, wound healing disturbances, pneumonia, urinary tract infections, sepsis, endocarditis, and peritonitis); cardiac complications (arrhythmias requiring medical treatment, pulmonary oedema, pulmonary embolism, myocardial infarction, and cardiovascular arrest); neurological complications (postoperative delirium and postoperative stroke); renal complications (increase of creatinine above twofold before surgery or need for dialysis); and haemorrhagic complications (postoperative bleeding with the need for postoperative red blood cell (RBC) transfusion).

Secondary outcome variables were postoperative need for vasopressors, postoperative complications, length of stay in the recovery room, post-anaesthesia care unit (PACU) or intensive care unit (ICU), the total length of hospital stay after surgery, and hospital mortality.

Statistical analysis

Due to deviations from the normal distribution (Kolmogorov-Smirnov test), all analyses were performed non-parametrically. Results were expressed as median with 25th to 75th percentiles. Mann-Whitney U test and exact Fisher's test were used for inter-group differences. Absolute and relative frequencies were used for categoric and dichotomous variables. Statistical analysis was carried out by using the Software Package for Social Sciences, 22.0 SPSS® for Macintosh (SPSS, Inc., Chicago, IL). A p value <0.05 was considered statistically significant.

The demographics and baseline covariates used for matching the GDFT group with an historical group were the age, the ASA score, and the P-POSSUM score, which are variables known to be independent predictors of postoperative morbidity and mortality. The ASA score and the P-POSSUM score were different between the groups when we analysed all the patients (GDFT group ($n = 130$) vs. control group ($n = 258$)) in favour of the control group. Several matching methods were excised in this study in order to find optimal balance using the identified baseline covariates. As a result, the individual matching method was chosen for this study and performed with the R package "optmatch" version 0.9-1.29 (Hansen and Klopfer 2006).

Results

Between December 1, 2012, and April 30, 2014, 130 patients were recruited as part of the prospective GDFT group. Two hundred and fifty-eight patients underwent hip revision arthroplasty surgery between 1/2011 and 08/2012, and 130 were finally used for analysis and comparison after matching (Fig. 2).

The basic characteristics from patients (before matching) showed significant difference regarding the ASA score and the P-POSSUM score between the groups (Additional file 1: Table S1). The matching was performed using different parameters (age, ASA score and P-POSSUM score) to achieve equal distributions of the basic characteristics and the perioperative risk factors.

Before surgery, the matched patients from the GDFT group and from the control group were comparable (Table 1).

During surgery, the GDFT protocol was properly followed 87.3% of the time. The overall fluid balance was comparable in both groups (Table 2). However, the GDFT group received more colloids and less crystalloids than the control group (Table 2). The GDFT group received more inotropes but not more vasopressors than the control group (Table 2).

Outcome variables

The postoperative morbidity rate was significantly lower in the GDFT group than in the control group (49.2 vs. 66.9%, $p = 0.006$) (Table 3). Postoperative LOS was significantly shorter in the GDFT group (11 days (9–15) vs. 9 days (8–12); $p = 0.003$) (Fig. 3). When patients were admitted in the ICU postoperatively, the patients from the control group stayed significantly longer in the ICU than the patients from the GDFT group (control group vs. GDFT group, 960 min (360–1210) vs. 400 min (207–825); $p < 0.001$). Other outcome variables are reported in Table 3 and Fig. 4.

Nevertheless, patients of the GDT group had significantly less postoperative cardiac complications (control group vs. GDT group, 7.7 vs. 1.5%; $p = 0.034$) (Table 3), especially as the new arrhythmias postoperatively occurred significantly more often in the control group (control group vs. GDT group, 6.9 vs. 0.8%; $p = 0.019$). The mortality rate was comparable between the groups (control group vs. GDT group, 0.8% (1) vs. 0.8% (1); 1.000).

Discussion

In this matched cohort study and quality improvement project, we implemented into clinical routine a goal-directed fluid therapy protocol in patients undergoing revision hip surgery. The implementation was successful with a high protocol compliance rate of 87%. Patients from the GDFT had a significantly reduced postoperative morbidity (relative decrease of 26.5% ($p = 0.006$)), as well as a 2-day shorter length of hospital stay ($p = 0.003$) and also a shorter ICU stay ($p < 0.001$, when the patients were admitted to the ICU postoperatively).

Many studies have demonstrated the ability of GDFT to improve postoperative outcome in patients undergoing major abdominal and vascular procedures. Recent meta-analysis of randomized controlled trials (RCTs) suggests a 25–50% reduction in postoperative morbidity that was associated with a 1–2-day reduction in hospital length of stay (Grocott et al. 2012; Hamilton et al. 2011; Pearse et al. 2014). However, only few studies were done in patients undergoing orthopaedic surgery. In 1996, Sinclair et al. showed in 40 patients undergoing repair of proximal femoral fractures that fluid loading to an optimal stroke volume resulted in a more rapid postoperative recovery and a significantly reduced hospital stay

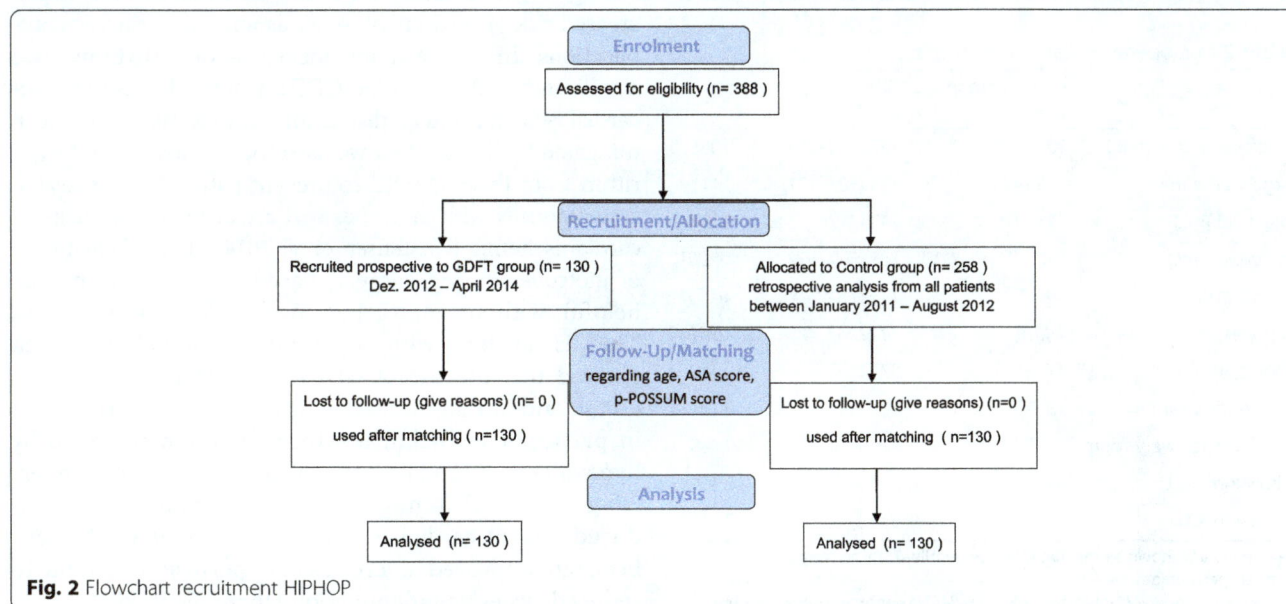

Fig. 2 Flowchart recruitment HIPHOP

Table 1 Characteristics of the study population before surgery

	Control group (n = 130)	GDFT group (n = 130)	p
Age (years)	72 (60–76)	71 (62–75)	0.643
Sex (w/m)	86/44	81/49	0.440
Body height (cm)	166 (160–171)	168 (163–175)	0.155
Body weight (kg)	76 (65–85)	79 (64–90)	0.177
BMI kg/m²	27.36 (24.69–30.06)	27.77 (23.80–32.11)	0.658
CCS	3 (2–5)	3 (2–4)	0.249
ASA score	2 (2–3)	2 (2–3)	0.730
P-POSSUM score	27.00 (23.00–31.00)	29.00 (24.00–33.00)	0.102

Parameters are shown as median and (25th percentile–75th percentile). CCS: The Charlson Comorbidity Score includes age, previous myocardial infarction or congestive heart failure, peripheral vascular disease, cerebrovascular disease, existing dementia, COPD, connective tissue disease, peptic ulcer disease, diabetes mellitus, moderate to severe chronic kidney disease, hemiplegia, leukaemia, malignant lymphoma, solid tumour, liver disease, and AIDS. Different points were distributed for the pre-existing diseases, and so, the survival rate during the first 2 years can be calculated

(Sinclair et al. 1997). In 2002, Venn et al. showed that an invasive intraoperative haemodynamic monitoring concept using fluid challenges during repair of femoral fracture reduced the recovery time and also length of hospital stay (Venn et al. 2002). More recently, Cecconi et al. reported that in patients undergoing primary hip replacement under regional anaesthesia a goal-directed haemodynamic therapy changes the intraoperative fluid management and reduces postoperative complications ($p = 0.05$) (Cecconi et al. 2011). As far as we know, our study is the first investigating the effects of GDFT in patients undergoing more complex hip revision surgery.

In sharp contrast to this overwhelming evidence coming from RCTs, only little attention has been put on clinical implementation at the bedside and the value of GDFT in real life. Kuper et al. published in 2011 a multicentre trial

Table 2 Intraoperative data of both groups

	Control group (n = 130)	GDFT group (n = 130)	p
Anaesthesia time (min)	185 (160–230)	197 (170–254)	0.056
Surgery time (min)	125 (99–159)	135 (107–171)	0.111
Total fluid (mL)	2210 (1658–3000)	2435 (1760–3480)	0.139
Crystalloids (mL)	1500 (1000–2000)	725 (500–1000)	<0.001
Colloids (mL)	500 (500–1000)	1250 (1000–1750)	<0.001
Inotropes	1 [0.8]	28 [21.5]	<0.01
Blood transfusion	47 [36.2]	57 [43.8]	0.255
NE at end of surgery	18 [13.8]	10 [7.7]	0.160
Admission recovery room	75 [57.7]	71 [54.6]	0.708
Admission PACU	44 [33.8]	53 [40.8]	0.305
Admission ICU	11 [8.5]	6 [4.6]	0.316

Parameters are shown as median (25th percentile–75th percentile) and number [percentage]
NE norepinephrine, ICU intensive care unit, PACU post-anaesthesia care unit

Table 3 Total morbidity and complication rates

	Control group (n = 130)	GDFT group (n = 130)	p
Total morbidity	87 [66.9%]	64 [49.2%]	0.006
Infectious complications	13 [10%]	10 [7.7%]	0.663
Cardiac complications	10 [7.7%]	2 [1.5%]	0.034
Postoperative arrhythmia	9 [6.9%]	1 [0.8%]	0.019
Neurological complications	6 [4.6%]	7 [5.4%]	1.000
Renal complications	2 [1.5%]	2 [1.5%]	1.000
Hemorrhagic complications	80 [61.5%]	56 [43.1%]	0.004

where they implemented GDFT into clinical practice. In spite of a lower than expected (65%) adoption rate during the implementation phase, they observed a significantly shorter length of hospital stay with GDFT. Cannesson et al. recently published another real-life implementation programme of GDFT in patients undergoing major abdominal procedures and observed a 14% decrease in postoperative morbidity associated with decrease in median hospital length of stay from 10 (6–16) days to 7 (5–11) days ($p = 0.0001$) (Cannesson et al. 2015). In line with these publications, our study shows that implementation of GDFT is not only possible in a tertiary university medical centre but also might be beneficial for patients in whom the postoperative morbidity rate decreased by 26.5% and hospital length of stay decreased from 11 (9–15) days to 9 (8–12) days during the implementation phase. Our protocol was pretty simple and part of a newly created standard operating procedure officially approved by the departments of anaesthesiology and orthopaedic surgery. Both factors may have contributed to the high compliance rate and the clinical benefits we observed.

One point of discussion is the increased use of inotropes during surgery that might put the GDFT patients at an increased risk of myocardial ischemia and other cardiac complications. In contrast, the incidence of arrhythmia was significantly reduced in the GDFT group. The risk of myocardial ischemia and cardiac complications might have been mitigated by the fact that we used the risk assessment algorithm from the ESA/ESC to prevent patients being treated systematically with inotropes that are at high risk for myocardial ischemia (Kristensen et al. 2014). The adequate use of inotropes during surgery, based on SV data, may be helpful without increasing myocardial complications. This is in line with a recent meta-analysis which showed that the use of GDFT is associated with a decrease and not an increase in cardiac complications and in particular arrhythmias which are often triggered by hypovolemia (Arulkumaran et al. 2014). Other underlying factors that might have contributed to the reduced rate of cardiovascular complications might have been an improved microvascular perfusion leading to reduced systemic inflammation (Jhanji et al. 2010).

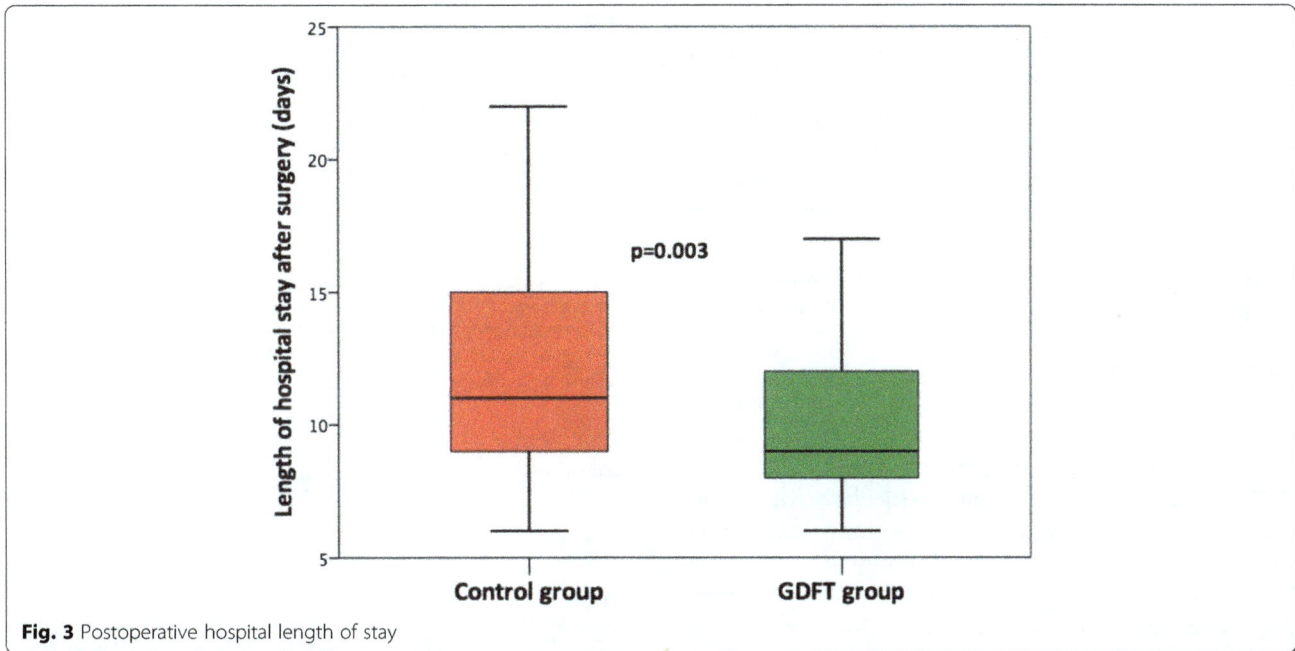

Fig. 3 Postoperative hospital length of stay

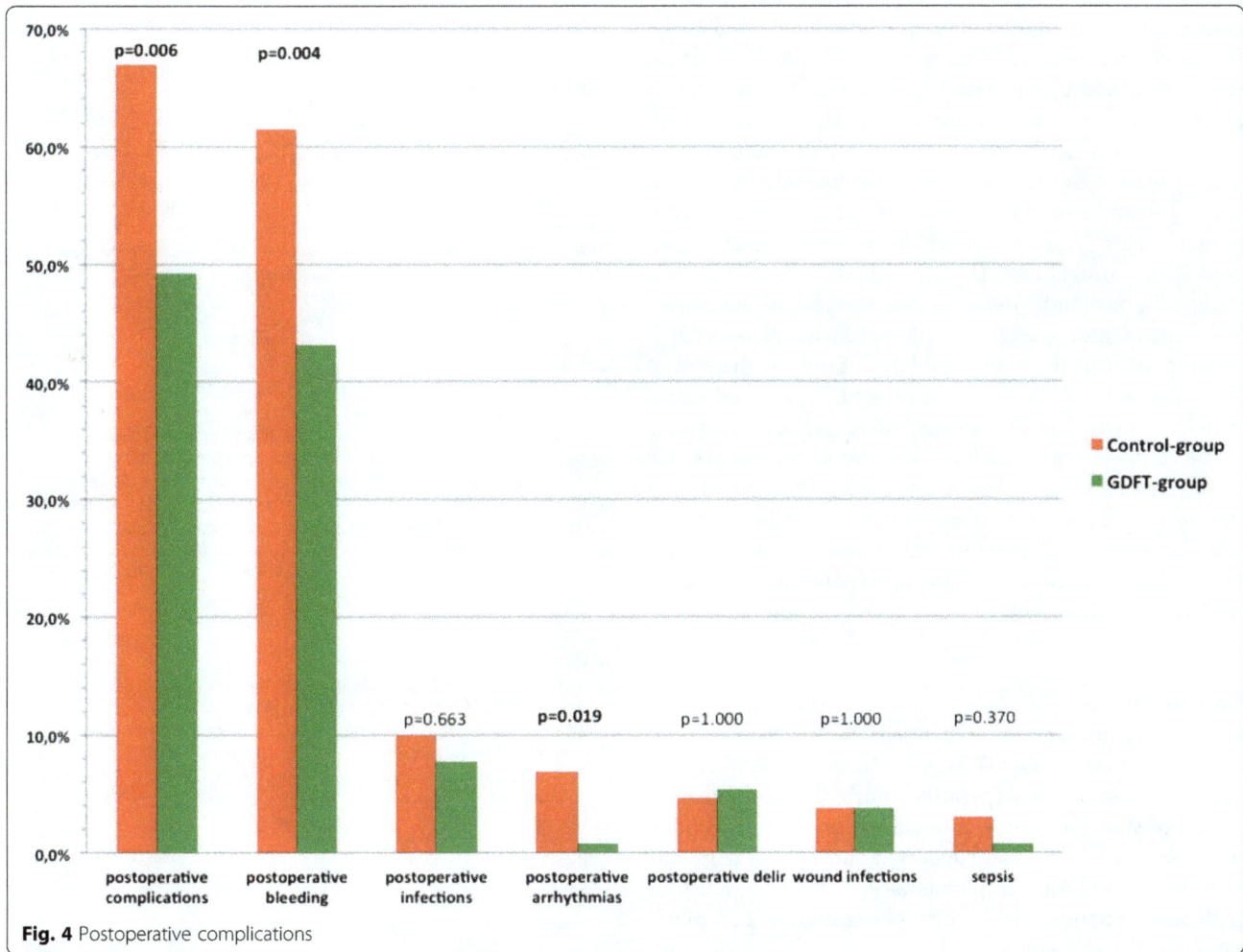

Fig. 4 Postoperative complications

Another interesting finding was the reduced transfusion rate after surgery seen in the GDFT group. We did not change our transfusion guidelines during the study period, so it is unlikely that a change in transfusion practice could have explained it. It could be speculated that due to an improved intraoperative microcirculation in the optimized group, early bleeding during surgery is better recognized by the surgeon, and therefore, surgical haemostasis might be performed more effectively preventing later bleeding complications. Nevertheless, this is speculative and needs to be reproduced by further research.

Our study has several limitations. Given its before-after design, we cannot claim causality between the GDFT intervention introduced as a new standard of care and the observed changes in postoperative outcome. However, RCTs also have their limitations, particularly when blinding is not possible, as is the case when studying changes in clinical behaviour. Indeed, when performing a RCT where fluid management is standardized by the use of a predefined treatment protocol, clinicians are inevitably sensibilized and trained about the risk of giving too little or too much fluid during the perioperative period. As a result, they may change their usual practice and the so-called control group may not reflect anymore what used to be standard management in their institution. This "training effect" will tend to decrease the likelihood to show a difference between the intervention and the control group. On the other hand, when performing RCTs, clinicians usually benefit from extra human and financial resources, helping them to ensure the new strategy is properly implemented. This "resource effect" tends in contrast to increase the probability to show a difference between groups. In our study, the fluid management of the historical control group was not influenced at all by GDFT training and use since we introduced it only at the end of 2012. And when GDFT was introduced, it was used for all patients undergoing hip revision surgery as part of a new standard operating procedure. As a result, we believe our quality improvement study provides a pretty fair idea of the impact of GDFT implementation in real-life conditions and is complementary of previous RCTs done in orthopaedic patients, showing a benefit in more controlled conditions.

Conclusions

In patients undergoing hip revision arthroplasty, the implementation of GDFT was associated with a significant decrease in postoperative morbidity and hospital length of stay. Our study confirms in real-life conditions what previous RCTs had suggested and is a clear invitation to expand our implementation to other surgical patient populations in whom postoperative complications remain an issue.

Additional file

Additional file 1: Table S1. With basic characteristics of all patients before matching. Table S2. Intraoperative data of both groups. Table S3. Length of ICU stay. Figure S1. shows the postoperative hospital length of stay of all patients before matching. Figure S2. shows the postoperative complications of all patients before matching. (DOCX 62 kb)

Abbreviations
GDFT: Goal-directed fluid therapy; ICU: Intensive care unit; PACU: Post-anaesthesia care unit; RBC: Red blood cells; SV: Stroke volume; SV_{opt}: Optimal stroke volume; $SV_{trigger}$: Trigger stroke volume

Acknowledgements
Not applicable.

Funding
The study was supported by Edwards Lifesciences (Edwards Lifesciences SA Route de l'Etraz 70 1260 Nyon). The sponsor had no access to the data and no role in the design and conduct of the study, collection and management of the data, approval of the manuscript, and decision to submit the manuscript for publication.

Authors' contributions
MH, MS, and MK outlined the study design and drafted parts of the manuscript. MH and JN performed the data collection and statistical analysis and drafted parts of the manuscript. FB performed the statistical analysis. VM and FB contributed to the "Discussion" section from the point of view of perioperative and intensive care medicine. MM and CP contributed from an orthopaedic's perspective. MH, MS, and FB were responsible for the design, coordination, and finalization of the manuscript. MH, FB, and MS had full access to the data. All authors read and approved the final manuscript.

Competing interests
FB, VM, MK, MM, and CP have nothing to disclose. MH received funding unrelated to this study from Edwards Lifesciences and Pulsion Medical Systems. MS received research funding for this study from Edwards Lifesciences (Edwards Lifesciences SA Route de l'Etraz 70 1260 Nyon). The sponsor had no direct access to the data and no role in the design and conduct of the study, collection and management of the data, approval of the manuscript, and decision to submit the manuscript for publication. MS received funding unrelated to this study from Masimo, Ratiopharm, Edwards Lifesciences, Pulsion Medical Systems, LMA, Fresenius Medical Care, and LidCO.

Author details
[1]Department of Anaesthesiology and Intensive Care Medicine, Charité University Hospital Berlin, Campus Charité Mitte and Campus Virchow-Klinikum, Berlin, Germany. [2]Centre for Musculoskeletal Surgery, Department of Orthopaedics, Charité University Hospital Berlin, Campus Charité Mitte and Campus Virchow-Klinikum, Berlin, Germany. [3]Department of Anaesthesiology, Intensive Care Medicine and Pain Therapy, Justus-Liebig-University, Giessen, Germany.

References

Arulkumaran N, Corredor C, Hamilton MA, Ball J, Grounds RM, Rhodes A, et al. Cardiac complications associated with goal-directed therapy in high-risk surgical patients: a meta-analysis. Br J Anaesth [Internet]. 2014;112(4):648–59.

Benes J, Chytra I, Altmann P, Hluchy M, Kasal E, Svitak R, et al. Intraoperative fluid optimization using stroke volume variation in high risk surgical patients: results of prospective randomized study. Crit Care. 2010;14(3):R118.

Cannesson M, Ramsingh D, Rinehart J, Demirjian A, Vu T, Vakharia S, et al. Perioperative goal-directed therapy and postoperative outcomes in patients undergoing high-risk abdominal surgery: a historical-prospective, comparative effectiveness study. Crit Care. 2015 Jul 22:1–11

Cecconi M, Fasano N, Langiano N, Divella M, Costa MG, Rhodes A, et al. Goal-directed haemodynamic therapy during elective total hip arthroplasty under regional anaesthesia. Crit Care. 2011;15(3):R132.

Gan TJ, Soppitt A, Maroof M, el-Moalem H, Robertson KM, Moretti E, et al. Goal-directed intraoperative fluid administration reduces length of hospital stay after major surgery. Anesthesiology. 2002;97(4):820–6.

Ghaferi AA, Birkmeyer JD, Dimick JB. Variation in hospital mortality associated with inpatient surgery. N Engl J Med [Internet] Mass Medical Soc. 2009;361(14):1368–75. Available from: http://www.nejm.org/doi/full/10.1056/NEJMsa0903048.

Grocott MP, Dushianthan A, Hamilton MA, Mythen MG, Harrison D, Rowan K, et al. Perioperative increase in global blood flow to explicit defined goals and outcomes following surgery. Cochrane Database Syst Rev (Online). 2012;11:CD004082.

Hamilton MA, Cecconi M, Rhodes A. A systematic review and meta-analysis on the use of preemptive hemodynamic intervention to improve postoperative outcomes in moderate and high-risk surgical patients. Anesth Analg. 2011;112(6):1392–402.

Hansen BB, Klopfer SO. Optimal full matching and related designs via network flows. J Comput Graph Stat. 2006;15(3):609–27.

Jhanji S, Vivian-Smith A, Lucena-Amaro S, Watson D, Hinds CJ, Pearse RM. Haemodynamic optimisation improves tissue microvascular flow and oxygenation after major surgery: a randomised controlled trial. Crit Care. 2010;14(4):R151.

Kristensen SD, Knuuti J, Saraste A, Anker S, Bøtker HE, De Hert S, et al. 2014 ESC/ESA guidelines on non-cardiac surgery: cardiovascular assessment and management: the Joint Task Force on non-cardiac surgery: cardiovascular assessment and management of the European Society of Cardiology (ESC) and the European Society of Anaesthesiology (ESA). Eur J Anaesthesiol. 2014;31(10):517–73.

Lopes MR, Oliveira MA, Pereira VOS, Lemos IPB, Auler JOC, Michard F. Goal-directed fluid management based on pulse pressure variation monitoring during high-risk surgery: a pilot randomized controlled trial. Crit Care. 2007;11(5):R100.

Pearse RM, Harrison DA, MacDonald N, Gillies MA, Blunt M, Ackland G, et al. Effect of a perioperative, cardiac output-guided hemodynamic therapy algorithm on outcomes following major gastrointestinal surgery: a randomized clinical trial and systematic review. JAMA. 2014;311(21):2181–90.

Pestaña D, Espinosa E, Eden A, Nájera D, Collar L, Aldecoa C, et al. Perioperative goal-directed hemodynamic optimization using noninvasive cardiac output monitoring in major abdominal surgery. Anesth Analg. 2014;119(3):579–87.

Scheeren TWL, Wiesenack C, Gerlach H, Marx G. Goal-directed intraoperative fluid therapy guided by stroke volume and its variation in high-risk surgical patients: a prospective randomized multicentre study. J Clin Monit Comput. 2013;27(3):225–33.

Sinclair S, James S, Singer M. Intraoperative intravascular volume optimisation and length of hospital stay after repair of proximal femoral fracture: randomised controlled trial. BMJ. 1997;315(7113):909–12.

Sury MRJ, Palmer JHMG, Cook TM, Pandit JJ. The state of UK anaesthesia: a survey of National Health Service activity in 2013. Br J Anaesth. 2014;113(4):575–84.

Venn R, Steele A, Richardson P, Poloniecki J, Grounds M, Newman P. Randomized controlled trial to investigate influence of the fluid challenge on duration of hospital stay and perioperative morbidity in patients with hip fractures. Br J Anaesth. 2002;88(1):65–71.

Vincent J-L. Logistics of large international trials: the good, the bad, and the ugly. Crit Care Med. 2009;37(Supplement):S75–9.

Weiser TG, Regenbogen SE, Thompson KD, Haynes AB, Lipsitz SR, Berry WR, et al. An estimation of the global volume of surgery: a modelling strategy based on available data. Lancet. 2008;372(9633):139–44.

Pre-operative anaemia is associated with total morbidity burden on days 3 and 5 after cardiac surgery

Julie Sanders[1], Jackie A. Cooper[2], Daniel Farrar[3], Simon Braithwaite[4], Updeshbir Sandhu[4], Michael G. Mythen[5] and Hugh E. Montgomery[6]*

Abstract

Background: Pre-operative anaemia is associated with mortality and red blood cell (RBC) transfusion requirement after cardiac surgery. However, the effect on post-operative total morbidity burden (TMB) is unknown. We explored the effect of pre-operative anaemia on post-operative TMB.

Methods: Data were drawn from the Cardiac Post-Operative Morbidity Score (C-POMS) development study ($n = 442$). C-POMS describes and quantifies (0–13) TMB after cardiac surgery by noting the presence/absence of 13 morbidity domains on days 3 (D3), 5 (D5), 8 (D8) and 15 (D15). Anaemia was defined as a haemoglobin concentration below 130 g/l for men and 120 g/l for women.

Results: Most patients were White British (86.1%) and male (79.2%) and underwent coronary artery bypass surgery (67.4%). Participants with pre-operative anaemia ($n = 137$, 31.5%) were over three times more likely to receive RBC transfusion (OR 3.08, 95%CI 1.88–5.06, $p < 0.001$), had greater D3 and D5 TMB (5 vs 3, $p < 0.0001$; 3 vs 2, $p < 0.0001$, respectively) and remained in hospital 2 days longer (8 vs 6 days, $p < 0.0001$) than non-anaemic patients. Transfused patients remained in hospital 5 days longer than non-transfused patients ($p < 0.0001$), had higher TMB on all days (all $p < 0.001$) and suffered greater pulmonary, renal, GI, neurological, endocrine and ambulation morbidities (p 0.026 to <0.001). Pre-operative anaemia and RBC transfusion were independently associated with increased C-POMS score.

Conclusions: Pre-operative anaemia and RBC transfusion are independently associated with increased post-operative TMB. Understanding TMB may assist in post-operative patient management to reduce morbidity. We recommend the use of the C-POMS tool as a standard outcome tool in further studies.

Keywords: Anaemia, Post-operative morbidity, Total morbidity burden, Red blood cell transfusion, Cardiac surgery

Background

Anaemia, defined as circulating haemoglobin (Hb) concentration level below 130 g/l for men and 120 g/l for women (World Health Organization 2008), affects 24.8% of the global population (World Health Organization 2008), and up to 54.4% of cardiac surgery patients (Hung et al. 2011) are anaemic prior to surgery.

Since Hb is the circulation's oxygen-carrying molecule, anaemia is associated with decreased blood oxygen content. Unless compensated for by increased blood flow, inadequate tissue oxygen delivery (Kurtz et al. 2010) may impair organ function. Furthermore, iron is not only essential for the synthesis of Hb's haem moiety but also plays an important role in oxidative metabolism (Dunn et al. 2007). Iron deficiency may thus directly impair mitochondrial oxidative metabolism and adenosine triphosphate (ATP) synthesis through direct mitochondrial effects, as well as through anaemia and resulting impairment of oxygen delivery (Davies et al. 1982). In pre-operative anaemic patients, these deficits follow the patient into surgery, which itself is associated with a substantial and sustained increase in metabolic activity

* Correspondence: h.montgomery@ucl.ac.uk
[6]Institute for Sport, Exercise and Health, University College London, 1st Floor 170 Tottenham Court Rd, London W1T 7HA, UK
Full list of author information is available at the end of the article

and hence in oxygen demand (Vallet and Futier 2010). By limiting the capacity to respond to this increased metabolic demand, pre-operative anaemia might thus be postulated to impair post-operative recovery.

Indeed, pre-operative anaemia has been associated with adverse outcome after cardiac surgery and has been associated with higher mortality (Hung et al. 2011; Zindrou et al. 2002; Cladellas et al.; van Straten et al. 2009; De Santo et al. 2009; Boening et al. 2011; Miceli et al. 2014), longer stay on the intensive care unit (ICU) (Hung et al. 2011; De Santo et al. 2009) and in hospital (Cladellas et al.; De Santo et al. 2009; Miceli et al. 2014; Kulier et al. 2007) and a higher incidence red blood cell (RBC) transfusion (De Santo et al. 2009; Boening et al. 2011). However, the evidence relating to the influence of pre-operative anaemia on post-operative morbidity is divided and only relates to specific outcomes, for example stroke (Cladellas et al.; Miceli et al. 2014; Fowler et al.) and renal dysfunction (Cladellas et al.; Miceli et al. 2014; Fowler et al.; Carrascal et al. 2010). Thus, whether anaemia is an independent risk factor for general morbidity after cardiac surgery (Fowler et al.) and the scale of this impact on total morbidity burden (TMB) has yet to be reported.

Thus, we explored the association between pre-operative anaemia and RBC transfusion requirement with TMB after cardiac surgery.

Methods

Participants

Patients were drawn from the Cardiac Post-Operative Morbidity Score (C-POMS) development and validation study; the methods describing how the C-POMS measurement tool was developed and validated are detailed elsewhere (Sanders et al.). In brief, patients undergoing any form of adult cardiac surgery (excluding cardiac surgery for a congenital heart condition or a cardiomyopathy) between January 2005 and November 2007 at the Heart Hospital, University College London Hospitals NHS Trust, UK, and who gave written informed consent were eligible for inclusion. Excluded were those <18 years old, undergoing emergency surgery, who were enrolled in clinical intervention trials or who died within 5 days of surgery.

Defining anaemia

Anaemia was defined as a haemoglobin (Hb) concentration below 130 g/l for men and 120g/l for women (Organisation WH 2008).

Outcome measurements

Post-operative morbidity and hence total morbidity burden were defined using the C-POMS tool (Table 1).

RBC transfusion

Allogenic RBC transfusions were defined as any RBC transfusion given to the participant in the intra- and post-operative period prior to discharge from hospital and were collected by staff using the C-POMS tool (Table 1).

At the time of data collection, there was no uniform protocol for blood transfusion, although the unit operated a generally restrictive transfusion policy. Trust guidelines stipulated that RBC transfusion was strongly indicated when the haemoglobin was below 70 g/l. Since November 1999, all allogeneic blood components produced in the UK have been subjected to leucocyte depletion (LD) whereby ≥99% of units have $<5 \times 10^6$ leucocytes and >90% $<1 \times 10^6$ leucocytes (Service UKBT and T 2007).

Total morbidity burden: C-POMS summary score

Post-operative morbidity was prospectively assessed on days 3 (D3), 5 (D5), 8 (D8) and 15 (D15) after cardiac surgery using the C-POMS tool (Sanders et al.). This represents TMB as a summary score (0–13), derived by noting the new or escalating presence or absence of 13 morbidity domains. Thus, the higher the score, the more morbidity experienced by the patient (Table 1).

Post-operative length of stay

Post-operative length of stay (LOS) was defined as the number of days from surgery (day of operation day 0) to discharge from hospital. This included any days spent in a receiving hospital following transfer from the operative hospital.

Other clinical data

Other clinical information including patient demographic details, relevant medical history, symptoms, risk factors, intra-operative details and general outcome variables (as shown in Table 2) were extracted from the C-POMS study. These were originally obtained from the medical and nursing records and the Society of Cardiothoracic Surgery of Great Britain and Ireland's local database.

Statistical analysis

All statistical analyses were performed in Stata version 13 (StataCorp Texas).

Baseline characteristics by anaemia were compared using Fisher's exact test for categorical variables and Mann-Whitney U test for continuous data. The association of transfusion with anaemia after adjustment for covariates (age, gender and EuroSCORE) was assessed using a logistic regression model, and the odds ratio and 95% confidence interval were obtained. Associations with individual C-POMS morbidities were examined

Table 1 The Cardiac Post-Operative Morbidity Score (C-POMS) (Sanders et al.)

Morbidity type	C-POMS criteria
Pulmonary	Presence of one or more of the following: ■ New requirement for oxygen or respiratory support (including nebuliser therapy or request for chest physiotherapy on or after D5) ■ Pleural effusion requiring drainage
Infectious	Presence of one or more of the following: ■ Currently on antibiotics ■ A temperature of >38 °C in the last 24 h ■ A white cell count/CRP level requiring in-hospital review or treatment
Renal	Presence of one or more of the following: ■ Decreased urine output requiring intervention (including IV furosemide) ■ Increased serum creatinine (>30% from pre-operative level) ■ Urinary catheter in situ ■ New urinary incontinence ■ Serum potassium abnormalities requiring treatment
Gastrointestinal	Presence of one or more of the following: ■ Unable to tolerate an enteral diet for any reason including nausea, vomiting and abdominal distension ■ The presence of a nasogastric tube ■ Diagnosis of a gastrointestinal bleed ■ Diarrhoea
Cardiovascular	Presence of one or more of the following: ■ The use of inotropic therapy for any cardiovascular cause ■ Pacing wires (on or after D5) and/or requiring temporary or new permanent pacing ■ Diagnostic tests or therapy within the last 24 h for any of the following: (1) new MI or ischaemia, (2) hypotension (requiring fluid therapy, pharmacological therapy or omission of pharmacological therapy), (3) atrial or ventricular arrhythmias, (4) cardiogenic pulmonary oedema, thrombotic event (requiring anticoagulation), (5) hypertension (pharmacological therapy or omission of pharmacological therapy)
Neurological	New neurological deficit (including confusion, delirium, coma, lack of coordination, drowsy/slow to wake, poor swallow, blurred vision, sedated, changing loss of consciousness)
Haematological	Presence of one or more of the following: ■ Untherapeutic INR requiring pharmacological therapy or omission of pharmacological therapy ■ Requirement for any of the following within the last 24 h: packed erythrocytes, platelets, fresh-frozen plasma or cryoprecipitate
Wound	Presence of one or more of the following: ■ Wound dehiscence requiring surgical exploration or drainage of pus from the operation wound with or without isolation of organisms ■ Chest drains ■ Wound pain significant enough to require continuing or escalating analgesic intervention
Pain	Post-operative pain significant enough to require parenteral opioids and/or continuing or additional analgesia.
Endocrine	New or additional requirements for blood sugar management
Electrolyte	Electrolyte (including sodium, urea, phosphate) imbalance requiring oral or intravenous intervention (not including potassium as included in renal category)
Review	Remaining in hospital for further review, investigation and/or procedure
Assisted ambulation	A new or escalated post-operative requirement for mobility assistance (including wheelchair, crutches, zimmer frame, walking sticks or assistance)
Non-C-POMS related reasons for delayed discharge on D5, D8 and D15 which the PDG decided should also be routine data collection in C-POMS on these days.	
Non-morbidity reason for delayed discharge	Where C-POMS is '0' but the patient remains in hospital, state the reason for lack of discharge: *Social reasons; Equipment at home; Mobility* (ongoing physic and OT needs); *Institutional failure* (transport not booked, OPA or follow-up not arranged); *Delayed discharge* (lack of rehab or other bed); *Discharge planned for today; Other medical reason*

CRP C-reactive protein, *IV* intravenous, *MI* myocardial infarction, *INR* international normalised ratio, *OPA* out-patient appointment, *OT* occupational therapy

using random intercept logistic regression models. p values were corrected for multiple comparisons over the 13 morbidities using the Bonferroni correction.

Hb concentration at each time point was divided into quintiles, and differences in C-POMS score were tested between quintiles using Kruskal-Wallis test and a non-parametric test for trend across ordered groups (Cuzick 1985). Differences in C-POMS by quintile over all time points were estimated using a random intercept model with time fitted as a fixed effect.

Correlations of Hb with LOS and C-POMS score were assessed by Spearman rank correlation, and multivariate

Table 2 Baseline characteristics (n = 442, unless otherwise stated). All values n(%) unless otherwise stated

	Overall (n = 442) Frequency (%)/mean ± SD	Anaemic (n = 139) Frequency (%)/mean ± SD	Not anaemic (n = 303) Frequency (%)/mean ± SD	P (anaemic vs not anaemic)
Demographics				
Age (mean/years)	66.5 ± 10.6	69.5 ± 10.5	65.11 ± 10.4	0.000
Female gender	92 (20.8)	32 (23.0)	60 (19.8)	0.451
Ethnicity (White British) (n = 438)	377 (86.1)	106 (76.8)	271 (90.3)	0.001
Medical history				
Renal (dialysis)	7 (1.6)	6 (4.3)	1 (0.3)	0.005
History of previous MI (n = 415)	147 (35.4)	49 (38.0)	98 (34.3)	0.375
Re-operation	18 (4.1)	8 (5.8)	10 (3.3)	0.299
Cerebrovascular accident	16 (3.6)	9 (6.5)	7 (2.3)	0.050
Gastrointestinal disease	50 (11.3)	23 (16.5)	2 (8.9)	0.023
Congestive heart failure (n = 415)	13 (3.1)	8 (6.2)	5 (1.7)	0.034
Symptoms				
NYHA class (n = 441)				
- I	114 (25.9)	32 (23.0)	82 (27.2)	0.245
- II	204 (46.3)	65 (46.8)	139 (46.0)	
- III	101 (22.9)	31 (22.3)	70 (23.2)	
- IV	22 (5.0)	11 (2.5)	11 (3.6)	
Cardiac risk factors				
Smoking				
- Current	49 (11.1)	14 (10.1)	35 (11.6)	0.891
- Ex	244 (55.2)	77 (55.4)	167 (55.1)	
- Never	149 (33.7)	48 (34.5)	101 (33.3)	
Hypertension	302 (68.3)	95 (68.3)	207 (68.3)	1.000
Hypercholesteraemia	341 (77.1)	101 (72.7)	240 (79.5)	0.142
Diabetes	103 (23.3)	53 (38.1)	50 (16.5)	0.000
BMI (kg/m²)/mean	28.6 ± 5.7	28.1 ± 6.0	28.8 ± 5.5	0.262
Examination and investigation				
LVEF (n = 434)				
- Good	323 (74.4)	101 (74.3)	222 (74.5)	0.167
- Fair	88 (20.3)	24 (17.6)	64 (21.5)	
- Poor	23 (5.3)	11 (8.1)	12 (4.0)	
Number diseased vessels (n = 435)				
- 0	79 (18.2)	28 (20.6)	51 (17.1)	0.799
- 1	34 (7.8)	10 (7.4)	24 (8.0)	
- 2	80 (18.4)	26 (19.1)	54 (18.1)	
- 3	242 (55.6)	72 (52.9)	170 (56.9)	
Pre-operative risk assessment				
EuroSCORE (median [IQR])	4 [1–5]	5 [2–6]	3 [1–4]	0.000
Intra-operative details				
Operative priority				
-Elective	308 (69.7)	73 (52.5)	235 (77.6)	0.000

Table 2 Baseline characteristics ($n = 442$, unless otherwise stated). All values n(%) unless otherwise stated *(Continued)*

Operation performed				
- CABG	298 (67.4)	86 (61.9)	212 (70.0)	0.103
- AVR	61 (13.8)	18 (12.9)	43 (14.2)	
- MVR	10 (2.3)	5 (3.6)	5 (1.7)	
- CABG + AVR	35 (7.9)	14 (10.1)	21 (6.9)	
- CABG + MVR	0 (0.0)	0 (0.0)	0 (0.0)	
- AVR + MVR	3 (0.7)	0 (0.0)	3 (1.0)	
- CABG + AVR + MVR	2 (0.5)	0 (0.0)	2 (0.7)	
- Other	33 (7.5)	16 (11.5)	17 (5.6)	
Duration of operation (min)	224.0 ± 54.1	230.3 ± 64.5	221.0 ± 48.3	0.098
Cardiopulmonary bypass used	410 (93.4)	139 (92.8)	281 (93.7)	0.837
Cardiopulmonary bypass time ($n = 428$)	79.0 ± 35.8	80.8 ± 41.6	78.2 ± 32.8	0.495
Aortic cross clamp time	51.0 ± 24.9	52.7 ± 29.5	50.26 ± 22.6	0.362
Outcome				
Number of hours ventilated (h) ($n = 392$)	9.84 ± 58.2	8.0 ± 6.6	10.6 ± 69.3	0.690
Length of ICU stay (mean/days) ($n = 416$)	2.0 ± 3.5	3.0 ± 5.7	1.6 ± 1.6	0.000
Readmitted to ICU	15 (3.4)	11 (8.4)	4 (1.4)	0.001
Return to theatre	21 (4.8)	13 (9.6)	8 (2.7)	0.003
Total length of hospital stay (mean/days)	11.8 ± 11.7	15.2 ± 17.2	10.2 ± 7.6	0.000

models were fitted for patient LOS and C-POMS score using ordinal logistic regression and random intercept models, respectively. Terms for both EuroSCORE and Hb were fitted as quintiles in the multivariate models as their distributions differed significantly from normality.

Results

Baseline characteristics

Of 748 potentially eligible patients undergoing cardiac surgery, 520 (69.5%) were screened (due to researcher availability) and 464 (89.2%) consented to participate. Fourteen participants subsequently became ineligible, leaving 450 who completed the study. Six participants declined for their data to be used outside the development of C-POMS, and a further two patients were without pre-operative Hb results, leaving 442 patients for analysis in this study.

Table 2 summarises the participants' characteristics. Overall, the majority were White British (377, 86.1%) and male (350, 79.2%) with a mean age of 66.5 years (range 19 to 91 years). Seven patients (1.6%) were receiving renal dialysis while 50 (11.3%) had gastrointestinal disease. Most underwent isolated coronary artery bypass graft (CABG) surgery (298, 67.4%) and received cardiopulmonary bypass (410, 93.4%). Overall, the patients remained in the ICU and hospital for 2.0 and 11.8 days, respectively.

Pre-operative anaemia

The overall median Hb was 135 (range 79 to 173). Pre-operative anaemia was present in 31.5% (139/442)

participants. The median Hb in the anaemic group was 116 (range 79 to 129 g/l) and 140 (range 120 to 173 g/l) in the non-anaemic groups ($p = 0.000$).

Table 2 shows the comparison of the pre-, intra- and post-operative characteristics between those with and without anaemia. Patients with pre-operative anaemia were older (69.5 vs 65.1 years, $p = 0.000$), less likely to be of White British ethnicity (76.8 vs 90.3%, $p = 0.001$) and more likely to be receiving pre-operative dialysis (4.3 vs 0.3%, $p = 0.005$) than non-anaemic participants. Those with anaemia were also more likely to have a history of cerebrovascular accident (6.5 vs 2.3%, $p = 0.05$), gastrointestinal (GI) disease (16.5 vs 8.9%, $p = 0.023$) or congestive heart failure (CHF) (6.2 vs 1.7%, $p = 0.034$) and to be diabetic (38.1 vs 16.5%, $p = 0.000$). Thus, as would be expected, anaemic patients had a higher EuroSCORE (5 vs 3, $p = 0.000$) and were more likely to be undergoing urgent (non-elective) surgery (47.5 vs 22.4%, $p = 0.000$). Furthermore, compared to non-anaemic patients, those with anaemia were more likely to return to theatre (9.6 vs 2.7%, $p = 0.003$), be readmitted to the ICU (8.4 vs 1.4%, $p = 0.001$) and so to stay longer in the ICU (3.0 vs 1.6 days, $p = 0.000$) and in hospital (15.2 vs 10.2 days, $p = 0.000$).

Pre-operative anaemia and RBC transfusion

Pre-operative anaemic patients were more likely to receive a RBC transfusion than non-anaemic patients (39.6 vs 14.5%, unadjusted odds ratio (OR) (95%CI)

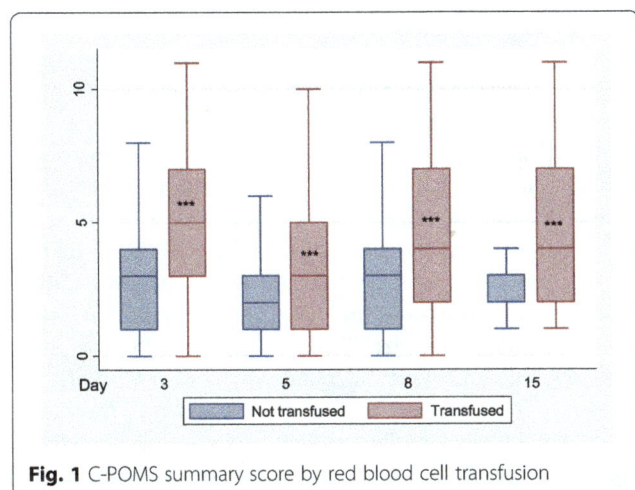

Fig. 1 C-POMS summary score by red blood cell transfusion

3.85 (2.42–6.15) $p < 0.0001$) and, if transfused, to receive more units (2 vs 1 unit, $p = 0.04$). The association between anaemia and transfusion remained after adjustment for age, gender, EuroSCORE and LOS. Overall, anaemic patients had over three times the odds (OR 3.08, 95%CI 1.88–5.06, $p < 0.001$) of requiring a RBC transfusion than non-anaemic patients (14.1 vs 33.6%).

Patients who received a RBC transfusion remained in hospital 5 days longer than those who did not (LOS 11 vs 6 days, $p < 0.0001$) and had a significantly higher C-POMS score on all days (D3 5 vs 3, D5 3 vs 2, D8 4 vs 3, D15 4 vs 2, all $p < 0.001$) (Fig. 1). Furthermore, RBC transfusion was associated with pulmonary, renal, GI, neurological, endocrine and ambulation morbidities (p 0.026 to <0.001), independent of Hb (Table 3).

Pre-operative anaemia and C-POMS score

Pre-operative Hb was correlated with C-POMS score on D3 (rho –0.28, $p < 0.0001$) and D5 (rho –0.18, $p = 0.0002$) but not D8 (rho –0.143, $p = 0.06$) or D15 (rho –0.28, $p = 0.06$). Patients with pre-operative anaemia had a significantly higher C-POMS score on D3 and D5 than non-anaemic patients (5 vs 3 and 3 vs 2, respectively, both $p < 0.0001$) but not on D8 (3 vs 3, $p = 0.32$) or D15 (3.5 vs 3, $p = 0.27$) (Fig. 2). Pre-operative anaemia was associated with renal ($p < 0.001$) and assisted ambulation ($p = 0.003$) but no other C-POMS domains (Table 4).

Both pre-operative anaemia and transfusion requirement were independently associated with an increased C-POMS score (Table 5). Pre-operative anaemia was associated with a 0.55 (se 0.20) $p = 0.005$ increase in score, while RBC transfusion requirement was associated with an increase score of 1.23 (se 0.22) ($p < 0.0001$). If Hb replaced anaemia in this statistical model, both Hb and transfusion are independently associated with C-POMS score. C-POMS score decreases with every one quintile increase in Hb (B (se) –0.18 (0.06) $p = 0.003$) and increases by 1.19 with transfusion (se 0.22) ($p < 0.0001$). Increased age was also independently associated with increased C-POMS score in both models.

Pre-operative anaemia and hospital LOS

Pre-operative Hb was correlated with hospital LOS (rho –0.32, $p < 0.00001$). When compared to patients with Hb >14.6 (quintile 5), those with Hb <12.1 (quintile 1) had a higher morbidity score on D3 (5 vs 2, $p < 0.0001$) and D5 (3 vs 2, $p = 0.007$) and stayed in hospital for an additional 4 days (LOS 10 vs 6 days, $p < 0.001$) (Table 6). Pre-operative anaemic patients

Table 3 Morbidity outcome by domain following RBC transfusion

C-POMS morbidity domain	OR (95%CI)[a]	p value	Bonferroni adjusted p value
Pulmonary	3.55 (1.87–6.73)	0.0001	0.001
Infectious	1.71 (0.71–4.15)	0.232	1.00
Renal	4.52 (1.88–10.83)	0.001	0.013
Gastrointestinal	2.58 (1.42–4.68)	0.002	0.026
Cardiovascular	4.14 (1.37–12.47)	0.012	0.156
Neurological	5.89 (2.65–13.09)	0.00001	0.0001
Haematological	2.98 (1.20–7.41)	0.019	0.247
Wound	1.89 (0.66–5.40)	0.237	1.000
Pain	1.39 (0.51–3.78)	0.514	1.000
Endocrine	4.40 (1.97–9.84)	0.0003	0.004
Electrolyte	0.66 (0.14–3.08)	0.594	1.000
Review	1.97 (1.06–3.64)	0.032	0.416
Assisted ambulation	6.49 (2.57–16.40)	0.00008	0.001

[a]Odds ratio for association of transfusion with domain after adjustment for age, gender, time point and Hb

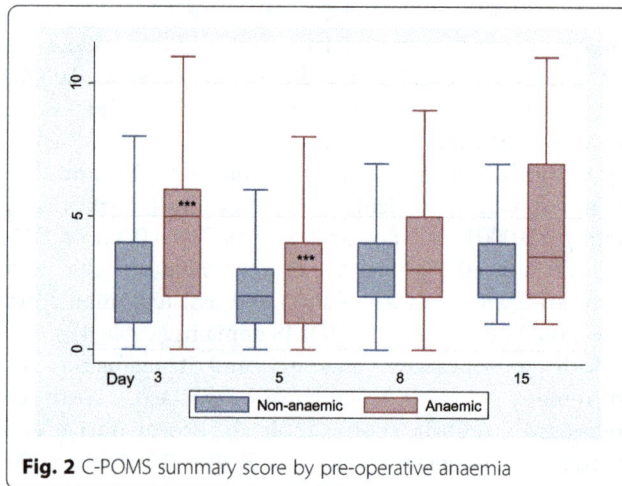

Fig. 2 C-POMS summary score by pre-operative anaemia

remained in hospital 2 days longer than non-anaemic patients (8 (inter-quartile range (IQR) 6–15) vs 6 (IQR 5–9) days, $p < 0.0001$, respectively).

Both pre-operative anaemia (OR 1.65, 95%CI 1.12–2.44, $p = 0.01$) and RBC transfusion requirement (OR 2.40, 95%CI 1.55–3.72, $p < 0.001$) were independently associated with increased hospital LOS (Table 7). If Hb level replaces pre-operative anaemia in the analysis model, there is a linear decrease in LOS over the five quintiles with odds ratios vs quintile 1 of 0.78, 0.64, 0.49 and 0.42 for quintiles 2 to 5. Lower Hb (OR per quintile of Hb 0.80, 95%CI 0.70–0.92, $p = 0.001$) and RBC transfusion requirement (OR 2.33, 95%CI 1.50–3.60, $p = 0.0002$) were independently associated with increased hospital LOS.

Discussion

Pre-operative anaemia has been associated with adverse outcome after cardiac surgery. However, whether anaemia is an independent risk factor for general morbidity after cardiac surgery (Fowler et al.) and the scale of this impact on total morbidity burden (TMB) has not previously been reported. Thus, our study explored the effect of pre-operative anaemia and RBC transfusion on total morbidity burden after cardiac surgery. Firstly, we found that compared to non-anaemic patients, pre-operative anaemic patients had significantly higher TMB (C-POMS scores) on D3 and D5, significantly more renal and ambulation morbidities and stayed in ICU and hospital an extra 1.4 days and an extra 2 days, respectively. As pre-operative anaemia was independently associated with increased TMB, reduction of post-operative morbidity might be achieved by treating pre-operative anaemia. Indeed, pre-operative optimization of anaemia in the UK is recommended (Service UKBT and T 2007; Department of Health 2007) as part of the patient blood management plan, with the use of intravenous (IV) iron if surgery may be delayed due to the time needed for oral iron to take effect (ERP Programme 2010). However, although IV iron therapy for anaemia has been shown to effectively treat anaemia in medical (Usmanov et al. 2008), and non-cardiac pre-operative settings (Munoz et al. 2009), the effect on cardiac surgical patients is not yet confirmed due to the low level of evidence available (Hogan et al. 2015). Thus, further prospective evidence in cardiac surgery patients is required before any recommendation for the use of IV iron to treat pre-operative anaemia in these patients can be made. Secondly, blood is a limited resource and is associated with high transfusion costs (Department of Health 2007), administration incidents and risks (Group SS 2014) and specifically poorer outcome in cardiac surgical patients (Galas et al. 2013). Our results found RBC transfusion to be independently associated with TMB, and patients spent an extra 5 days in hospital. Thus, strategies

Table 4 Pre-operative anaemia and morbidity outcome by domain

C-POMS morbidity domain	OR (95%CI)[a]	p value	Bonferroni adjusted p value
Pulmonary	1.60 (0.93–2.76)	0.088	1.00
Infectious	1.87 (0.84–4.17)	0.125	1.00
Renal	6.88 (2.97–15.92)	0.000006	0.00008
Gastrointestinal	0.89 (0.52–1.53)	0.674	1.000
Cardiovascular	1.64 (0.62–4.31)	0.319	1.000
Neurological	0.81 (0.40–1.66)	0.571	1.000
Haematological	1.35 (0.60–3.03)	0.467	1.000
Wound	2.12 (0.80–5.62)	0.133	1.000
Pain	1.53 (0.63–3.75)	0.349	1.000
Endocrine	2.83 (1.38–5.80)	0.005	0.065
Electrolyte	2.73 (0.70–10.68)	0.150	1.000
Review	1.22 (0.68–2.20)	0.510	1.000
Assisted ambulation	4.96 (2.16–11.38)	0.0002	0.0026

[a]Odds ratio for association of anaemia with domain after adjustment for age, gender, time point and transfusion

Table 5 Multivariate models for associations with C-POMS

		Model including anaemia		Model including Hb	
		B (se)	p value	B (se)	p value
Age	10-year increase	−0.15 (0.10)	0.13	−0.16 (0.10)	0.11
Gender	Female/male	−0.15 (0.22)	0.49	−0.34 (0.23)	0.13
EuroSCORE	Per quintile	0.48 (0.08)	<0.0001	0.48 (0.08)	<0.0001
Anaemia	Yes/no	0.55 (0.20)	0.005	–	–
Hb	1 SD increase	–	–	−0.29 (0.10)	0.003
Transfusion	Yes/no	1.23 (0.22)	<0.0001	1.19 (0.22)	<0.0001

to reduce RBC use may reduce transfusion errors, reduce healthcare costs and improve patient well-being. However, although there are considerable differences in transfusion triggers across UK cardiac surgery centres (Murphy et al. 2013), restrictive transfusion protocols (Ternström et al. 2014) and patient blood management systems (Gross et al. 2015) do not appear to reduce post-operative morbidity in all instances, with the TITRe2 trial suggesting liberal transfusion may actually be superior after cardiac surgery (Murphy et al. 2015). This again raises the question on whether it is anaemia or RBC transfusion that carries the greatest risk (Vincent 2015; Du Pont-Thibodeau et al. 2014), and hence, exploring TMB in future anaemia and transfusion studies in cardiac surgery is needed. Adding further complexity to our understanding of pre-operative anaemia, treatment strategies and outcome, hepcidin, the principal regulator of systemic iron homeostasis, has been found to be an independent risk factor for poor outcome (Hung et al. 2015). This provides a new variable for consideration in further work, which is much needed before any conclusions can be made.

Where evidence exists, our study is comparable to other studies in terms of incidence of anaemia (De Santo et al. 2009; Kulier et al. 2007) and medical history (De Santo et al. 2009; Kulier et al. 2007). Our results were also consistent with others identifying pre-operative anaemia as a risk factor for post-operative renal complications (Cladellas et al.; Miceli et al. 2014; Fowler et al.)

but not for cardiovascular complications (Cladellas et al.; Miceli et al. 2014; Fowler et al.; Carrascal et al. 2010). However, our findings did not suggest pre-operative anaemia to be associated with stroke (Miceli et al. 2014; Fowler et al.), infection (Cladellas et al.; Fowler et al.) or respiratory failure (Carrascal et al. 2010) as has been found previously. This is likely to be due to difference in definitions used between the studies, and thus the use of a standardised framework, like C-POMS, is advocated for future morbidity outcome after cardiac surgery studies.

There are four main limitations with our study. Firstly, pre-operative baseline characteristics obtained from the Society of Cardiothoracic Surgery of Great Britain and Ireland local database were 93.9% complete. It is possible the small amount of missing data may have had an influence on comparisons on the baseline characteristics. Secondly, although C-POMS is a validated tool for the description and quantification of morbidity after cardiac surgery (Sanders et al.), there are limitations to its use (Sanders et al.). This includes transient morbidities which may be missed on non-data collection days and that fluctuations cannot be tracked. Thirdly, as it is recommended that treatment of pre-operative anaemia should rely on the diagnosis of the type of anaemia, identifying the underlying cause or disease (Weiss and Goodnough 2005), we had intended to explore outcome by type of anaemia. However, since only 1.4% (2/139) of anaemic patients in our study had pre-operative

Table 6 Median C-POMS score and hospital length of stay by quintile of Hb

Quintile	D3	D5	D8	D15	All time points	Hospital LOS
	Median [IQR]	Median [IQR]	Median [IQR]	Median [IQR]	B^{a} (se)	Median [IQR]
1 (≤121)	5 [2–6] 90	3 [1–5] 87	4 [2–6] 54	4 [2–7.5] 20	0	10 [6–17.5] 88
2 (122–131)	4 [2–5] 93	2 [1–4] 90	3 [2–4] 43	3 [2–3] 7	−0.82 (0.29)	7.5 [6–11] 90
3 (132–138)	2 [1–5] 82	2 [1–3] 80	3 [1–4] 31	2 [2–6] 7	−1.34 (0.30)	6.5 [5–10] 82
4 (139–146)	3 [1–5] 89	2 [1–3] 82	3 [2–5] 29	3 [1–4] 6	−1.25 (0.29)	6 [5–9] 88
5 (>146)	2 [1–4] 85	2 [1–3] 78	3 [1–4] 19	2.5 [1.5–3] 4	−1.71 (0.29)	6 [5–8] 86
p value	<0.0001	0.007	0.28	0.67	<0.0001	<0.0001
p value (trend)	<0.0001	0.001	0.16	0.15	<0.0001	<0.0001

IQR inter-quartile range

[a]Difference in C-POMS score for each quintile compared to quintile 1 after adjustment for day of follow-up

Table 7 Multivariate models for length of stay

		Model including anaemia		Model including Hb	
		OR (95%CI)	p value	OR (95%CI)	p value
Age	10-year increase	0.77 (0.64–0.94)	0.009	0.76 (0.63–0.92)	0.006
Gender	Female/male	1.24 (0.80–1.91)	0.34	1.01 (0.65–1.57)	0.95
EuroSCORE	Per quintile	1.85 (1.57–2.19)	<0.0001	1.83 (1.55–2.16)	<0.0001
Hb	Yes/no	–	–	0.71 (0.59–0.86)	0.001
Anaemia	1 SD increase	1.65 (1.12–2.44)	0.01	–	–
Transfusion	Yes/no	2.40 (1.55–3.72)	<0.0001	2.25 (1.45–3.49)	0.0003

haematinic profiles available, this was not feasible. Finally, we cannot prove that the associations we report are causal. Investigating this issue will require interventional studies to mitigate against pre-operative anaemia and post-operative transfusion, and we would advocate for such trials to take place.

Conclusions

In conclusion, while previous evidence is inconclusive on the effect of pre-operative anaemia-specific morbidity outcome (for example stroke and renal dysfunction) after cardiac surgery, our study suggests that pre-operative anaemia and RBC transfusion use are independently associated with significant overall total morbidity burden following cardiac surgery. Thus, strategies to reduce pre-operative anaemia and RBC transfusion need are important. However, understanding that TMB (at the level of detail that the C-POMS tool permits) associated with pre-operative anaemia and RBC transfusion may assist in post-operative patient management to reduce morbidity, especially if it is not possible to ascertain whether it is anaemia or RBC transfusion that carries the greatest risk to patient well-being and recovery. We would recommend the use of the C-POMS tool as a standard morbidity outcome measurement tool in further studies to explore this and whether interventions implemented to reduce post-operative morbidity burden actually do reduce TMB as measured using the C-POMS tool.

Abbreviations

ATP: Adenosine triphosphate; AVR: Aortic valve replacement; BMI: Body mass index; CABG: Coronary artery bypass graft; CHF: Congestive heart failure; C-POMS: Cardiac Post-Operative Morbidity Score; CRP: C-reactive protein; D3 (D5, D8, D15): Day 3 (day 5, day 8, day 15); GI: Gastrointestinal; Hb: Haemoglobin; ICU: Intensive care unit; INR: International normalised ratio; IQR: Inter-quartile range; IV: Intravenous; LD: Leucocyte depletion; LOS: Length of stay; LVEF: Left ventricular ejection fraction; MI: Myocardial infarction; MVR: Mitral valve replacement; NYHA: New York Heart Association; OPA: Out-patient appointment; OR: Odds ratio; OT: Occupational therapy; RBC: Red blood cell; TMB: Total morbidity burden; UK: United Kingdom

Acknowledgements

The authors would like to thank all members of the protocol development group (PDG) and to the patients who generously gave their time and consent to participate in the C-POMS study.

Funding

This work was unfunded, but Professors Hugh Montgomery and Michael Mythen were supported by the National Institute for Health Research University College London Hospitals Biomedical Research Centre.

Authors' contributions

Each author has fulfilled the ICMJE guidelines to qualify as an author. According to the ICMJE guidelines, to qualify as an author, one should have (1) made substantial contributions to the conception and design (JS, DF, HM), acquisition of data (JS, SB, US), or analysis (JC) and interpretation of data (JS, DF, HM, MM); (2) been involved in drafting the manuscript or revising it critically for important intellectual content (ALL), and (3) given final approval of the version to be published (ALL). Each author has participated sufficiently in the work to take public responsibility for appropriate portions of the content and has agreed to be accountable for all aspects of the work in ensuring that questions related to the accuracy or integrity of any part of the work are appropriately investigated and resolved. All authors read and approved the final manuscript.

Authors' information

Not included.

Competing interests

The authors declare that they have no competing interests.

Author details

[1]St Bartholomew's Hospital, Barts Health NHS Trust, London, UK. [2]Centre for Cardiovascular Genetics, University College London, London, UK. [3]Department of Cardiac Anaesthesia and Critical Care, University College London Hospitals NHS Foundation Trust, London, UK. [4]UCL Medical School, University College London, London, UK. [5]University College London Hospitals NHS Trust, London, UK. [6]Institute for Sport, Exercise and Health, University College London, 1st Floor 170 Tottenham Court Rd, London W1T 7HA, UK.

References

Boening A, Boedeker R-H, Scheibelhut C, Rietzschel J, Roth P, Schönburg M. Anemia before coronary artery bypass surgery as additional risk factor increases the perioperative risk. Ann Thorac Surg. 2011;92:805–10.

Carrascal Y, Maroto L, Rey J, Arevalo A, Arroyo J, Echevarria JR, Arce N, Fulquet E. Impact of preoperative anemia on cardiac surgery in octogenarians. Interact Cardiovasc Thorac Surg. 2010;10:249–255.

Cladellas M, Bruguera J, Comin J, Vila J, de JE, Marti J, Gomez M. Is pre-operative anaemia a risk marker for in-hospital mortality and morbidity after valve replacement? Eur Heart J. 2006;(27):1093–1099.

Cuzick J. A Wilcoxon-type test for trend. Stat Med. 1985;4:87–90.

Davies KJ, Maguire JJ, Brooks GA, Dallman PR, Packer L. Muscle mitochondrial bioenergetics, oxygen supply, and work capacity during dietary iron deficiency and repletion. Am J Physiol. 1982;242:E418–E427.

Department of Health: Better Blood Transfusion. Safe and Appropriate Use of Blood. Volume HSC 2007/0. London: Department of Health; 2007.

De Santo L, Romano G, Della Corte A, de Simone V, Grimaldi F, Cotrufo M, de Feo M. Preoperative anemia in patients undergoing coronary artery bypass grafting predicts acute kidney injury. J Thorac Cardiovasc Surg. 2009;138:965–70.

Du Pont-Thibodeau G, Harrington K, Lacroix J. Anemia and red blood cell transfusion in critically ill cardiac patients. Ann Intensive Care. 2014;4:16.

Dunn LL, Suryo RY, Richardson DR. Iron uptake and metabolism in the new millennium. Trends Cell Biol. 2007;17:93–100.

ERP Programme. Delivering enhanced recovery. Helping patients to get better sooner after surgery. Department of Health; 2010. Archived and accessible via http://www.dh.gov.uk/prod_consum_dh/groups/dh_digitalassets/@dh/@en/@ps/documents/digitalasset/dh_115156.pdf.

Fowler AJ, Ahmad T, Phull MK, Allard S, Gillies MA, Pearse RM. Meta-analysis of the association between preoperative anaemia and mortality after surgery. Br J Surg. 2015;102:1314–1324.

Galas FR, Almeida JP, Fukushima JT, Osawa EA, Nakamura RE, Silva CM, de Almeida EP, Auler Jr. JO, Vincent JL, Hajjar LA. Blood transfusion in cardiac surgery is a risk factor for increased hospital length of stay in adult patients. J Cardiothorac Surg. 2013;8:54.

Gross I, Seifert B, Hofmann A, Spahn DR. Patient blood management in cardiac surgery results in fewer transfusions and better outcome. Transfusion. 2015;55:1075–81.

Group SS. Annual Serious Hazards of Transfusion (SHOT) Report 2014. 2014.

Hogan M, Klein AA, Richards T. The impact of anaemia and intravenous iron replacement therapy on outcomes in cardiac surgery. Eur J Cardiothorac Surg. 2015;47:218–226.

Hung M, Besser M, Sharples LD, Nair SK, Klein AA. The prevalence and association with transfusion, intensive care unit stay and mortality of pre-operative anaemia in a cohort of cardiac surgery patients. Anaesthesia. 2011;66:812–818.

Hung M, Ortmann E, Besser M, Martin-Cabrera P, Richards T, Ghosh M, Bottrill F, Collier T, Klein AA. A prospective observational cohort study to identify the causes of anaemia and association with outcome in cardiac surgical patients. Heart. 2015;101:107–112.

Kulier A, Levin J, Moser R, Rumpold-Seitlinger G, Tudor IC, Snyder-Ramos SA, Moehnle P, Mangano DT. Impact of preoperative anemia on outcome in patients undergoing coronary artery bypass graft surgery. Circulation. 2007;116:471–9.

Kurtz P, Schmidt JM, Claassen J, Carrera E, Fernandez L, Helbok R, Presciutti M, Stuart RM, Connolly ES, Badjatia N, Mayer SA, Lee K. Anemia is associated with metabolic distress and brain tissue hypoxia after subarachnoid hemorrhage. Neurocrit Care. 2010;13:10–16.

Miceli A, Romeo F, Glauber M, de Siena PM, Caputo M, Angelini GD. Preoperative anemia increases mortality and postoperative morbidity after cardiac surgery. J Cardiothorac Surg. 2014;9:137.

Munoz M, Garcia-Erce JA, Diez-Lobo AI, Campos A, Sebastianes C, Bisbe E. Usefulness of the administration of intravenous iron sucrose for the correction of preoperative anemia in major surgery patients. Med Clin (Barc). 2009;132:303–306.

Murphy M, Murphy G, Gill R, Herbertson M, Allard S, Grant-Casey J. National comparative audit of blood transfusion: 2011 audit of blood transfusion in adult cardiac surgery. Available at http://hospital.blood.co.uk/audits/national-comparative-audit/national-comparative-audit-reports/.

Murphy GJ, Pike K, Rogers CA, Wordsworth S, Stokes EA, Angelini GD, Reeves BC, TITRe2 Investigators. Liberal or restrictive transfusion after cardiac surgery. N Engl J Med. 2015;372:997–1008.

Sanders J, Keogh BE, Van der Meulen J, Browne JP, Treasure T, Mythen MG, Montgomery HE. The development of a postoperative morbidity score to assess total morbidity burden after cardiac surgery. J Clin Epidemiol. 2012;65: 423–433.

Service UKBT and T. Guidelines for the blood transfusion services in the UK. 7th ed. 2007.

Ternström L, Hyllner M, Backlund E, Schersten H, Jeppsson A. A structured blood conservation programme reduces transfusions and costs in cardiac surgery. Interact Cardiovasc Thorac Surg. 2014;19:788–94.

Usmanov RI, Zueva EB, Silverberg DS, Shaked M. Intravenous iron without erythropoietin for the treatment of iron deficiency anemia in patients with moderate to severe congestive heart failure and chronic kidney insufficiency. J Nephrol. 2008;21:236–242.

Vallet B, Futier E. Perioperative oxygen therapy and oxygen utilization. Curr Opin Crit Care. 2010;16:359–364.

van Straten AH, Hamad MA, van Zundert AJ, Martens EJ, Schonberger JP, de Wolf AM. Preoperative hemoglobin level as a predictor of survival after coronary artery bypass grafting: a comparison with the matched general population. Circulation. 2009;120:118–125.

Vincent J-L. Which carries the biggest risk: anaemia or blood transfusion? Transfus Clin Biol J la Société Fr Transfus Sang. 2015;22:148–50.

Weiss G, Goodnough LT. Anemia of chronic disease. N Engl J Med. 2005;352: 1011–1023.

World Health Organization. Worldwide Prevalence of Anaemia 1993–2005. WHO Global Database on Anaemia. 2008.

Zindrou D, Taylor KM, Bagger JP. Preoperative haemoglobin concentration and mortality rate after coronary artery bypass surgery. Lancet. 2002;359:1747–1748.

Predictors of total morbidity burden on days 3, 5 and 8 after cardiac surgery

Julie Sanders[1,2], Jackie Cooper[3], Michael G. Mythen[2,4] and Hugh E. Montgomery[2*]

Abstract

Background: Post-operative morbidity affects up to 36% of cardiac surgical patients. However, few countries reliably record morbidity outcome data, despite patients wanting to be informed of all the risks associated with surgery. The Cardiac Post-Operative Morbidity Score (C-POMS) is a new tool for describing and scoring (0–13) total morbidity burden after cardiac surgery, derived by noting the presence/absence of 13 morbidity domains on days 3, 5, 8 and 15. Identifying modifiable C-POMS risk factors may suggest targets for intervention to reduce morbidity and healthcare costs. Thus, we explored the association of C-POMS with previously identified predictors of post-operative morbidity.

Methods: A systematic literature review of pre-operative risk assessment models for post-operative morbidity was conducted to identify variables associated with post-operative morbidity. The association of those variables with C-POMS was explored in patients drawn from the original C-POMS study ($n = 444$).

Results: Seventy risk factors were identified, of which 56 were available in the study and 49 were suitable for analysis. Numbers were too few to analyse associations on D15. Thirty-three (67.3%) and 20 (40.8%) variables were associated with C-POMS on at least 1 or 2 days, respectively. Pre-operative albumin concentration, left ventricular ejection fraction and New York Heart Association functional class were associated with C-POMS on all days. Of the 16 independent risk factors, pre-operative albumin and haemoglobin concentrations and weight are potentially modifiable.

Conclusions: Different risk factors are associated with total morbidity burden on different post-operative days. Pre-operative albumin and haemoglobin concentrations and weight were independently predictive of post-operative total morbidity burden suggesting therapeutic interventions aimed at these might reduce both post-operative morbidity risk and health-care costs in patients undergoing cardiac surgery.

Keywords: Risk factor, Cardiac surgery, Morbidity outcome, C-POMS

Background

In surgery, post-operative mortality is the most commonly cited outcome variable and to date has been considered the standard measure of quality of care. However, while cardiac operative mortality has fallen (currently 2.1% in the USA (Society of Thoracic Surgeons) and 1.5% in the UK (Bridgewater et al. 2008)), post-operative morbidity remains common affecting between 4.3% (Fortescue et al. 2001) and 36% (Magovern et al. 1996) of cardiac patients and significantly prolonging length of stay (LOS) (Dupuis et al. 2001). Such morbidity has substantial impact on healthcare resources, with the average in-hospital incremental cost of experiencing any complication at $15,468 per patient (Brown et al. 2008). Thus, strategies to identify and reduce post-operative morbidity might reduce both patient well-being and healthcare costs.

However, few countries reliably record morbidity outcome data (Weiser et al. 2008). Previously, morbidity definitions included death (Fortescue et al. 2001), focused on major morbid events only (Huijskes et al. 2003), or used surrogate markers of morbidity (for example post-operative LOS (Magovern et al. 1996; Dupuis et al. 2001)). Likewise, many national cardiac surgical registers collect only 30-day mortality outcome and in some cases hospital LOS. Contrastingly, although the Society of Thoracic Surgeons national database contains 49 variables related to post-operative events, a composite metric aimed at defining post-operative

* Correspondence: h.montgomery@ucl.ac.uk
[2]Institute for Sport, Exercise and Health, University College London, 1st Floor 170 Tottenham Court Rd, London W1T 7HA, UK
Full list of author information is available at the end of the article

morbidity includes in-hospital death and only five severe specific morbidities (Shahian et al. 2010).

The Cardiac Post-Operative Morbidity Score (C-POMS) (Sanders et al. 2012) is a simple, validated score (0–13) by which to identify and quantify total morbidity burden (TMB) after adult cardiac surgery (Table 1) on multiple post-operative days. We have previously reported that every unit increase in C-POMS is associated with a 1.7, 2.2 and 4.5-day increase in subsequent LOS on days 3 (D3), 5 (D5) and 8 (D8) (Sanders et al. 2012), which has significant associated health-care costs, organisational and resource implications. Efforts to identify the risk factors associated with this post-operative TMB score may not only assist in identifying modifiable risk factors for which therapeutic interventions can be implemented to reduce the post-operative risk, but also serve to potentially further validate C-POMS as a useful clinical tool in cardiac surgery post-operative morbidity assessment.

Thus, we sought to identify risk factors associated with post-operative TMB, as assessed by the C-POMS tool, with an aim of identifying potentially modifiable risk factors that could be therapeutic targets to reduce post-operative cardiac surgical morbidity.

Methods

The National Research Ethics Committee London-Bentham (Chair Professor David Katz) gave ethics permission for this study (protocol amendment 7) on 6 September 2011 (reference 04/Q0502/73). All patients included in this study gave written informed consent to participate.

Participants

Patients were drawn from the development and validation of the C-POMS study, detailed elsewhere (Sanders et al. 2012). In brief, patients undergoing any form of adult cardiac surgery (excluding cardiac surgery for a congenital heart condition or a cardiomyopathy) between January 2005 and November 2007 at the Heart Hospital, University College London Hospitals NHS Trust, UK, and who gave written informed consent were eligible for inclusion. Excluded were those <18 years old, undergoing emergency surgery, who were enrolled in clinical intervention trials or who died within 5 days of surgery.

C-POMS

The development and validation of the C-POMS tool and score is detailed elsewhere (Sanders et al. 2012). In brief, The McMaster Framework (Kirshner and Guyatt, 1985; Guyatt et al. 1992) for constructing and assessing health indices for discriminative instruments, comprising item selection, item scaling, item reduction and determination of reliability and validity processes, was used.

The C-POMS represents TMB as a summary score (0–13), derived by noting the presence or absence of 13 morbidity domains on days 3 (D3), 5 (D5), 8 (D8) and 15 (D15) after cardiac surgery (Table 1).

Pre- and intra-operative clinical data

A protocol development group, comprising 15 representatives from cardiac nursing, surgery, intensive care and anaesthesia, determined the pre-, intra-, and post-operative variables to be collected prior to commencement of the study. In brief, these included demographic details, past and current medical history, coronary heart disease risk factors, routine biochemistry and haematology measurements, anaesthesia details, operative details and a detailed record of the first 24 h in the intensive care unit. Variables were either obtained from the Society of Cardiothoracic Surgery national database or prospectively from the medical and nursing records by a dedicated, experienced research nurse using a standardised proforma.

Identification and categorisation of potential risk factors

To identify pre-operative risk prediction models of post-operative morbidity following cardiac surgery, a systematic literature review was conducted using the basic framework for conducting systematic reviews from the Centre for Reviews and Dissemination (Dissemination Centre for Reviews and Dissemination 2001). Three methodological quality filters were utilised. Firstly, the study population was defined as an adult population undergoing any form of cardiac surgery (excluding transplantation and grown-up congenital heart surgery); only methodologies that constructed a pre-operative risk assessment tool were included; valid outcomes were mortality and morbidity. There were no exclusions on the basis of the definition of either outcome. Search terms included cardiac surgery score, cardiac surgery risk score, pre-operative risk; cardiac surgery and risk prediction score; cardiac surgery, coronary artery bypass graft (CABG), surgery morbidity and surgery outcome. In addition to publication databases (the National Centre for Biotechnology Information, Entrez retrieval system and the Web of Science ISI Citation Databases), sources of on-going and recently completed studies (The National Research Register, The Cochrane Library of Systematic Reviews) were also interrogated to identify eligible papers. In total, the abstracts of 1067 papers were scrutinised. Backward and forward citation searches were conducted on all identified eligible papers. Overall, a total of 21 pre-operative risk prediction models were identified.

All pre- and intra-operative variables obtained within the C-POMS study were classified with respect to these models into one of two tiers (results in Additional file 1):

Table 1 The Cardiac Post-Operative Morbidity Score (C-POMS) (as reported in Sanders et al. 2012)

Morbidity type	C-POMS criteria
Pulmonary	Presence of one or more of the following: • New requirement for oxygen or respiratory support (including nebuliser therapy or request for chest physiotherapy on or after D5) • Pleural effusion requiring drainage
Infectious	Presence of one or more of the following: • Currently on antibiotics • Has had a temperature of >38 °C in the last 24 h • Has a white cell count/CRP level requiring in-hospital review or treatment
Renal	Presence of one or more of the following: • Presence of decreased urine output requiring intervention (including IV furosemide) • Increased serum creatinine (>30% from pre-operative level) • Urinary catheter in situ • New urinary incontinence • Serum potassium abnormalities requiring treatment
Gastrointestinal	Presence of one or more of the following: • Unable to tolerate an enteral diet for any reason including nausea, vomiting and abdominal distension • Nasogastric tube • Diagnosis of a gastrointestinal bleed • Diarrhoea
Cardiovascular	Presence of one or more of the following: • The use of inotropic therapy for any cardiovascular cause • Pacing wires (on or after D5) and/or requiring temporary or new permanent pacing • Diagnostic tests or therapy within the last 24 h for any of the following: (1) new MI or ischaemia, (2) hypotension (requiring fluid therapy, pharmacological therapy or omission of pharmacological therapy), (3) atrial or ventricular arrhythmias, (4) cardiogenic pulmonary oedema, thrombotic event (requiring anticoagulation), (5) hypertension (pharmacological therapy or omission of pharmacological therapy)
Neurological	New neurological deficit (including confusion, delirium, coma, lack of coordination, drowsy/slow to wake, poor swallow, blurred vision, sedated, changing loss of consciousness)
Haematological	Presence of one or more of the following: • Untherapeutic INR requiring pharmacological therapy or omission of pharmacological therapy • Requirement for any of the following within the last 24 h: packed erythrocytes, platelets, fresh-frozen plasma, or cryoprecipitate
Wound	Presence of one or more of the following: • Wound dehiscence requiring surgical exploration or drainage of pus from the operation wound with or without isolation of organisms • Chest drains • Wound pain significant enough to require continuing or escalating analgesic intervention
Pain	Postoperative pain significant enough to require parenteral opioids and/or continuing or additional analgesia
Endocrine	New or additional requirements for blood sugar management

Table 1 The Cardiac Post-Operative Morbidity Score (C-POMS) (as reported in Sanders et al. 2012) *(Continued)*

Electrolyte	Electrolyte (including sodium, urea, phosphate) imbalance requiring oral or intravenous intervention (not including potassium as included in renal category)
Review	Remaining in hospital for further review, investigation and/or procedure
Assisted ambulation	A new or escalated post-operative requirement for mobility assistance (including wheelchair, crutches, zimmer frame, walking sticks or assistance)

CRP C-reactive protein, *IV* intravenous, *MI* myocardial infarction, *INR* international normalised ratio, *OPA* out-patient appointment, *OT* occupational therapy

Tier 1 variables were those which had been associated with morbidity risk in three or more separate papers (significant evidence), while tier 2 variables were those identified in one or two papers (some evidence).

Statistical methods

Baseline characteristics are presented as mean ± SD or n (%). For the univariate analysis, C-POMS is presented as the median score and compared over categories using the Kruskal-Wallis test. The association of continuous variables with C-POMS was assessed using the Spearman rank correlation. For the multivariate analysis, variables with $p < 0.25$ on univariate analysis were considered for inclusion into the models and stepwise regression with backwards elimination and a threshold of $p < 0.05$ was run. Validation of the models was performed by running 1000 bootstrap samples. Variables selected in at least 60% of the bootstrap samples were included in the final model. For the data on all time points combined, the models used were random intercept models with time fitted as a fixed effect.

Results

Baseline participant characteristics

Of 748 potentially eligible patients undergoing cardiac surgery, 520 (69.5%) were screened (due to researcher availability) and 464 (89.2%) consented to participate. Fourteen participants subsequently became ineligible, leaving 450 who completed the study. Six participants declined for their data to be used outside the development of C-POMS.

Table 2 summarises participant characteristics. The majority were White British (379, 85.4%), male (351, 79.1%) with a mean age of 66.6 years (range 19–91 years). Most had triple vessel disease (243, 54.7%), a good (>50%) left ventricular ejection fraction (LVEF) (323, 74.1%) and were of moderate mortality risk (mean EuroSCORE 4.1). The majority had elective surgery (69.6%), using cardiopulmonary bypass (412, 93.4%) and stayed on intensive care unit (ICU) for an average of 2.0 days while remaining in the operating hospital for

Table 2 Baseline characteristics (n = 444). All values n (%) unless otherwise stated

	Frequency/mean ± SD
Demographics	
Age (mean/years)	66.6 ± 10.7
Female gender	93 (20.9)
Ethnicity (White British)	379 (85.4)
Medical history	
Renal (dialysis)	7 (1.6)
History of previous MI	148 (33.3)
Re-operation	18 (4.1)
Symptoms	
NYHA Class	
I	115 (26.0)
II	205 (46.3)
III	101 (22.8)
IV	22 (5.0)
Cardiac risk factors	
Smoking	
Current	49 (11.0)
Ex	245 (55.2)
Never	150 (33.8)
Hypertension	303 (68.2)
Hypercholesteraemia	343 (77.4)
Diabetes	103 (23.2)
Body mass index (kg/m²)/mean	28.5 ± 5.6
Examination and investigation	
LVEF	
Good	323 (74.1)
Fair	90 (20.6)
Poor	23 (5.3)
Pre-operative risk assessment	
EuroSCORE	4.1 ± 2.8
Intra-operative details	
Operative priority—elective	309 (69.6)
Operation performed	
CABG	299 (67.3)
AVR	61 (13.7)
MVR	10 (2.3)
CABG + AVR	36 (8.1)
CABG + MVR	0 (0.0)
AVR + MVR	3 (0.7)
CABG + AVR + MVR	2 (0.5)
Other	33 (7.4)
Cardiopulmonary bypass used	412 (93.4)

Table 2 Baseline characteristics (n = 444). All values n (%) unless otherwise stated (Continued)

Outcome	
Length of ICU stay (mean/days)	2.0 ± 3.5
Return to theatre	21 (4.8)
Total length of hospital stay (mean/days)	11.8 ± 11.7

9.5 days. The observed in-hospital mortality rate was 1.3%. Overall, 444 (100.0%) were in-patients on D1 and D3, 420 (94.6%) on D5, 178 (40.1%) on D8 and 45 (10.1%) on D15. Subsequent risk factor analysis was only appropriate on D3, D5 and D8 due to low numbers on D15.

Tier 1 and 2 analysis

Univariate analysis Fifty-six variables were identified in tiers 1 and 2. The incidence of seven (12.5%) pre-operative variables (cardiogenic shock, catheter-induced coronary closure, intra-aortic balloon pump, intubation, permanent pacemaker, immunosuppressant medications and inotropes) was too small for analysis, resulting in 49 variables (23 tier 1; 26 tier 2) for analysis. Thirty-three of the 49 (67.3%) variables previously identified to be associated with post-operative morbidity were found to be associated with C-POMS on at least one post-operative day (Table 3). Of those, 10 variables were associated with C-POMS summary score on 1 day only, on either D3 (smoking, body mass index, urgency of operation, use of cardiopulmonary bypass, total drainage within the first 12 h and D1 inotropes) or D5 (ethnicity, neurological history, pre-operative heart rate and dialysis). No variables were solely predictive of D8 C-POMS summary score. Twenty variables (40.8%) were associated with C-POMS summary score on 2 days, while 3 variables (pre-operative albumin and New York Heart Association (NYHA) class and LVEF) were associated with C-POMS summary score on all days.

Overall, 8/23 (34.7%) tier 1 variables and 8/26 (34.7%) tier 2 variables were not associated with C-POMS summary score on any post-operative day (results in Additional file 2).

Multivariate analysis Of the 49 variables, 16 (32.7%) were independent risk factors of C-POMS summary score on one or more post-operative days, while no variables were associated with C-POMS outcome on all three post-operative days (Table 4).

There were eight tier 1 variables, all of which (with the exception of renal dysfunction) were associated with TMB on D3. Diabetes, LVEF, CABG surgery and renal dysfunction were also associated with D5 C-POMS summary score. However, only tier 2 variables (pre-operative

Table 3 Univariate analysis: tier 1 and 2 predictors of C-POMS summary score on D3, D5 and D8

Variable	D3 ($n = 441$)		D5 ($n = 419$)		D8 ($n = 177$)	
	Median C-POMS/Rho	p	Median C-POMS/Rho	p	Median C-POMS/Rho	p
Tier 1 variables						
Demographics						
Age	0.188	0.000	0.110	0.025	0.133	0.078
Age quartiles						
1 (0–59)	2.0	0.002	2.0	0.010	2.0	0.300
2 (60–68)	3.0		2.0		3.0	
3 (69–74)	3.0		2.0		4.0	
4 (≥75)	4.0		2.5		3.0	
Age grp 2						
<65	2.0	0.000	2.0	0.044	2.5	0.083
65–74	3.0		2.0		3.0	
≥75	4.0		2.5		3.0	
Age grp 3						
<70	3.0	0.001	2.0	0.426	3.0	0.225
70–79	3.0		2.0		3.0	
>80	5.0		2.0		3.0	
Gender						
M	3.0	0.024	2.0	0.016	3.0	0.215
F	3.0		3.0		2.5	
Medical history						
Diabetes						
Y	4.0	0.000	2.5	0.015	3.0	0.308
N	3.0		2.0		3.0	
Cerebrovascular disease						
Y	4.0	0.028	3.0	0.023	4.0	0.219
N	3.0		2.0		3.0	
Neurological history						
Y	4.0	0.103	3.0	0.016	4.0	0.553
N	3.0		2.0		3.0	
Congestive heart failure						
Y	4.0	0.009	4.0	0.025	4.0	0.310
N	3.0		2.0		3.0	
COPD/lung disease						
Y	4.0	0.005	3.0	0.012	3.0	0.380
N	3.0		2.0		3.0	
Renal disease						
Y	5.0	0.064	5.0	0.001	5.0	0.025
N	3.0		2.0		3.0	

Table 3 Univariate analysis: tier 1 and 2 predictors of C-POMS summary score on D3, D5 and D8 *(Continued)*

POSSUM ECG						
Normal	3.0	0.000	2.0	0.000	3.0	0.200
Sinus abnormal	5.0		4.0		–	
AF	4.0		3.0		3.0	
Any other abnormal	5.0		2.5		2.0	
Paced						
Y	5.0	0.005	4.0	0.014	2.5	0.875
N	3.0		2.0		3.0	
Dialysis						
Y	5.5	0.073	7.5	0.006	5.5	0.064
N	3.0		2.0		3.0	
Pre-operative measurements						
Body mass index(kg/m^2)	0.100	0.043	0.077	0.130	0.099	0.206
LVEF						
Good	3.0	0.013	2.0	0.011	3.0	0.013
Fair	3.0		2.0		4.0	
Poor	5.0		5.0		4.0	
Intra-operative						
Type of surgery						
CABG	3.0	0.000	2.0	0.000	3.0	0.718
AVR	4.0		3.0		3.0	
MVR	5.0		3.0		3.5	
CABG + AVR	4.0		2.0		3.0	
AVR + MVR	3.0		3.0		4.5	
CABG + MVR + AVR	5.0		5.0		6.0	
Other	5.0		3.0		3.0	
Urgency of op						
Elective	3.0	0.002	2.0	0.061	3.0	0.327
Urgent	4.0		2.0		3.0	
Within first 12 h						
Systolic blood pressure (highest)	0.002	0.959	0.026	0.599	−0.089	0.238
Tier 2 variables						
Demographics						
Ethnicity						
Caucasian	3.0	0.052	2.0	0.008	3.0	0.532
Asian	2.0		1.0		3.0	
Black	5.0		3.0		3.0	
Other	2.0		3.0		1.0	
Medical history						
Smoking						
Current	2.0	0.048	2.0	0.395	3.0	0.753
Ex	3.0		2.0		3.0	
Never	3.0		2.0		3.0	

Table 3 Univariate analysis: tier 1 and 2 predictors of C-POMS summary score on D3, D5 and D8 *(Continued)*

	D3		D5		D8	
Family Hx CAD						
Y	3.0	0.002	2.0	0.019	3.0	0.686
N	4.0		2.0		3.0	
Atrial arrhythmia						
Y	4.0	0.021	3.0	0.007	3.0	0.781
N	3.0		2.0		3.0	
Pre-operative measurements						
Albumin	−0.210	0.000	−0.144	0.004	−0.183	0.019
Haemoglobin	−0.279	0.000	−0.180	0.000	−0.143	0.058
Heart rate	0.090	0.058	0.179	0.000	0.080	0.294
Weight	0.044	0.369	0.042	0.399	0.101	0.186
No diseased vessels						
0	4.0	0.011	3.0	0.000	3.0	0.203
1	3.0		2.0		2.0	
2	3.0		2.0		2.0	
3	3.0		2.0		3.0	
NYHA class						
1	2.0	0.001	1.0	0.002	3.0	0.001
2	3.0		2.0		3.0	
3	4.0		3.0		3.0	
4	5.0		2.5		5.0	
CCSC class						
0	3.0	0.041	3.0	0.042	3.0	0.317
1	2.0		2.0		2.0	
2	3.0		2.0		3.0	
3	3.0		2.0		3.0	
4	4.0		2.0		4.0	
Cardiomegaly						
Y	5.0	0.000	3.0	0.000	4.0	0.141
N	3.0		3.0		3.0	
Not stated	3.0		3.0		3.0	
Extracardiacarteriopathy						
Y	5.0	0.003	3.0	0.004	4.5	0.147
N	3.0		2.0		3.0	
Current medications						
Diuretic						
Y	4.0	0.003	3.0	0.003	3.0	0.780
N	3.0		2.0		3.0	
Intra-operative						
Cardiopulmonary bypass						
Y	3.0	0.001	2.0	0.072	3.0	0.098
N	2.0		1.0		1.0	

Table 3 Univariate analysis: tier 1 and 2 predictors of C-POMS summary score on D3, D5 and D8 *(Continued)*

Within 1st 12 h after surgery						
Total drainage	0.139	0.004	0.030	0.542	0.031	0.679
Post-operative (D1)						
Heart rhythm						
Sinus rhythm	3.0	0.000	2.0	0.002	3.0	0.473
Sinus tachycardia	2.5		2.0		2.5	
Sinus bradycardia	4.0		2.0		4.0	
Atrial fibrillation	5.0		3.0		4.0	
Other	3.0		2.0		3.0	
Inotropes						
Y	4.0	0.004	3.0	0.070	3.0	0.923
N	3.0		2.0		3.0	

albumin, number of diseased vessels and number of saphenous vein grafts) were independently predictive of D8 score and these variables were not independent risk factors for any other post-operative day. Pre-operative haemoglobin, 12 h drainage, pre-operative weight and extra cardiacarteriopathy were tier 2 risk factors associated with D3 and D5 morbidity score, while pre-operative cardiomegaly and NYHA class were associated with D5 score only. Considering all time points, 12-h total drainage, pre-operative weight, extra-cardiac arteriopathy, age, diabetes, CABG surgery, pre-operative cardiomegaly and pre-operative albumin level were independently predictive of C-POMS-defined post-operative morbidity outcome.

Discussion

We found that over two thirds (67.3%) of variables, previously reported as a risk factor for post-operative morbidity, were associated with the new C-POMS (denoting TMB) on at least one post-operative day, with 40% being significant risk factors for two post-operative days and three (6.1%) associated on all three post-operative days. From these results, there are four main findings of note. Firstly, we aimed to identify independent modifiable C-POMS risk factors amenable to therapeutic intervention. These were found to be pre-operative albumin and haemoglobin levels and weight—all tier 2 variables. Previously, pre-operative hypoalbuminaemia has been identified as a risk factor for post-operative delirium (Rudolph et al. 2009), reoperation for bleeding (Engelman et al. 1999), requirement for renal replacement therapy need (Engelman et al. 1999; Sato et al. 2015), increased ICU and hospital LOS (Engelman et al. 1999; Koertzen et al. 2013) and increased mortality (Engelman et al. 1999; Koertzen et al. 2013) cardiac surgery. While hypoalbuminaemia may be directly harmful, it may also mark other pathological states, such as anaemia, since pre-operative hypoalbuminaemia and anaemia are independently

associated (Carrascal et al. 2010). Similarly, in cardiac surgery, pre-operative anaemia is associated with in-hospital (De Santo et al. 2009; Hung et al. 2011) or 30-day (Boening et al. 2011) mortality, post-operative blood transfusion rate (De Santo et al. 2009; Hung et al. 2011; Boening et al. 2011), ICU (De Santo et al. 2009; Hung et al. 2011) and in-hospital LOS (De Santo et al. 2009), major adverse cardiovascular events (Boening et al. 2011), and renal complications (De Santo et al. 2009; Boening et al. 2011) than non-anaemic patients. However, evidence relating to whether pre-operative anaemia is associated with infection (Boening et al. 2011) or not (De Santo et al. 2009) is conflicting. There is less evidence relating pre-operative weight to post-operative outcome. Weight loss after bariatric surgery improves hypertension, diabetes and dyslipidaemia (Batsis et al. 2007), although unintended pre-operative weight loss (≥10%) is also associated with prolonged hospital LOS (van Venrooij et al. 2008). Evidence of association is, of course, not the same as proof of causation. However, overall, taken with associated literature, our findings suggest pre-operative albumin, haemoglobin and weight to be candidates for pre-operative interventional studies with the aim of improving post-operative morbidity.

Secondly, we identified 17 *independent* risk factors for TMB on at least one post-operative day. Interestingly, except for renal dysfunction, the other seven tier 1 variables were all associated with D3 morbidity, with only three (diabetes, LVEF and CABG surgery) also being associated on D5 and none with D8 morbidity. Independent risk factors for D8 TMB lay entirely in tier 2. Such findings perhaps suggest that different risk factors are associated with outcome on different post-operative days and that well-accepted risk factors may only be useful for predicting morbidity risk in the first few days of recovery. Patterns of morbidity are well-recognised to differ with time after surgery, and it is likely that their drivers (whether they be intrinsic, environmental, or related to nascent morbidities) will also vary. Such factors

Table 4 Tier 1 and 2 (combined) independent predictors of C-POMS summary score

Variable	D3			D5			D8			Combined over all time points	
	Effect	B(se)	p	Effect	B(se)	p	Effect	B(se)	p	B(se)	p
Pre-operative haemoglobin	1 SD increase	−0.42 (0.11)	<0.0001		−0.29 (0.12)	0.01					
12-h total drainage	1 SD increase	0.47 (0.10)	<0.001		0.35 (0.10)	0.001				0.31 (0.09)	0.001
Pre-operative weight	1 SD increase	0.34 (0.10)	0.001		0.27 (0.11)	0.02				0.26 (0.09)	0.004
Extra-cardiac arteriopathy	Yes: no	0.73 (0.34)	0.03		0.87 (0.35)	0.01				0.66 (0.31)	0.03
Age	Per year	0.03 (0.009)	0.001							0.024 (0.009)	
Diabetes	Yes: no	0.75 (0.23)	0.002		0.64 (0.27)	0.02				0.92 (0.22)	<0.0001
Left ventricular ejection fraction	Poor: good/fair	0.88 (0.43)	0.04		1.38 (0.45)	0.003					
CABG surgery	Yes: no	−1.17 (0.24)	<0.0001		−1.02 (0.25)	<0.0001				−1.06 (0.21)	<0.0001
MVR surgery	Yes: no	1.40 (0.54)	0.01								
Operative urgency	Urgent: elective	0.48 (0.22)	0.03								
Chronic obstructive pulmonary disease	Yes: no	0.77 (0.30)	0.01								
NYHA class				1 category increase	0.47 (0.24)	0.05					
Renal				Yes: no	2.46 (0.74)	0.001					
Pre-operative cardiomegaly				Yes: no	0.66 (0.32)	0.04				0.66 (0.28)	0.02
Pre-operative albumin							1 SD increase	−0.43 (0.20)	0.04		
Number of diseased vessels							Increase of 1	1.04 (0.36)	0.005	−0.38 (0.09)	<0.0001
Number of saphenous vein grafts							1 SD increase	−0.66 (0.31)	0.04		

are likely to explain the fact that correlations between D3 and D5 with D8 data differed. Furthermore, this study adds to the evidence that pre-operative haemoglobin concentration, pre-operative weight, extra-cardiac arteriopathy, pre-operative cardiomegaly, NYHA class, pre-operative albumin, number of diseased vessels, and number of saphenous vein grafts are independently associated with morbidity outcome.

Thirdly, as expected, the majority of tier 1 variables (those with significant evidence of association with post-operative morbidity) were associated with TMB on at least one post-operative day. While this is not clinically surprising, it does further validate C-POMS as a useful clinical tool in outcome assessment following cardiac surgery. In relation to the eight tier 1 variables that were not associated with TMB on any post-operative day, combining cerebrovascular accident and transient ischaemic attack to a combined cerebrovascular disease variable was associated with a higher C-POMS on D3 and D5, in line with other morbidity risk assessment models (Magovern et al. 1996; Huijskes et al. 2003; Higgins et al. 1992; Tuman et al. 1992). Furthermore, while hypertension has been independently associated with post-operative morbidity in some studies (for example, Fortescue et al. (2001) and Ivanov et al. (2006)), this has been disputed by others (Higgins et al. 1992; Hattler et al. 1994). However, our results pertaining to systolic blood pressure, previous cardiac surgery and diagnosed peripheral vascular disease are at odds with the literature.

Finally, this study also adds to the more limited data relating to some variables (those in tier 2) and their association with post-operative morbidity after cardiac surgery. Of these, 65.4% were associated with C-POMS TMB score on at least one post-operative day, while pre-operative albumin measurement and NYHA class were risk factors for all three post-operative days. Furthermore, this study also confirmed the findings of previous studies suggesting that unstable angina or recent myocardial infarction (Tuman et al. 1992; Hattler et al. 1994) and pre-existing liver disease (Higgins et al. 1992) are not associated with post-operative morbidity. However, while our study corroborated that of Magovern et al. (Magovern et al. 1996) showing that pre-operative atrial arrhythmia and cardiomegaly are associated with morbidity outcome (Magovern et al. 1996), such results conflict with those found by Hattler and colleagues (Hattler et al. 1994).

There are four main limitations of this study. Firstly, there was no consistent definition of post-operative morbidity used in the pre-operative risk assessment models reported by others. Thus, a wide-range of variables to predict such diversely described outcomes were identified. However, over two-thirds of all variables were found to be associated with TMB, as defined by C-POMS, on at least one post-operative day suggesting that C-POMS is a valid measure of morbidity. Secondly,

from the pre-operative risk assessment models, it is difficult to assess what variables were not found to be associated with post-operative morbidity. Most studies did not report variables for which no association with morbidity was identified, due to the often large number (>100) of variables included. We have made our statistically non-significant results available to redress this balance and to aid in the evaluation of this (and other) tools. Thirdly, 14 risk factors identified in the pre-operative risk assessment models were available within this study dataset. Some variables, such as transplantation and ventricular-septal defect, were not available as these surgery types were not included in the study, while the others were non-routinely recorded items. Aside from catastrophic states, the variables not included were all tier 2 variables and in the main were only associated with outcome in one previous study. Finally, analysis to identify risk predictors for C-POMS TMB on D15 could not be conducted due to there being too few participants remaining in the hospital on D15 ($n = 45$). However, this could be the subject of future work.

Conclusions

Post-operative morbidity is increasingly accepted as an independent quality of care indicator, with approximately 80% of patients wanting to be informed of all the risks associated with surgery (Larobina et al. 2007). Thus, in obtaining operative consent, patients should be told about 'less serious side effects and complications' (General Medical Council 2008). C-POMS is a tool that permits such morbidity assessment and TMB scoring at several time points after cardiac surgery, allowing both broad and detailed tracking of morbidities. We have found that pre-operative albumin, haemoglobin and weight are potentially modifiable risk factors for which the investigation of the effect of therapeutic interventions on C-POMS outcome is warranted. Furthermore, we have identified, for the first time, that risk factors differ for different post-operative days. Further work should include the identification of novel risk factors of C-POMS TMB score for each post-operative day, and the identification of risk factors associated with each C-POMS morbidity type to identify the risk factors associated with D15 C-POMS summary score. Additionally, further validation of these results could be sought in a subsequent C-POMS dataset. Such identification of risk factors for C-POMS TMB may aid patient group and individual risk stratification and potentially reduce healthcare costs.

Abbreviations

AVR: Aortic valve replacement; CABG: Coronary artery bypass graft; CAD: Coronary artery disease; CCSC: Canadian cardiovascular score; COPD: Chronic obstructive pulmonary disease; C-POMS: Cardiac Post-Operative Morbidity Score; CRP: C-reactive protein; D3 (D5, D8, D15): Day 3, (day 5, day 8, day 15); ICU: Intensive care unit; INR: International normalised ratio; IV: Intravenous; LOS: Length of stay;

LVEF: Left ventricular ejection fraction; MI: Myocardial infarction; MVR: Mitral valve replacement; NYHA: New York Heart Association; OPA: Out-patient appointment; OT: Occupational therapy; TMB: Total morbidity burden; UK: United Kingdom; USA: United States of America

Acknowledgements
The authors would like to thank all members of the protocol development group (PDG) and the patients who generously gave their time and consent to participate in the C-POMS study.

Funding
This work was unfunded, but Professors Hugh Montgomery and Michael Mythen were supported by the National Institute for Health Research University College London Hospitals Biomedical Research Centre.

Authors' contributions
Each author has fulfilled the ICMJE guidelines to qualify as an author. According to the ICMJE guidelines, to qualify as an author, one should have made substantial contributions to conception and design (JS, MM, HM) or acquisition of data (JS), or analysis (JC) and interpretation of data (JS, MM, HM); been involved in drafting the manuscript or revising it critically for important intellectual content (ALL); and given final approval of the version to be published (ALL). Each author has participated sufficiently in the work to take public responsibility for the appropriate portions of the content and have agreed to be accountable for all aspects of the work in ensuring that questions related to the accuracy or integrity of any part of the work are appropriately investigated and resolved.

Competing interests
The authors declare that they have no competing interests.

Authors' information
Not included.

Author details
[1]St Bartholomew's Hospital, Barts Health NHS Trust, London, UK. [2]Institute for Sport, Exercise and Health, University College London, 1st Floor 170 Tottenham Court Rd, London W1T 7HA, UK. [3]Centre for Cardiovascular Genetics, University College London, London, UK. [4]Department of Anaesthesia, University College London Hospitals NHS Trust, London, UK.

References
Batsis JA, Romero-Corral A, Collazo-Clavell ML, Sarr MG, Somers VK, Brekke L, Lopez-Jimenez F. Effect of weight loss on predicted cardiovascular risk: change in cardiac risk after bariatric surgery. Obesity.(Silver.Spring). 2007;15(3):772–84.

Boening A, Boedeker RH, Scheibelhut C, Rietzschel J, Roth P, Schonburg M. Anemia before coronary artery bypass surgery as additional risk factor increases the perioperative risk. AnnThoracSurg. 2011;92:805–10.

Bridgewater B, Kinsman R, Ireland on behalf of the S for CS in GB and: Demonstrating quality: the sixth National Adult Cardiac Surgical database report. Henley-on-Thames, UK: Dendrite Clinical Systems Ltd; 2008.

Brown PP, Kugelmass AD, Cohen DJ, Reynolds MR, Culler SD, Dee AD, Simon AW. The frequency and cost of complications associated with coronary artery bypass grafting surgery: results from the United States Medicare program. Ann Thorac Surg. 2008;85(6):1980–6.

Carrascal Y, Maroto L, Rey J, Arévalo A, Arroyo J, Echevarría JR, Arce N, Fulquet E. Impact of preoperative anemia on cardiac surgery in octogenarians. Interact Cardiovasc Thorac Surg. 2010;10:249–55.

De Santo L, Romano G, Della Corte A, de Simone V, Grimaldi F, Cotrufo M, de Feo M. Preoperative anemia in patients undergoing coronary artery bypass grafting predicts acute kidney injury. J Thorac Cardiovasc Surg. 2009;138:965–70.

Dissemination Centre for Reviews and Dissemination. CRD Report 4 (2nd Edition). Undertaking systematic reviews of research on effectiveness:CRD's guidance for those carrying out or commissioning reviews. 2001.

Dupuis JY, Wang F, Nathan H, Lam M, Grimes S, Bourke M: The cardiac anesthesia risk evaluation score: a clinically useful predictor of mortality and morbidity after cardiac surgery. Anesthesiology. 2001;94(2):194–204.

Engelman DT, Adams DH, Byrne JG, Aranki SF, Collins Jr. JJ, Couper GS, Allred EN, Cohn LH, Rizzo RJ. Impact of body mass index and albumin on morbidity and mortality after cardiac surgery. J Thorac Cardiovasc Surg. 1999;118(5):866–73.

Fortescue EB, Kahn K, Bates DW. Development and validation of a clinical prediction rule for major adverse outcomes in coronary bypass grafting. Am J Cardiol. 2001;88(11):1251–8.

General Medical Council. Consent: patients and doctors making decisions together. 2008.

Guyatt GH, Kirshner B, Jaeschke R. Measuring health status: what are the necessary measurement properties? J Clin Epidemiol. 1992;45(1):1341–5.

Hattler BG, Madia C, Johnson C, Armitage JM, Hardesty RL, Kormos RL, Pham SM, Payne DN, Griffith BP. Risk stratification using the Society of Thoracic Surgeons Program. Ann Thorac Surg. 1994;58(5):1348–52.

Higgins TL, Estafanous FG, Loop FD, Beck GJ, Blum JM, Paranandi L. Stratification of morbidity and mortality outcome by preoperative risk factors in coronary artery bypass patients. A clinical severity score. JAMA. 1992;267(17):2344–8.

Huijskes RV, Rosseel PM, Tijssen JG. Outcome prediction in coronary artery bypass grafting and valve surgery in the Netherlands: development of the Amphiascore and its comparison with the Euroscore. Eur J Cardiothorac Surg. 2003;24(5):741–9.

Hung M, Besser M, Sharples LD, Nair SK, Klein AA. The prevalence and association with transfusion, intensive care unit stay and mortality of pre-operative anaemia in a cohort of cardiac surgery patients. Anaesthesia. 2011;66:812–8.

Ivanov J, Borger MA, Rao V, David TE. The Toronto Risk Score for adverse events following cardiac surgery. Can J Cardiol. 2006;22(3):221–7.

Kirshner B, Guyatt G. A methodological framework for assessing health indices. J Chronic Dis. 1985;38(1):27–36.

Koertzen M, Punjabi P, Lockwood G. Pre-operative serum albumin concentration as a predictor of mortality and morbidity following cardiac surgery. Perfusion. 2013;28:390–4.

Larobina ME, Merry CJ, Negri JC, Pick AW. Is informed consent in cardiac surgery and percutaneous coronary intervention achievable? ANZ J Surg. 2007;77(7):530–4.

Magovern JA, Sakert T, Magovern GJ, Benckart DH, Burkholder JA, Liebler GA, Magovern Sr. GJ. A model that predicts morbidity and mortality after coronary artery bypass graft surgery. J Am Coll Cardiol. 1996;28(5):1147–53.

Rudolph JL, Jones RN, Levkoff SE, Rockett C, Inouye SK, Sellke FW, Khuri SF, Lipsitz LA, Ramlawi B, Levitsky S, Marcantonio ER. Derivation and validation of a preoperative prediction rule for delirium after cardiac surgery. Circulation. 2009;119(2):229–36.

Sanders J, Keogh BE, Van der Meulen J, Browne JP, Treasure T, Mythen MG, Montgomery HE. The development of a postoperative morbidity score to assess total morbidity burden after cardiac surgery. J Clin Epidemiol. 2012;65:423–33.

Sato Y, Kato TS, Oishi A, Yamamoto T, Kuwaki K, Inaba H, Amano A. Preoperative factors associated with postoperative requirements of renal replacement therapy following cardiac surgery. Am J Cardiol. 2015;116:294–300.

Shahian DM, O'Brien SM, Normand SL, Peterson ED, Edwards FH. Association of hospital coronary artery bypass volume with processes of care, mortality, morbidity, and the Society of Thoracic Surgeons composite quality score. J Thorac Cardiovasc Surg. 2010;139(2):273–82.

Society of Thoracic Surgeons: Online STS risk calculator. http://riskcalc.sts.org/stswebriskcalc/#/. Accessed 01 Feb 17.

Tuman KJ, McCarthy RJ, March RJ, Najafi H, Ivankovich AD. Morbidity and duration of ICU stay after cardiac surgery. A model for preoperative risk assessment. Chest. 1992;102(1):36–44.

van Venrooij LM, De VR, Borgmeijer-Hoelen MM, Haaring C, de Mol BA. Preoperative unintended weight loss and low body mass index in relation to complications and length of stay after cardiac surgery. Am J Clin Nutr. 2008; 87(6):1656–61.

Weiser TG, Regenbogen SE, Thompson KD, Haynes AB, Lipsitz SR, Berry WR, Gawande AA. An estimation of the global volume of surgery: a modelling strategy based on available data. Lancet. 2008;372(9663):139–44.

Surgeons' views on preoperative medical evaluation

Kevin R. Riggs[1], Zackary D. Berger[2], Martin A. Makary[3], Eric B. Bass[2] and Geetanjali Chander[2*]

Abstract

Background: There is substantial variation in the practice of preoperative medical evaluation (PME) and limited evidence for its benefit, which raises concerns about overuse. Surgeons have a unique role in this multidisciplinary practice. The objective of this qualitative study was to explore surgeons' practices and their beliefs about PME.

Methods: We conducted of semi-structured interviews with 18 surgeons in Baltimore, Maryland. Surgeons were purposively sampled to maximize diversity in terms of practice type (academic vs. private practice), surgical specialty, gender, and experience level. General topics included surgeons' current PME practices, perceived benefits and harms of PME, the surgical risk assessment, and potential improvements and barriers to change. Interviews were audio-recorded and transcribed. Transcripts were analyzed using content analysis to identify themes, which are presented as assertions. Transcripts were re-analyzed to identify supporting and opposing instances of each assertion.

Results: A total of 15 themes emerged. There was wide variation in surgeons' described PME practices. Surgeons believed that PME improves surgical outcomes, but not all patients benefit. Surgeons were cognizant of the financial cost of the current system and the potential inconvenience that additional tests and office visits pose to patients. Surgeons believed that PME has minimal to no risk and that a normal PME is reassuring to them and patients. Surgeons were confident in their ability to assess surgical risk, and risk assessment by non-surgeons rarely affected their surgical decision-making. Hospital and anesthesiology requirements were a major driver of surgeons' PME practices. Surgeons did not receive much training on PME but perceived their practices to be similar to their colleagues. Surgeons believed that PME provides malpractice protection, welcomed standardization, and perceived there to be inadequate evidence to significantly change their current practice.

Conclusions: Views of surgeons should be considered in future research on and reforms to the PME process.

Keywords: Preoperative care, Risk assessment, Medical overuse

Background

Patients often undergo extensive, multidisciplinary evaluation prior to elective surgery. Initially, the evaluation is aimed at determining whether patients indeed have a surgical condition. Once this has been determined and a tentative decision to proceed with surgery has been made, patients often undergo additional preoperative medical evaluation (PME)—testing and evaluation aimed at assessing and minimizing surgical risk (Riggs and Segal 2016). There is substantial variation in this practice of PME (Thilen et al. 2013; van Gelder et al. 2012; Wijeysundera et al. 2012) and limited evidence for benefit (Balk et al.

2014; Wijeysundera et al. 2010), which has raised concerns about overuse (Baxi and Lakin 2015; Brateanu and Rothberg 2015; Smetana 2015).

The perioperative process is complex and includes diverse provider types, including surgeons, anesthesiologists, primary care and medical specialists, and spans multiple settings, including the outpatient clinic, operating room, and hospital. Surgeons are uniquely situated as they follow patients through the entirety of this process, from prior to surgery to the hospital to the postoperative follow-up. This unique vantage point may give surgeons important insights regarding the processes of PME that can assist with improving the efficiency of the system. However, knowledge of surgeons' views on PME is limited. Several recent qualitative studies focused

* Correspondence: gchande1@jhmi.edu
[2]Division of General Internal Medicine, Johns Hopkins University School of Medicine, 1830 E. Monument Street, Room 8060, Baltimore, MD 21287, USA
Full list of author information is available at the end of the article

narrowly on preoperative testing in low-risk situations (Brown and Brown 2011; Patey et al. 2012), and several quantitative surveys focused on preoperative consultations (Katz et al. 1998; Pausjenssen et al. 2008). The objective of this study was to more broadly explore surgeons' modern practices and beliefs about PME.

Methods
Study design
We conducted a qualitative study consisting of semi-structured interviews with surgeons. Because the preoperative process is complex and so little is known about surgeons' practices and what motivates those practices, we felt that a qualitative approach would allow us to explore that complexity better than a quantitative survey.

Setting and participants
Surgeons were recruited from clinical practices in Baltimore, Maryland. We purposively recruited surgeons to maximize the diversity of our sample with the goal of hearing a wide range of practices and opinions. We recruited an approximately equal mix of academic and private practice surgeons, and a mix of general (including colorectal, vascular, oncologic, thoracic, endocrine, breast, and plastic) and non-general (including orthopedic, urologic, and otolaryngologic) surgical specialties. Additionally, we oversampled women and sought a mix of early-, mid-, and late-career surgeons.

We contacted surgeons from two local academic institutions via publically available email addresses. We were unable to locate publically available email addresses for local private practice surgeons, so we obtained their contact information with the assistance of the Johns Hopkins Clinical Research Network, a research consortium of area hospitals and health systems. All surgeons were located in and around Baltimore, Maryland. Surgeons were offered a small monetary incentive for participating, and they were interviewed in-person in a private setting that was convenient for them, typically their offices.

Interview guide
General topics for questioning included surgeons' current PME practices and related training, surgical risk assessment, potential benefits and potential downsides for patients and others in the health care system, and ideas for improving the system. Each author was involved in developing the initial interview guide. As the study progressed, the interview guide underwent revisions to allow further exploration of new topics that had been raised in prior interviews. Additionally, semi-structured interviews allowed for topics not included in the guide to emerge and be explored. The final interview guide is shown in the Appendix.

Data collection and analysis
One investigator (KRR) conducted the interviews in person between June 2015 and May 2016. Just prior to the interview, participant characteristics were collected using a brief questionnaire. Interviews were audio-recorded and the recordings were transcribed verbatim. Identifying information was removed from interview transcripts.

The transcripts were initially analyzed using conventional thematic content analysis (Hsieh and Shannon 2005). A codebook of descriptive codes (also known as topical codes) was developed collaboratively by two authors (KRR and GC) as the transcripts were reviewed. The transcripts were coded using textual data analysis software (ATLAS.ti version 7, Scientific Software Development), which allowed coded segments to be compared to all other segments with the same code to look for emerging themes. The outcome of this type of thematic analysis is the identification of general themes (e.g., reassurance as a benefit of preoperative medical evaluation), which can then be used to construct new theory (e.g., as with grounded theory methodologies). The goal of our analysis was not to develop theory but to identify themes in the form of specific assertions representing practices and beliefs (Erickson 1986; Saldaña 2013). The initial stage of coding was ongoing during the time interviews were being conducted, and helped guide the determination that enough data had been collected (a concept known as thematic saturation) (Guest et al. 2006).

After the initial stage of thematic analysis, each of the transcripts was then re-coded for supporting and opposing instances of each theme (except for "practice variation" which we just described). We tabulated the number of interviews in which instances of each theme appeared (not necessarily mutually exclusive, as supporting and opposing instances of a theme could each appear in an interview). Each transcript was independently coded by two team members to enhance reliability, and discrepancies were resolved by consensus. The institutional review board at the Johns Hopkins University School of Medicine approved the study.

Results
We interviewed a total of 18 surgeons, whose demographic characteristics are shown in Table 1. One-third of the surgeons were female, and the mean age and mean time since finishing their training was 43.4 years and 9.7 years, respectively. Surgeons were evenly split between academic and private practice, and slightly more than half (11/18) were general surgery specialties.

Practice variation
The variation in surgeons' descriptions of their PME practices was striking. Each surgeon said they required an evaluation and some testing for a majority of their

Table 1 Surgeon characteristics

	(n = 18)
Gender, female	6
Age, mean (range)	43.4 (32–66)
Years since completed training, mean (range)	9.7 (1–36)
Practice setting	
Academic	9
Private practice	9
Surgery type	
General	
Colorectal	4
Vascular	2
Oncologic	1
Thoracic	1
Endocrine	1
Breast	1
Plastic	1
Non-general	
Orthopedic	5
Urologic	1
Otolaryngologic	1

patients, typically directed by primary care physicians (PCPs) or preoperative clinics run by anesthesiology. However, some surgeons were selective about who would require these additional visits based on patient factors and operation factors, while others required these visits in all of their patients with no exceptions. Surgeons were split on whether they preferred PCPs or anesthesiologists direct the PME, and while most surgeons felt that either was adequate, some required patients to be seen separately by both. Some surgeons ordered necessary tests themselves, while others had consultants order them (sometimes at the discretion of the consultants, and other times dictated by the surgeons). Some surgeons required specialist involvement (e.g., cardiology) in certain cases, while others left that determination to the discretion of the clinician performing the PME. Some surgeons would require visits with several specialists in addition to a PCP visit for some patients, while others said that a specialist visit should obviate the need for a PCP visit. Most surgeons initiated the process of evaluation after the tentative decision for surgery had been made, and they added patients to the operating room schedule at that point. However, a few surgeons said they waited for the results of preoperative consults or tests before adding patients to the operating room schedule to make sure they were "cleared."

Patient benefits and harms

Themes related to the benefits and harms of PME and representative quotations are shown in Table 2. Universally, surgeons believed that PME provided some benefit to at least some patients. The primary benefit that surgeons cited was the identification of occult conditions. Many shared stories of patients who appeared well but had serious pathology incidentally discovered in the PME, which was either able to be addressed (making surgery safer) or required surgery to be canceled (saving the patient an unnecessary or unsafe surgery). Surgeons also indicated that they believed the PME resulted in optimization or "fine tuning" of chronic conditions, although they were less specific in their evidence supporting this belief.

Surgeons generally agreed that PME was overall beneficial, though many acknowledged that the benefits typically accrue to a minority of patients and that most patients did not derive a direct medical benefit. Some surgeons pointed out that it is not possible to identify who will benefit ahead of time, and so PME that ends up not being beneficial is ultimately justified by the minority of cases where patients derive a medical benefit.

Even when the results of the PME are normal and do not alter the surgical plan, some surgeons believed that they were still worthwhile. In some cases, this was just because the surgeons like to "have those numbers." In addition, they believed that normal test results and "another pair of eyes" reviewing the case were reassuring to patients as well as surgeons and anesthesiologists. Other potential patient benefits were mentioned less frequently, including as opportunities for education or to increase patient engagement, or just a reason for people who might not otherwise see a primary care doctor to do so.

The majority of surgeons denied that there could possibly be any medical harms from PME. While many of the surgeons explicitly recognized that PME essentially represents "screening" that patients may not otherwise receive if they were not considering surgery, they believed that anything identified through this screening (e.g., lab abnormalities or lung nodules) ultimately represented a benefit to patients. However, one surgeon cited the potential of falsely abnormal results to delay surgery and another specifically cited "overtreatment."

Surgeons generally downplayed potential medical harms of the PME, but they largely recognized the inconvenience to patients of extra office visits and tests. Some mentioned that visits in preoperative clinics the day before surgery would require out-of-town patients to spend a night in a hotel. A number of surgeons mentioned that patients had brought up the inconvenience of the PME to them, although only one had ever heard a

Table 2 Themes related to benefits and harms of preoperative medical evaluation

Theme	Number of interviews supporting theme, representative quote	Number of interviews opposing theme, representative quote
The preoperative medical evaluation can improve surgical outcomes by identifying treatable occult conditions and/or optimizing chronic conditions.	12 interviews "I think it prevents catastrophes. I mean, you wouldn't want to carry someone to the operating room and have the stress test on the operating room table. But by doing a preoperative evaluation you might uncover, whether it's the EKG, whether it's laboratory findings, you might uncover something that suggests this person is at high risk for cardiovascular disease which might lead to other evaluation which could prevent a misadventure, so to speak, in the operating room." -Academic urologic surgeon	2 interviews "I mean if you believe the trials, you know, the CARP trial being the classic one, there is no benefit for preoperative evaluation." -Academic vascular surgeon
Many patients do not medically benefit from the preoperative medical evaluation	8 interviews "How many pre-ops do you have to do before you find something really wrong? Because most people, you are not going to find anything in that kind of situation." -Private practice colorectal surgeon	0 interviews
A normal preoperative medical evaluation before surgery is reassuring to patients and physicians	6 interviews "There is a peace of mind I get from it, because if I have those numbers and objective data in front of me then it makes me feel more confident that the patient is going to be safe." -Academic endocrine surgeon	0 interviews
The preoperative medical evaluation has minimal to no medical risk for patients	12 interviews "I don't see an overt downside to a preoperative evaluation other than the logistics of it, frankly." -Academic vascular surgeon	2 interviews "It's sort of like screening for most conditions, where if they're not symptomatic and you find something, you are forced- you're not forced, but the standard of care at that point is to pursue it, and sometimes that even postpones surgery because something has been discovered that may or may not be clinically important, and so I think it's just a lot of extra engagement with the health care system." -Academic otolaryngologic surgeon
Additional office visits and tests can be an inconvenience for patients	16 interviews "It's cumbersome. I mean it's difficult. They have to come back on a separate day. A lot of my out-of-towners, it's difficult, right, because let's say you live in Kansas and you are coming here for surgery and you see me and we schedule surgery. You go home and see your family, and now you've got to come back a couple of days before the surgery to go to the [preoperative clinic]. And so it's an inconvenience for sure." -Academic oncologic surgeon	1 interviews "But, interestingly enough, the patients accept it very willingly. Almost expected, not just accepted." -Academic colorectal surgeon
The financial cost to the patient and/or healthcare system is a downside of the preoperative medical evaluation.	14 interviews "It's expensive and most of it is not necessary. And it's expensive both from the standpoint of true monetary cost of doing testing but also there's a time expense for everybody." -Academic endocrine surgeon	3 interviews "And I think there is a benefit in that if you can prevent a complication, there is a huge benefit not only clinically, but also financially." -Academic oncologic surgeon

patient bring up out-of-pocket costs for extra office visits or tests.

Surgical risk assessment

Themes related to risk assessment and representative quotations are shown in Table 3. Universally, surgeons indicated that in their initial evaluation of patients, they performed their own assessment of patients' surgical risk. For the most part, these assessments were informal, described as "a gestalt," "the eyeball test," or "spit balling." Few had ever used a formal risk assessment tool or calculator, and none reported using them regularly. However, surgeons were generally confident in their ability to estimate risk. Two surgeons mentioned research

Table 3 Themes related to risk assessment

Theme	Number of interviews supporting theme, representative quote	Number of interviews opposing theme, representative quote
Surgeons are confident in their ability to assess patients' surgical risk.	13 interviews "I think we get a good gestalt of the patients overall by the time you get through the H&P. The longest assessment is the initial visit. Once you can confirm their medical history and the medications you get a good sense of their risk." -Academic orthopedic surgeon	5 interviews "I don't really have the expertise to figure out their cardiac risk whereas the other providers generally do… I mean, qualitatively I can tell. Some patients are probably going to be higher risk than others, but beyond that I'm not really trained in what to specifically look for." -Private practice orthopedic surgeon
The risk assessment provided by non-surgeons is viewed primarily as either clearing or not clearing the patient for surgery.	11 interviews "I'll generally make sure there's no glaringly abnormal laboratory studies and make sure at least the note from PCP says the patient is cleared for surgery or moderate—make sure it doesn't say they're at extremely high risk or really not cleared for surgery. If that were the case, then they probably would have notified me beforehand, so I'm not going to read [the note] in detail." -Private practice orthopedic surgeon	4 interviews "If I was about to do a big operation on someone and the preop says, "whoa, whoa, whoa, hold on, this is a really sick person," sometimes there's a lesser option. If they uncover things that I wasn't aware of, I might go with, for obstructing colon cancer, I might go with a stoma. Just give them a bag, a quick operation, rather than trying to take it out and do this five hour operation." -Academic colorectal surgeon

indicating that surgeons' gestalt is as good as a more formal risk assessment, and one even said that if their assessment differed from the consultant's assessment that "I still trust myself more."

Some surgeons found the risk assessment provided by the consultants performing the PME to be helpful, but most reported that it rarely affected their surgical plan. Most surgeons viewed the PME a task that had to be completed, and a majority of surgeons spontaneously used the terminology "cleared" or "clearance" to describe the assessment of the clinicians performing PME, reflecting this belief. This view is driven in part by the timing of the PME, which typically occurs after a tentative decision to have surgery has been made, so surgeons have already made an assessment that the benefits outweigh the risks. To this end, some surgeons explicitly said that they do not routinely review the notes provided by consulting clinicians, and that when there are problems that are going to delay or prevent surgery, they are contacted directly about them. So while other clinicians' risk assessment is not routinely incorporated in the decision to have surgery, unanticipated problems discovered during the PME often result in the surgery being reconsidered.

Drivers of current PME practice, potential improvements, and barriers to change

Themes related to drivers of current PME practice, potential improvements, and barriers to change and representative quotations are shown in Table 4. Most surgeons indicated that their requirements for preoperative testing and medical office visits were driven by hospital or anesthesiology requirements, although they were not always able to describe the specifics of those requirements. Many surgeons were focused on ensuring that

anesthesiology's requirements were met to ensure that cases were not canceled at the last minute, sometimes driving surgeons to order or request more than they thought was actually needed.

Most surgeons reported receiving very little formal training in how to perform the PME. Some of the general surgeons indicated that during their training, they were responsible for performing PME, so they gained some expertise and comfort in doing so, even if they had to "muddle through and figure it out." On the other hand, most of the specialty surgeons indicated that they outsourced PME to primary care or anesthesia during their training, and so they never gained any experience or comfort with it.

Despite the variation and lack of training, most surgeons perceived that their practice was very similar to their colleagues'. In part, this related to hospital requirements that essentially standardized both their practice and their colleagues' practice. However, several explicitly stated that they developed their current practice by observing and adopting that of their colleagues.

Many surgeons felt the PME reduced their malpractice risk, although this was not universal. Some indicated that the reduced risk was due to the PME leading to fewer complications, but many indicated that even in the case of non-preventable complications, the fact that another physician had "cleared" the patient for surgery would be protective.

Several surgeons indicated that they welcomed more standardization of the PME. Toward this end, several thought consensus guidelines would be helpful because they would reduce their uncertainty as to whether the patient had received an adequate PME and may even reduce the malpractice risk. However, several surgeons expressed skepticism that there was adequate evidence

Table 4 Themes related to drivers of current practice, potential improvements and barriers to change

Theme	Number of interviews supporting theme, representative quote	Number of interviews opposing theme, representative quote
Hospital and/or anesthesiology requirements (including informal or perceived requirements) are a major driver of surgeons' use of preoperative services.	14 interviews "For major surgery, everybody needs to get a set of pre-operative tests, and the standards are set mostly by the hospital where the surgery is going to take place. Some of these hospitals send us a grid and on one side there are patient's characteristics like age, whether they are a smoker, whether they have certain medical conditions. On the other end, based on the response to the first set of questions, it tells us whether we should get an electrocardiogram, a chest X-ray, some blood work, etc. What we do most of the time, because it's always better to have more than have your surgeries get delayed because you didn't get enough, we go ahead and get more extensive blood work. Let's say they request basic chemistry, we may go ahead and get some liver function tests as well." -Private practice colorectal surgeon	2 interviews "I get coags on everybody and I think that some people push back and say you don't need to do that unless somebody has some history of a bleeding problem or something along those lines. [Even if anesthesia didn't require them], I would still get them." -Academic orthopedic surgeon
Surgeons receive minimal formal training on performing preoperative medical evaluations.	13 interviews You know, my residency didn't really—we do kind of general surgery time and stuff like that, but certainly in medical school, I never really learned "here's how to properly preop the patient." We sort of encountered it a lot as you would, for example, consult medicine to see if you can fix some old lady's hip. You'd sort of learn indirectly by seeing how they would clear them, but I guess I never really learned formally the right ways to do it. -Private practice orthopedic surgeon	1 interview I did [get specific training about what to order on who and why] for disease processes that could produce intraoperative problems. So hyperthyroidism, pheochromocytoma, those sorts of things. Did I get training about more subtle things? Like, for example, this person is taking Plavix, here are the things you need to do about those patients. Not really. -Academic endocrine surgeon
Surgeons' preoperative medical evaluation practices are similar to their colleagues' practices.	14 interviews "My senior partners had been doing this for 30 years, and so I kind of just picked up the flow of how the office works and how they do [the preoperative medical evaluation]." -Private practice breast surgeon	4 interviews "I think my colleague probably does fewer testings, like in terms of cardiac clearance. I think that he may, for example, instead of having a cardiology work them up, he says, I'll just go ahead and order an ECHO or a stress test. And if those look fine then he clears them." -Private practice thoracic surgeon
The preoperative medical evaluation reduces surgeons' malpractice risk.	12 interviews "I guess it probably would give you a little defense if patient develop post-op medical issue. Then it probably will be a help defensively to say hey, I got the medical opinion on that. There's no question that's part of the deal when you get a medical clearance." -Private practice vascular surgeon	2 interviews "I guess it could go both ways in the sense that I mean in theory [the preoperative medical evaluation] should lower [the malpractice risk], but in reality if you do not read the note, it may increase it." -Private practice colorectal surgeon
Surgeons welcome standardization of preoperative medical evaluation protocols.	6 interviews "I think there were sort of national or at least sort of acceptable agreed upon standards between institutions, I think that would just be a lot easier because then theoretically it would be more interchangeable. Like if we just agreed that, you know, this is the definitive article and here's this grid. Wherever you fall on this grid, this is how we've decided as a medical community that people are cleared for surgery. Then you can go anywhere and do it and you know what people are going to get, and it kind of takes the guesswork out." -Private practice orthopedic surgeon	2 interviews "It would be nicer if things weren't mandatory, because in some cases–especially in the hospital–if a patient is coming in two months later, and their pre-op was done 75 days ahead, and you know that there hasn't been a whole lot of change in the interim, it would be nice if we could kind of use our judgment. But, they don't allow room for that, because I guess they don't want to trust people's judgment." -Private practice plastic surgeon
There is inadequate evidence regarding the benefits of preoperative medical evaluation.	3 interviews I definitely don't know if it is absolutely necessary to preop my young 20-year olds. I	0 interviews

Table 4 Themes related to drivers of current practice, potential improvements and barriers to change *(Continued)*

Theme	Number of interviews supporting theme, representative quote	Number of interviews opposing theme, representative quote
	mean is there a possibility that something could pop up during some of their routine blood work or something? Of course. But you know that from a cost analysis standpoint I don't know if it is really needed. More studies that need to look into that. -Private practice orthopedic surgeon	

that a less resource-intensive PME process would be safe, although they indicated that more evidence could persuade them to change their practice.

Discussion

In this qualitative study, we elicited a comprehensive picture of surgeons' views on PME. This study supplements prior studies, which were more narrowly focused either on testing in low-risk situations (Brown and Brown 2011; Patey et al. 2012) or medical consultations (Katz et al. 1998; Pausjenssen et al. 2008). For example, Brown and Brown (Brown and Brown 2011) conducted qualitative interviews with a diverse group of clinicians involved with preoperative testing (which included 7 surgeons out of 23 participants), and reported themes similar to ours with respect to satisfying hospitals' and anesthesiologists' requirements to avoid delays and cancellations, the potential medicolegal benefit of preoperative testing, and clinicians' desire to have more standardization. However, most of our themes were not reported in these previous studies.

The results of this study have several important implications for future efforts to improve the process of PME. First, the PME should not primarily be viewed as simply providing a "risk assessment" or "risk stratification." Surgeons are generally confident in their ability to estimate surgical risk, and since a tentative decision to proceed with surgery has already been made, simply providing another risk estimation will not routinely cause those decisions to be reconsidered. Rather, surgeons are looking for confirmation of their assessment (i.e., that they did not miss something important). Surgeons also want to assure that patients' chronic conditions are being appropriately treated (i.e., "optimization" (Riggs and Segal 2016)), although how often conditions are actively being managed during this process is uncertain. Additionally, more research on who is best suited to direct the PME (i.e., PCPs or dedicated preoperative clinics) may be helpful, though as described by several surgeons in the study, it is likely unnecessarily redundant to have more than a single preoperative assessment.

Second, surgeons recognize that not every patient benefits from the PME, but they do believe that the process improves surgical outcomes overall. Further, while they are aware of the potential inconvenience of the process for patients, they do not believe that current evidence is adequate to justify changing their practice to require fewer tests or office visits. While some commentators have argued that evidence is sufficient to limit preoperative testing in many situations (Brateanu and Rothberg, 2015; Smetana 2015), high-quality evidence demonstrating the safety of less intensive PME is generally lacking (Balk et al. 2014) (with the exception of cataract surgery (Schein et al. 2000)). High-quality evidence demonstrating the safety of forgoing certain preoperative services and research examining the effect of less intensive PME on patient experience has the potential to change practices.

Finally, surgeons were very clear that one of their primary concerns is satisfying anesthesia and hospital requirements in order to avoid last minute cancellations. In part, this problem arises from the current workflow, where anesthesiologists may be assigned to cases on the day before or the day of surgery. Variation in the anesthesiologists' opinion of what constitutes an appropriate PME may drive surgeons to be more exhaustive in terms of preoperative tests and consultations than they otherwise would be, in order to avoid last-minute delays and cancellations. More uniformity about what anesthesiologists expect would be welcomed by surgeons, as it would decrease anxiety about delays and cancellations and may lead to a less intensive PME. Consensus guidelines, even in the absence of more high-quality evidence, could drive more standardization and could even allay surgeons' concerns about malpractice liability (Kirkpatrick and Burkman 2010). However, surgeons seem more attentive to local hospital policies than to national clinical guidelines, so future guidelines would likely have more impact if targeted at hospitals and anesthesiologists rather than surgeons or internists who perform PME.

This study has several limitations. First, we presented our themes as assertions, although qualitative research is not meant to be hypothesis testing, so these assertions warrant further quantitative testing in more representative samples. Second, all surgeons were currently practicing in a small geographic region, so their practices and beliefs could be specific to that region. Finally, we tried to avoid any specific focus on overuse or low-value care, though surgeons may have perceived that to be an implicit subject and tailored their interviews to avoid describing some low-value practices.

Conclusion

Surgeons' PME practices vary dramatically, even within a single geographic area. While overuse in PME may be a legitimate concern, surgeons generally view PME as beneficial, so future research on PME and future reforms to the PME process should take into account surgeons' views on the topic. More research into the safety of forgoing certain preoperative services and patient satisfaction with less intensive PME, and increasing standardization of the process through consensus guidelines may be options to decrease unwarranted variation and increase the value of PME.

Appendix
Final interview guide

1. What are the operations you most commonly perform?
2. What is your typical patient population like?
3. What is your standard practice for "preops"? (Or whichever term is familiar.)
4. Who usually performs those preops?
5. What tests do you recommend or require be obtained as part of the preop?
6. Do you order those tests? Why or why not?
7. Do you request specialists to be involved in the preop? If so, how do you make that decision?
8. How do you request a preop?
9. How do you process preop notes and test results?
10. Is there something specific in the preop note that you are looking for?
11. (If not everyone gets a pre-op) How do you decide who doesn't need a pre-op?
12. Does your practice or institution have rules about preops? If so, what are they?
13. Are there any clinical guidelines for preops that affect your practice? If so, what are they?
14. How were you trained about doing preops?
15. How does your current practice differ from the way you were trained?
16. How do you think your practice differs from your colleagues? Others in your community?
17. In your opinion, what are the benefits to the patients from preops?
18. What are the potential downsides for the patients?
19. Do you ever change your surgical plan based on the preop? If so, how?
20. What are the benefits to you, the other providers involved, or the health system from preops? How do preops affects a surgeon's risk of malpractice?
21. What are the potential downsides to you or the health system from preops?
22. Do anesthesiologists ever cancel cases because of inadequate preop? If so, examples?
23. How comfortable do you feel in estimating a patient's operative risk?
24. How do you estimate a patient's operative risk?
25. Do patients express preferences or expectations regarding preops? If so, how?
26. Do you have any memorable anecdotes about a patient who was impacted positively or negatively by a preop?
27. Do you think there would be any way to make the preop system better?
28. Anything else?

Abbreviations
PCP: Primary care physician; PME: Preoperative medical evaluation

Funding
Dr. Riggs's work on this study was funded by the Society of General Internal Medicine Founders' Grant and by NIH grant T32 HL007180.

Authors' contributions
KR and GC conceived the study. All authors contributed to the study design. KR, GC, and ZB undertook the data analysis. KR drafted the manuscript which underwent revision by all other authors. All authors read and approved the final manuscript.

Competing interests
The authors declare that they have no competing interests.

Author details
[1]Division of Preventive Medicine, University of Alabama at Birmingham, Birmingham, AL, USA. [2]Division of General Internal Medicine, Johns Hopkins University School of Medicine, 1830 E. Monument Street, Room 8060, Baltimore, MD 21287, USA. [3]Department of Surgery, Johns Hopkins University School of Medicine, Baltimore, MD, USA.

References
Balk EM, Earley A, Hadar N, Shah N, Trikalinos TA. Benefits and Harms of Routine Preoperative Testing: Comparative Effectiveness. Rockville, MD: Agency for Healthcare Research and Quality; 2014.

Baxi SM, Lakin JR. Preoperative testing—a bridge to nowhere: a teachable moment. JAMA Intern Med. 2015;175(8):1272–3.

Brateanu A, Rothberg MB. Why do clinicians continue to order 'routine preoperative tests' despite the evidence? Cleve Clin J Med. 2015; 82(10):667–70.

Brown SR, Brown J. Why do physicians order unnecessary preoperative tests? A qualitative study. Fam Med. 2011;43(5):338–43.

Erickson F. Qualitative methods in research on teaching. In: Wittrock M, editor. Handbook of research on teaching. New York: Macmillan; 1986. p. 119–61.

Guest G, Bunce A, Johnson L. How many interviews are enough? Field Methods. 2006;18(1):59–82.

Hsieh HF, Shannon SE. Three approaches to qualitative content analysis. Qual Health Res. 2005;15(9):1277–88.

Katz RI, Barnhart JM, Ho G, Hersch D, Dayan SS, Keehn L. A survey on the intended purposes and perceived utility of preoperative cardiology consultations. Anesth Analg. 1998;87(4):830–6.

Kirkpatrick DH, Burkman RT. Does standardization of care through clinical guidelines improve outcomes and reduce medical liability? Obstet Gynecol. 2010;116(5):1022–6.

Patey AM, Islam R, Francis JJ, Bryson GL, Grimshaw JM, Canada PPT. Anesthesiologists' and surgeons' perceptions about routine pre-operative testing in low-risk patients: application of the Theoretical Domains Framework (TDF) to identify factors that influence physicians' decisions to order pre-operative tests. Implement Sci. 2012;7:52.

Pausjenssen L, Ward HA, Card SE. An internist's role in perioperative medicine: a survey of surgeons' opinions. BMC Fam Pract. 2008;9:4.

Riggs KR, Segal JB. What is the rationale for preoperative medical evaluations? A closer look at surgical risk and common terminology. Br J Anaesth. 2016;117(6):681–4.

Saldaña J. The coding manual for qualitative researchers. 2nd ed. London: Sage; 2013.

Schein OD, Katz J, Bass EB, et al. The value of routine preoperative medical testing before cataract surgery. Study of medical testing for cataract surgery. N Engl J Med. 2000;342(3):168–75.

Smetana GW. The conundrum of unnecessary preoperative testing. JAMA Intern Med. 2015;175(8):1359–61.

Thilen SR, Bryson CL, Reid RJ, Wijeysundera DN, Weaver EM, Treggiari MM. Patterns of preoperative consultation and surgical specialty in an integrated healthcare system. Anesthesiology. 2013;118(5):1028–37.

van Gelder FE, de Graaff JC, van Wolfswinkel L, van Klei WA. Preoperative testing in noncardiac surgery patients: a survey amongst European anaesthesiologists. Eur J Anaesthesiol. 2012;29(10):465–70.

Wijeysundera DN, Austin PC, Beattie W, Hux JE, Laupacis A. Outcomes and processes of care related to preoperative medical consultation. Arch Intern Med. 2010;170(15):1365–74.

Wijeysundera DN, Austin PC, Beattie WS, Hux JE, Laupacis A. Variation in the practice of preoperative medical consultation for major elective noncardiac surgery: a population-based study. Anesthesiology. 2012;116(1):25–34.

Comparison of risk-scoring systems in the prediction of outcome after liver resection

S. Ulyett[1,2]* , G. Shahtahmassebi[2,3], S. Aroori[1], M. J. Bowles[1], C. D. Briggs[1], M. G. Wiggans[1], G. Minto[1,2] and D. A. Stell[1,2]

Abstract

Background: Risk prediction techniques commonly used in liver surgery include the American Society of Anesthesiologists (ASA) grading, Charlson Comorbidity Index (CCI) and cardiopulmonary exercise tests (CPET). This study compares the utility of these techniques along with the number of segments resected as predictive tools in liver surgery.

Methods: A review of a unit database of patients undergoing liver resection between February 2008 and January 2015 was undertaken. Patient demographics, ASA, CCI and CPET variables were recorded along with resection size. Clavien-Dindo grade III–V complications were used as a composite outcome in analyses. Association between predictive variables and outcome was assessed by univariate and multivariate techniques.

Results: One hundred and seventy-two resections in 168 patients were identified. Grade III–V complications occurred after 42 (24.4%) liver resections. In univariate analysis of CPET variables, ventilatory equivalents for CO_2 (VEqCO$_2$) was associated with outcome. CCI score, but not ASA grade, was also associated with outcome. In multivariate analysis, the odds ratio of developing grade III–V complications for incremental increases in VEqCO$_2$, CCI and number of liver segments resected were 1.09, 1.49 and 2.94, respectively.

Conclusions: Of the techniques evaluated, resection size provides the simplest and most discriminating predictor of significant complications following liver surgery.

Keywords: Preoperative assessment, Liver resection, Surgical complications, Cardiopulmonary exercise testing

Background

Despite the technical advances, liver resection remains potentially dangerous and is associated with a morbidity rate of 18.2–32.4% (Ulyett et al. 2015; Wiggans et al. 2014; Poon et al. 2004) and mortality rate of 1.4–5.3% (Nygard et al. 2012; Belghiti et al. 2000; Dimick et al. 2004). Preoperative estimation of risk allows counselling of patients regarding treatment options and helps in operative planning. A number of techniques are commonly used preoperatively to estimate risk including the American Society of Anesthesiology (ASA) grade, Charlson Comorbidity Index (CCI) and Cardiopulmonary Exercise Tests (CPET). The ASA grading system is a subjective assessment of the degree of systemic disease made at the time

of surgery (Saklad 1941). CCI is a 22-point scoring matrix based on comorbid diagnoses (Charlson et al. 1987), which was originally designed to predict long-term survival in an unselected population but has also been shown to be of value in predicting outcome after surgery (Backemar et al. 2015; Schmolders et al. 2015). CPET provides an objective measurement of cardiorespiratory fitness, where the volume of oxygen consumption at peak (VO$_{2 peak}$) and at anaerobic threshold (AT), ventilatory efficiency in the elimination of carbon dioxide (CO_2) (VEeqCO$_2$), heart rate (HR) and oxygen (O_2) pulse (a surrogate measure of cardiac output) are measured. This technique was initially used to predict mortality in patients undergoing a range of abdominal procedures (Older et al. 1993) and has been shown to be of value in predicting outcomes in patients undergoing pancreatic (Chandrabalan et al. 2013) and vascular (Thompson et al. 2011) surgery.

* Correspondence: simon.ulyett@nhs.net
[1]Derriford Hospital, Plymouth PL6 8DH, UK
[2]Peninsula Schools of Medicine and Dentistry, Plymouth University, Plymouth PL6 8BU, UK
Full list of author information is available at the end of the article

Data on the use of these tools in the context of liver surgery is scarce. The ASA grade has been shown to influence the development of postoperative complications after liver resection (Belghiti et al. 2000), and CCI has been assessed in the prediction of short-term outcomes (Schroeder et al. 2006). Data on the use of CPET before liver surgery is conflicting, with one study showing a useful correlation with complications (Junejo et al. 2012) and another showing only minimal association (Dunne et al. 2014). None of the tools takes into account the extent of the proposed operation, and no comparison between the techniques has been undertaken.

The aim of this study is to determine the relative value of these risk prediction tools in patients undergoing liver surgery and also to assess their value compared to risk prediction based on the extent of the surgical procedure undertaken.

Methods

A review of a prospectively maintained database of all patients undergoing resection of parenchymal liver lesions between February 2008 and January 2015 was undertaken. Follow up was completed in June 2015. The primary endpoint was development of Clavien-Dindo (CD) grade III–V complications.

To reduce heterogeneity of the study population, patients undergoing synchronous bowel resection or surgery for obstructing lesions of the proximal hepatic duct or in the presence of liver cirrhosis were excluded, as surgery in these situations is associated with higher risk (Wiggans et al. 2014; Belghiti et al. 2000; Das et al. 2001). Liver resection was undertaken using Cavitron Ultrasonic Surgical Aspirator (CUSA). General anaesthetic was administered by specialist liver anaesthetists. Low central venous pressures (CVP) were maintained although invasive CVP monitoring was not undertaken. The extent of liver resection was described according to the Brisbane Classification (Pang 2002). Radiofrequency ablation (RFA) was used where major liver resections were performed leaving a residual contralateral disease. Where subsegmental resections were undertaken, these were rounded up to the nearest integer in analyses. Postoperatively, all patients undergoing major resection were cared for in a critical care unit. Retrieved data include age, gender, indication for surgery and use of preoperative chemotherapy. ASA grade was determined at the time of surgery by the responsible anaesthetist, and CCI was calculated postoperatively from clinical records. The use of perioperative blood transfusion was also recorded.

CPET was introduced as a preoperative assessment tool in February 2008 and was initially available at the discretion of referring consultants for patients considered to be at higher risk of surgical complications. After November 2013, CPET has been undertaken in the majority of patients. CPET was undertaken using a cycle ergometer (nSpire™ Zan® 600, Colorado, USA, or MGC Diagnostics®, MN, USA). The protocol consists of 2 mins of rest, 1 min of cycling without resistance, and then a ramped protocol of between 10 and 25 watts/min. CPET variables measured included $VO_{2\ peak}$, anaerobic threshold (AT), O_2 pulse, relative O_2 pulse, resting (rHR) and peak heart rate (pHR) and ventilatory equivalents for CO_2 (VEqCO$_2$). AT was calculated using the V-slope method and $VO_{2\ peak}$ was averaged over the last 30 s of the test. CPET were undertaken and interpreted by three specialist liver anaesthetists. In patients where AT was not achieved, a nominal low value of 8 ml/kg/min was assigned as this group have been shown to have poor outcomes (Lai et al. 2013; Challand et al. 2012).

Postsurgical outcomes occurring within 30 days of surgery were classified according to the CD system (Dindo et al. 2004). Broadly, grade I–II complications include minor variations in the patient pathway including the use of anti-emetics and antibiotics, grade III complications require postoperative intervention (commonly for bile leaks), grade IV complications are determined by organ failure and grade V complication is death. In this study, grade III–V complications were used as a composite outcome of significant adverse postoperative events. Patients may develop complications in more than one grade, particularly as grade III and IV complications may have different aetiology. Liver failure was classified according to the International Study Group for Liver Surgery consensus definition of post-hepatectomy liver failure (PHLF) (Rahbari et al. 2011) and renal failure according to the RIFLE scoring system (Bellomo et al. 2004). For the purposes of this study, heart failure was defined as the requirement for inotropic medication to treat hypotension of suspected cardiac cause, after removal of epidural catheter. Respiratory failure was defined as a return to critical care unit for respiratory support.

Statistical analyses were carried out using chi-square and Mann-Whitney U tests for categorical and continuous data, respectively. Binary logistic regression was used to assess the effect of risk factors on outcome. Repeat resections in individual patients were analysed separately where separate CPET were performed.

Confirmation was obtained from the South-West Health Research Authority that Research Ethics Committee review was not required because patient data were collected prospectively as a normal part of hospital care, and all data were anonymised. No patient consent was required for this study. This study was registered with the Research Registry (unique identification 464) (Research Registry) and conforms with the STROBE guidelines (von Elm et al. 2008).

Results

Details of patients selected for the study are shown in Fig. 1. Nine (5%) patients had repeat resections. Patient and operative characteristics, CPET parameters and ASA and CCI scores are shown in Table 1. $VEqCO_2$ results were unavailable in five patients. Intraoperative RFA was used in addition to resection in 11 patients and portal vein embolization prior to resection in three patients. Laparoscopic resection was performed on 32 (18.6%) occasions.

A surgeon estimated that the intraoperative blood loss was less than 500 ml in 81 (47%) and more than 1000 ml in 31 (18%) resections. Forty-four patients required a blood transfusion intraoperatively with a median transfusion of 2 units (1–18) for those transfused. Clavien-Dindo grade III to V complications occurred following 42 (24%) of 172 resections (Table 2). Eleven patients suffered both III and IV/V complications. One patient developed heart failure secondary to cardiac arrhythmia requiring cardiac pacing. There were no cases of postoperative respiratory failure. The proportion of patients suffering grade III–V complications in the selective and non-selective CPET periods was similar (22 and 27%, respectively).

Demographic details, ASA, CCI, use of pre-operative chemotherapy, CPET variables and the number of liver segments resected in patient groups with and without significant postoperative complications are shown in Table 3. In univariate analysis CCI score, but not ASA grade, was associated with grade III–V complications ($P = 0.02$). Of the CPET variables, $VEeqCO_2$ was associated with the development of grade III–V complications ($P = 0.005$). AT was not detectable in three patients due to very limited exercise tolerance, and none of whom suffered grade III–V complications. The number of liver segments resected was strongly associated with outcome (Fig. 2). The use of preoperative chemotherapy was not associated with postoperative complications.

Multivariate analysis of predictive scores and the extent of liver resection shows that the extent of resection, $VEqCO_2$ and CCI are independently associated with the development of grade III–V complications (Table 4). ASA grade was not associated with outcome. The strongest association with complications was shown to be with the extent of liver resection, where each extra segment of liver resected increased the odds of developing CD grade III–V complications by a factor of 2.94 (1.86–4.66). The greatest range of predictive values (17–50) was noted for $VEqCO_2$, where an incremental increase of 1.09 was noted in the OR of developing grade III–V complications.

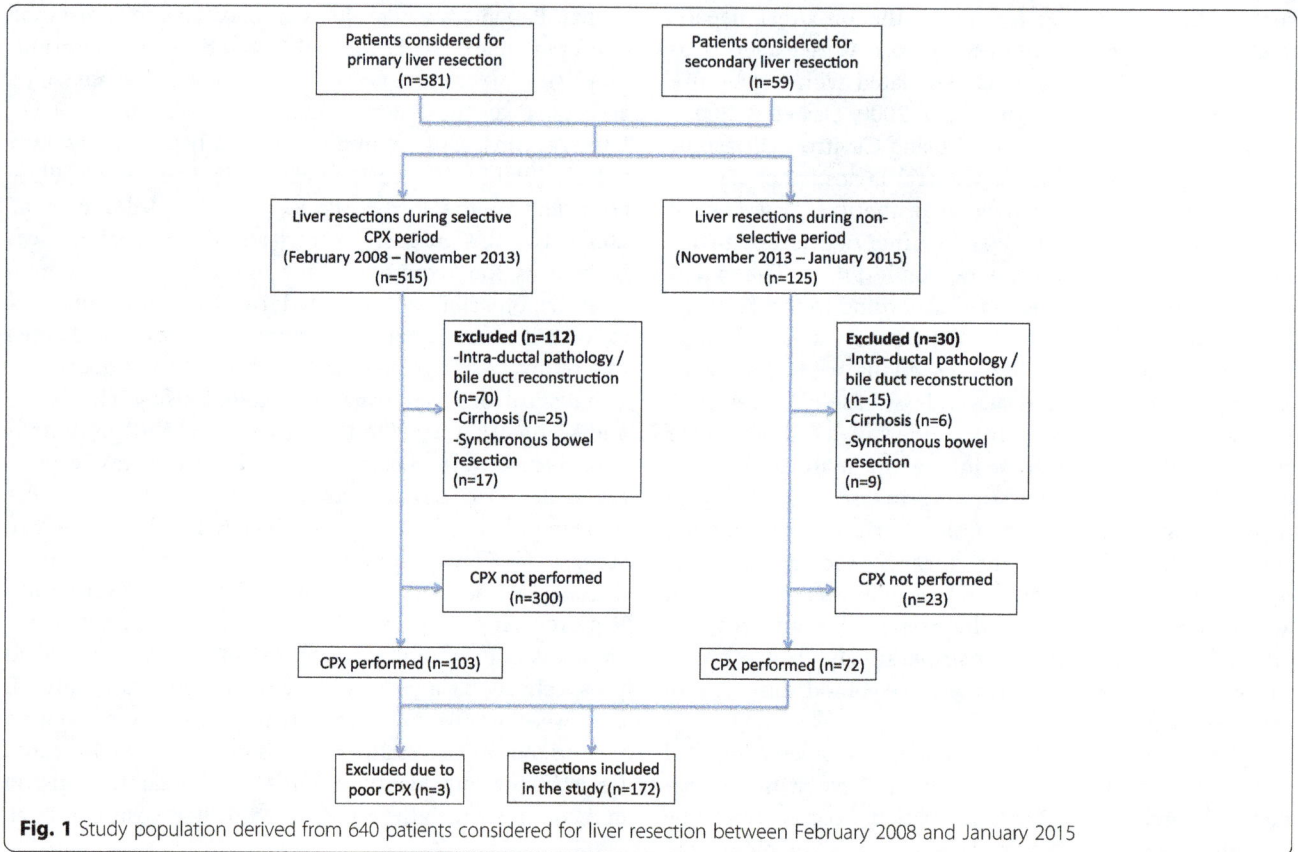

Fig. 1 Study population derived from 640 patients considered for liver resection between February 2008 and January 2015

Table 1 Baseline patient characteristics

Age (median [range])	69 (22–90)	CPET parameters	
Gender (%)			
Male	119 (69.2)	VO$_2$ at AT (ml/kg/min, [range])	12.5 (5.6–23.1)
Female	53 (30.8)		
Diagnosis (%)			
Colorectal metastases	134 (77.9)	VO$_{2 peak}$ (ml/kg/min, [range])	18.9 (6.4–35.5)
Hepatoma	12 (7)		11.8 (5–25.3)
Neuroendocrine tumour	6 (3.5)	Oxygen pulse (ml/beat, [range])	
Other	20 (11.6)		
ASA (%)			
I	8 (4.7)		14.9 (7.8–26.6)
II	93 (54.1)	Relative oxygen pulse (100 ml/beat/kg, [range])	
III	70 (40.7)		
IV	1 (0.6)		
CCI (median [range])	4 (0–9)	Resting heart rate (beats/min, [range])	77 (39–119)
Preoperative chemotherapy (%)		Peak heart rate (beats/min, [range])	132 (79–180)
Yes	62 (36)		29.6 (17.1–49.9)
No	94 (54.7)		
Unknown	16 (9.3)	VEeqCO$_2$ at AT (range)	
RFA used (%)			
Yes	11 (6.4)		
No	161 (93.6)		
Number of segments resected (%)			
1	46 (26.7)		
2	13 (7.6)		
3	14 (8.1)		
4	64 (37.2)		
5	31 (18)		
6	4 (2.3)		

Demographic and operative characteristics of 172 liver resections in 168 patients who had preoperative CPET
RFA radiofrequency ablation

Table 2 Summary of complications after liver resection

Grade III complications (%)	15 (8.6)
• Bile leak requiring ERCP	3 (1.7)
• Bile leak requiring drain	4 (2.3)
• Infected collection requiring drain	1 (0.6)
• Further surgery required	2 (1.1)
• Open drainage of collection following colonic injury,	
• Laparotomy undertaken for ileus	
• Pneumothorax requiring drain	1 (0.6)
• Cardiac pacing	1 (0.6)
• Ascites requiring drain	1 (0.6)
• Pleural effusion requiring drain	1 (0.6)
• Gastric burn secondary to radiofrequency ablation	1 (0.6)
Grade IV and V complications (%)	37 (21.3)
• Liver failure alone	24 (13.8)
• Renal failure alone	6 (3.4)
• Liver and renal failure	6 (3.4)
• Heart failure	2 (1.1)
• Death	2 (1.1)

Summary of Clavien-Dindo grade III–V postoperative complications following 172 liver resections in 168 patients. Some patients suffered more than one complication

Discussion

The main finding of this study is the very significant association between postoperative complications in liver surgery and the extent of the liver resection undertaken. There is a weaker association between postoperative complications and risk scores formulated by assessment of recorded comorbidity (CCI) and CPET parameters. Subjective assessment of a patient's fitness at the time of surgery by ASA score is not predictive of postoperative complications.

The scoring systems under assessment in this study were chosen because they assess risk by different techniques. CPET is an objective measure of cardiovascular fitness,

CCI scores are derived from recorded comorbidity, ASA grade is a subjective assessment of overall health and the number of liver segments resected provides a simple measure of operative extent. Assessment of the techniques in parallel allows a comparison of their relative utility.

The role of CPET in liver surgery is yet to be established, with conflicting outcomes from the two published studies investigating the technique (Junejo et al. 2012; Dunne et al. 2014). CPET is useful in surgery where cardiorespiratory complications form a major part of adverse outcomes, such as vascular (Thompson et al. 2011; Elkouri et al. 2004) and cardiothoracic (Van Diepen et al. 2014) surgery. As the main cause of morbidity and death after liver surgery is liver failure (Poon et al. 2004; Belghiti et al. 2000; Jarnagin et al. 2002), the degree of cardiovascular fitness is likely to have a weaker association with outcome. In our series, significant cardiovascular complications were rare, occurring in only two patients. Also, patients undergoing liver resection may be a selected group with better physical function, as many will have previously undergone, and recovered from, primary colorectal surgery. AT was originally shown to be useful in predicting mortality in a large, unselected population undergoing a range of elective abdominal procedures including vascular surgery, in which 24% of patients had evidence of pre-existing cardiovascular disease (Older et al. 1993), and mortality in this context is more likely to be related to cardiovascular health.

Table 3 Comparison of potential risk factors for developing complications

Variable (median)	CD 0–II ($n = 130$)	CD III–V ($n = 42$)	P value
Age (range)	69 (22–90)	70 (49–88)	0.47
Gender (%)			0.057
Male	85 (65.4)	34 (81)	
Female	45 (34.6)	8 (19)	
ASA (%)			0.187
I–II	80 (61.5)	21 (50)	
III–IV	50 (38.5)	21 (50)	
CCI (range)	4 (0–7)	5 (1–9)	0.021
Preoperative chemotherapy (%)			0.85
Yes	46 (35.4)	16 (38.1)	
No	71 (54.6)	23 (54.8)	
Unknown	13 (10)	3 (7.1)	
Number of segments resected (range)	3 (1–6)	4 (3–6)	< 0.001
VO_2 at AT (ml/kg/min, [range])	12.8 (6.4–22.9)	12.5 (5.6–23.1)	0.84
$VO_{2\ peak}$ (ml/kg/min, [range])	18.8 (6.4–35.5)	19.2 (11.8–30.8)	0.65
Oxygen pulse (ml/beat, [range])	11 (5–20.5)	12.3 (5–25.3)	0.39
Relative oxygen pulse (100 ml/beat/kg, [range])	15 (7.8–26.6)	14.9 (10–24.5)	0.52
Resting heart rate (beats/min, [range])	74 (39–115)	80 (43–119)	0.54
Peak heart rate (beats/min, [range])	131.5 (79–180)	133.5 (85–172)	0.89
$VEeqCO_2$ at AT (range)	29.1 (17.1–49.9)	31.7 (24.4–46.2)	0.005

Univariate analysis of association of age, gender, diagnosis, ASA grade, CCI, preoperative chemotherapy, extent of resection and CPET values with Clavien-Dindo 0–II and III–V complications following 172 liver resections

Of the CPET parameters under study, $VEqCO_2$ was shown to be predictive of postoperative complications, in keeping with earlier findings (Junejo et al. 2012). Although the incremental OR for predicting CD grade III–V complications is low (1.09), this effect is noted over a large range of values (17–50). Despite other studies demonstrating the value of AT in the prediction of outcomes after liver resection (Dunne et al. 2014), this parameter was not

shown to be of value in this series, although many of the CPET variables are mathematically related, and the difference in predictive value between them may be less than is apparent in a multivariate analysis. In a similar manner to CCI, the median $VEqCO_2$ was very similar between groups with CD grade 0–II and III–V complications (29.1 vs 31.7) with significant overlap in range, and this may limit the usefulness of this test. ASA was not shown to

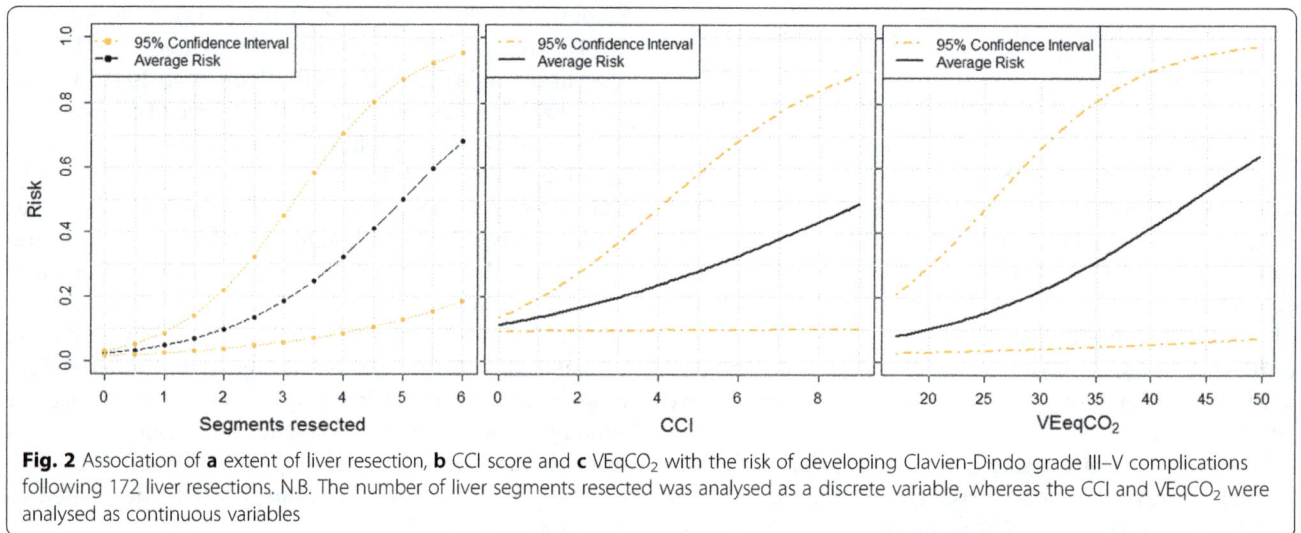

Fig. 2 Association of **a** extent of liver resection, **b** CCI score and **c** $VEqCO_2$ with the risk of developing Clavien-Dindo grade III–V complications following 172 liver resections. N.B. The number of liver segments resected was analysed as a discrete variable, whereas the CCI and $VEqCO_2$ were analysed as continuous variables

Table 4 Comparison of risk assessment techniques

	OR	95% CI	P value	Range of predictive values
ASA grade	0.85	0.37–1.94	0.7	1–4
CCI score	1.49	1.09–2.04	0.01	0–9
VEeqCO$_2$ at AT	1.09	1.01–1.17	0.04	17–50
Number of liver segments resected	2.94	1.86–4.66	< 0.001	1–6

Multivariate analysis of risk assessment techniques in the prediction of CD grade III–V complications compared with grade 0–II complications following 172 liver resections

predict outcome in multivariate analysis compared with the other measures. ASA is known to be a highly subjective tool, with significant inter-observer variation (Mak et al. 2002; Ranta et al. 1997). In practice, this is also too blunt a tool to be of value, as 95% of patients have ASA score of II or III.

The CCI is a well-researched measure used to weight outcomes in cancer surgery (Dobbins et al. 2015). The tool has also been used in registry data when comparing outcomes between individual hospitals (Dobbins et al. 2015) and clinicians (Ugolini and Nobilio 2004). Its role in predicting specific surgical complications is variable. It has not been shown to be associated with complications in gynaecologic or colorectal surgery (Suidan et al. 2015; Krarup et al. 2015), but is associated with outcome in orthopaedic surgery (Schmolders et al. 2015). While CCI is associated with complications in this study, it is less predictive of outcome over the range of measured values than either the number of liver segments resected or VEqCO$_2$ (Fig. 2). Although CCI provides a simple measure that can be easily calculated with knowledge of a patient's medical history, the median score of patients suffering grade III–V complications is only one point higher than those with grade 0–II complications, with a large overlap in the score range which limits the usefulness of the technique. Also, the CCI system records comorbidity rarely relevant in the context of elective liver surgery, including AIDS and lymphoma, while other more common potential risk factors, such as extremes of BMI (Vigano et al. 2011; Balzan et al. 2010) and NAFLD (Wakai et al. 2011), are not included.

The factor with the greatest predictive value for outcome in this analysis is the extent of the liver resection undertaken, which may be expected as liver failure due to insufficient liver volume is the major cause of death after liver surgery (Wiggans et al. 2013). The high odds ratio of 2.94 in the prediction of grade III–V complications for increasing number of resected segments make this a factor of high clinical relevance and easily utilised, as the extent of liver resection to be undertaken is usually known preoperatively. Of note, the increased risk of liver resection with increasing number of resected segments is non-

linear, with the largest absolute increase in risk being experienced by patients undergoing resection of five and six liver segments.

Each of the three techniques shown to be of value has very wide confidence intervals in the prediction of outcome (Fig. 2). The potential risk faced by patients undergoing liver surgery is affected by all of the factors under study (comorbidity, physical functioning and extent of liver resection), and each of the tests used individually therefore will be limited in their predictive value. Other factors are also likely to influence operative risk, particularly the presence of a coexisting liver disease. A useful area of further study would be to develop a compound risk scoring system based on all these factors.

The study may be subject to bias due to patient selection. Throughout the series, CPET has been undertaken on patients perceived to be less healthy, which accounts for the male predominance of the population under study. It is unlikely however that CPET parameters would be more predictive of complications in a healthier population. A potential limitation of this study is the degree of confounding caused by prior awareness of CPET results by clinicians, as it is possible that patients with low levels of fitness were treated differently. Preoperative medication which may affect CPET results has not been recorded. However, in undertaking CPET, it is important to estimate functional parameters as they would be at the time of surgery, including the influence of medication.

Conclusions

This study represents a large case-series, which attempts to answer the question of how best to assess risk in patients undergoing liver resection. The simplest factor to consider is the extent of the planned liver resection. CCI and CPET parameters may be useful discriminators for potential risk in patients undergoing the same resection type and may also contribute to decision-making in patients who require extended liver resections.

Abbreviations
AIDS: Acquired immunodeficiency syndrome; ASA: American Society of Anesthesiology; AT: Anaerobic threshold; BMI: Body mass index; CCI: Charlson Comorbidity Index; CD: Clavien-Dindo; CPET: Cardiopulmonary Exercise Testing; HR: Heart rate; NAFLD: Non-alcoholic fatty liver disease; O$_2$: Oxygen; PHLF: Post-hepatectomy liver failure; RFA: Radiofrequency ablation; VEeqCO$_2$: Ventilatory efficiency in the elimination of carbon dioxide; VO$_2$ peak: Volume of oxygen consumption at peak

Acknowledgements
None.

Funding
None.

Authors' contributions

SU is responsible for the study design, data collection and interpretation and manuscript preparation. GS contributed to the data interpretation, production of Fig. 2 and review of the statistical methods. SA, MJB, CDB and MGW took part in the data collection. GM did the setup of the CPET service and helped with the CPET data collection and interpretation. DAS contributed to the study design, data collection and interpretation and manuscript preparation. All authors read and approved the final manuscript.

Competing interests

The authors declare that they have no competing interests.

Author details

¹Derriford Hospital, Plymouth PL6 8DH, UK. ²Peninsula Schools of Medicine and Dentistry, Plymouth University, Plymouth PL6 8BU, UK. ³Nottingham Trent University, Nottingham NG1 4BU, UK.

References

Backemar L, et al. Comorbidities and risk of complications after surgery for esophageal cancer: a Nationwide cohort study in Sweden. World J Surg. 2015;39:2282–8.

Balzan S, et al. Safety of liver resections in obese and overweight patients. World J Surg. 2010;34:2960–8.

Belghiti J, et al. Seven hundred forty-seven hepatectomies in the 1990s: an update to evaluate the actual risk of liver resection. J Am Coll Surg. 2000;191:38–46.

Bellomo R, et al. Acute renal failure: the second international consensus conference of the acute dialysis quality initiative (ADQI) group. Crit Care. 2004;8:R204–12.

Challand C, et al. Randomized controlled trial of intraoperative goal-directed fluid therapy in aerobically fit and unfit patients having major colorectal surgery. Br J Anaesth. 2012;108:53–62.

Chandrabalan VV, et al. Pre-operative cardiopulmonary exercise testing predicts adverse post-operative events and non-progression to adjuvant therapy after major pancreatic surgery. HPB (Oxford). 2013;15:899–907.

Charlson ME, et al. A new method of classifying prognostic comorbidity in longitudinal studies: development and validation. J Chronic Dis. 1987;40:373–83.

Das BC, et al. Analysis of 100 consecutive hepatectomies: risk factors in patients with liver cirrhosis or obstructive jaundice. World J Surg. 2001;25:266–72. discussion 72-3

Dimick JB, et al. National trends in the use and outcomes of hepatic resection. J Am Coll Surg. 2004;199:31–8.

Dindo D, et al. Classification of surgical complications: a new proposal with evaluation in a cohort of 6336 patients and results of a survey. Ann Surg. 2004;240:205–13.

Dobbins TA, et al. Assessing measures of comorbidity and functional status for risk adjustment to compare hospital performance for colorectal cancer surgery: a retrospective data-linkage study. BMC Med Inform Decis Mak. 2015;15:55.

Dunne DF, et al. Cardiopulmonary exercise testing before liver surgery. J Surg Oncol. 2014;110:439–44.

Elkouri S, et al. Perioperative complications and early outcome after endovascular and open surgical repair of abdominal aortic aneurysms. J Vasc Surg. 2004;39:497–505.

Jarnagin WR, et al. Improvement in perioperative outcome after hepatic resection: analysis of 1,803 consecutive cases over the past decade. Ann Surg. 2002;236:397–406. discussion -7

Junejo MA, et al. Cardiopulmonary exercise testing for preoperative risk assessment before hepatic resection. Br J Surg. 2012;99:1097–104.

Krarup PM, et al. Association of Comorbidity with Anastomotic leak, 30-day mortality, and length of stay in elective surgery for colonic cancer: a Nationwide cohort study. Dis Colon rectum. 2015;58:668–76.

Lai CW, et al. Patients' inability to perform a preoperative cardiopulmonary exercise test or demonstrate an anaerobic threshold is associated with inferior outcomes after major colorectal surgery. Br J Anaesth. 2013;111:607–11.

Mak PH, et al. The ASA physical status classification: inter-observer consistency. American Society of Anesthesiologists. Anaesth Intensive Care. 2002;30:633–40.

Nygard IE, et al. Mortality and survival rates after elective hepatic surgery in a low-volume centre are comparable to those of high-volume centres. ISRN Surgery. 2012;2012:783932.

Older P, et al. Preoperative evaluation of cardiac failure and ischemia in elderly patients by cardiopulmonary exercise testing. Chest. 1993;104:701–4.

Pang YY. The Brisbane 2000 terminology of liver anatomy and resections. HPB 2000; 2:333–39. HPB (Oxford). 2002;4(2):99.

Poon RT, et al. Improving perioperative outcome expands the role of hepatectomy in management of benign and malignant hepatobiliary diseases: analysis of 1222 consecutive patients from a prospective database. Ann Surg. 2004;240:698–708.

Rahbari NN, et al. Posthepatectomy liver failure: a definition and grading by the international study Group of Liver Surgery (ISGLS). Surgery. 2011;149:713–24.

Ranta S, et al. A survey of the ASA physical status classification: significant variation in allocation among Finnish anaesthesiologists. Acta Anaesthesiol Scand. 1997;41:629–32.

Research Registry. editor^, editors " City. http://www.researchregistry.com/.

Saklad M. Grading of patients for surgical procedures. Anesthesiology. 1941;2:281–4.

Schmolders J, et al. Validation of the Charlson comorbidity index in patients undergoing revision total hip arthroplasty. Int Orthop. 2015;39:1771–7.

Schroeder RA, et al. Predictive indices of morbidity and mortality after liver resection. Ann Surg. 2006;243:373–9.

Suidan RS, et al. Predictive value of the age-adjusted Charlson Comorbidity index on perioperative complications and survival in patients undergoing primary debulking surgery for advanced epithelial ovarian cancer. Gynecol Oncol. 2015;138:246–51.

Thompson AR, et al. Cardiopulmonary exercise testing provides a predictive tool for early and late outcomes in abdominal aortic aneurysm patients. Ann R Coll Surg Engl. 2011;93:474–81.

Ugolini C, Nobilio L. Risk adjustment for coronary artery bypass graft surgery: an administrative approach versus EuroSCORE. Int J Qual Health Care. 2004;16:157–64.

Ulyett S, et al. Clinical assessment prior to hepatectomy identifies high-risk patients. J Surg Res. 2015;198:87–92.

Van Diepen S, et al. Predicting cardiovascular intensive care unit readmission after cardiac surgery: derivation and validation of the Alberta provincial project for outcomes assessment in coronary heart disease (APPROACH) cardiovascular intensive care unit clinical prediction model from a registry cohort of 10,799 surgical cases. Crit Care. 2014;18:651.

Vigano L, et al. Liver resection in obese patients: results of a case-control study. HPB (Oxford). 2011;13:103–11.

von Elm E, et al. The strengthening the reporting of observational studies in epidemiology (STROBE) statement: guidelines for reporting observational studies. J Clin Epidemiol. 2008;61:344–9.

Wakai T, et al. Surgical outcomes for hepatocellular carcinoma in nonalcoholic fatty liver disease. J. Gastrointest. Surg. 2011;15:1450–8.

Wiggans MG, et al. Renal dysfunction is an independent risk factor for mortality after liver resection and the main determinant of outcome in posthepatectomy liver failure. HPB Surg. 2013;2013:875367.

Wiggans MG, et al. The interaction between diabetes, body mass index, hepatic Steatosis, and risk of liver resection: insulin dependent diabetes is the greatest risk for major complications. HPB Surg. 2014;2014:586159.

Association of postoperative nausea/vomiting and pain with breastfeeding success

Ramon Abola*⑩, Jamie Romeiser, Suman Grewal, Sabeen Rizwan, Rishimani Adsumelli, Ellen Steinberg and Elliott Bennett-Guerrero

Abstract

Background: Successful breastfeeding is a goal set forth by the World Health Organization to improve neonatal care. Increasingly, patients express the desire to breastfeed, and clinicians should facilitate successful breastfeeding. The primary aim of this study is to determine if postoperative nausea and vomiting (PONV) or postoperative pain are associated with decreased breastfeeding success after cesarean delivery.

Methods: This is a historical cohort study using the Stony Brook Elective Cesarean Delivery Database. Self-reported breastfeeding success at 4 weeks postoperative was analyzed for associations with postoperative antiemetic use and postoperative pain scores. Breastfeeding success was also analyzed for associations with patient factors and anesthetic medications.

Results: Overall, 86% of patients (n = 81) who intended on breastfeeding reported breastfeeding success. Breastfeeding success was not associated with postoperative nausea or vomiting as measured by post anesthesia care unit antiemetic use (15% use in successful vs. 18% use in unsuccessful, p = 0.67) or 48-h antiemetic use (28% use in successful group vs 36% use in unsuccessful group, p = 0.732). Pain visual analog scale scores at 6, 12 and 24 h postoperatively were not significantly different between patients with or without breastfeeding success. Breastfeeding success was associated with having had at least 1 previous child (86% vs 36%, p < 0.001). Patients with asthma were less likely to have breastfeeding success (45% vs 4%, p = 0.002).

Conclusions: Efforts to improve PONV and pain after cesarean delivery may not be effective in improving breastfeeding success. To possibly improve breastfeeding rates, resources should be directed toward patients with no previous children and patients with asthma.

Keywords: Breastfeeding, Postoperative pain, Postoperative nausea and vomiting (PONV), Prelabor cesarean delivery

Background

Successful breastfeeding is a goal set forth by the World Health Organization to improve neonatal care (WHO, 2011). The American Academy of Pediatrics (AAP) recommends that children are exclusively breastfed for the first six months of life (So, 2012). Increasingly, patients express the desire to breastfeed, and clinicians should facilitate successful breastfeeding. Previous studies have reported that cesarean deliveries were associated with a lower breastfeeding rate compared to vaginal deliveries (Prior et al., 2012). This is important because cesarean delivery rates have steadily increased over the past three decades in the United States. Most recently, the Centers for Disease Control reported a cesarean delivery rate of 32.2% in the United States (Osterman & Martin, 2014).

After cesarean delivery, routine postoperative care can delay maternal bonding with the infant. A delay in initial breastfeeding has been associated with less successful breastfeeding (Lin et al., 2011; Wallwiener et al., 2016). Our primary objective was to determine if postoperative nausea and vomiting (PONV) after cesarean delivery is

* Correspondence: Ramon.abola@stonybrookmedicine.edu
Stony Brook Medicine, Department of Anesthesiology, HSC-4-060, Stony Brook, NY 11794, USA

negatively associated with breastfeeding success. We also evaluated if postoperative pain affects breastfeeding success. We hypothesized that patients who had more PONV and pain would be less successful at breastfeeding.

Methods

After institutional and ethics approval, a registry was created for patients who presented for prelabor (elective or scheduled) cesarean delivery. Information collected included patient demographics and comorbidities, indications for cesarean delivery, intraoperative management and postoperative outcomes including length of stay, pain scores and use of antiemetics. Patients were contacted by telephone 4 weeks after delivery in order to complete a brief telephone survey. Two questions related to breastfeeding were asked: 1. Did you intend on breastfeeding? 2. Were you successful with breastfeeding? Successful breastfeeding was subjectively defined by each individual patient.

At our institution, patients who present for elective/scheduled cesarean delivery typically receive a spinal anesthetic with bupivacaine (12 mg), fentanyl (10 mcg) and morphine (0.2 mg). A phenylephrine infusion and a fluid bolus of lactated ringer's are used to decrease the incidence of spinal hypotension. Antiemetics and supplemental intravenous analgesics or sedatives are given as needed. After delivery, patients receive an infusion of oxytocin (20 units over 1 h and then 5 units/h for 4 h). In our post anesthesia care unit (PACU), patients can receive ketorolac (30 mg) for postoperative pain. The postoperative analgesia regimen includes intrathecal morphine from the spinal anesthetic, oral acetaminophen, oral ibuprophen and oxycodone as needed.

The data were collected prospectively by anesthesia providers and entered into a Microsoft Access database. This project was authorized by the Stony Brook Medicine Division of Medical and Regulatory Affairs Office as part of the Surgical Quality Improvement Program (SQIP). Following de-identification and extraction of all SQIP patient records, a data analysis was performed as part of the Surgical Quality Data Users Group (SQDUG). The SQIP/SQDUG protocols were approved by our institution's investigational review board (Committees on Research Involving Human Subjects [CORIHS] #170753-9 – Stony Brook University).

Fisher's exact tests and Wilcox rank sum tests were used to examine association between breastfeeding success and the following variables: comorbidities, ASA classification, intraoperative sedative and analgesic medications, PACU antiemetics, 48 h antiemetics, parity, and Visual analog scale (VAS) score at 6, 12 and 24 h after surgery. All calculations were performed at an alpha of 0.05 using SAS 9.4 Software © (SAS Institute Inc., Cary, NC).

Results

Information was collected for 391 patients who presented to Stony Brook University Medical Center between October 2013 and September 2014 for elective or scheduled cesarean delivery. Overall, 132 patients completed a post-discharge telephone survey 4 weeks after surgery (34% survey completion). Ninety-four surveyed patients (71%) stated that they intended to breastfeed. Further analysis was performed on this cohort who intended to breastfeed. Eighty one patients (86%) reported successful breastfeeding and 11 patients (11%) reported they were unsuccessful with breastfeeding; two did not report on their success (2%).

With regard to our primary objective, breastfeeding success was not associated with PONV. Breastfeeding success was not associated with PACU antiemetic use (15% use in successful vs. 18% use in unsuccessful, $p = 0.67$). Breastfeeding success was not found to be associated with 48-h antiemetic use (28% use in successful vs. 36% use in unsuccessful, $p = 0.73$, Table 1). Pain visual analog scale scores (VAS) at 6, 12 and 24 h postop were not significantly different between patients with or without breastfeeding success (Table 2).

Breastfeeding success was positively associated with having previous children: 86% of those who reported success had at least one previous child; just 36% of those who were unsuccessful had at least one previous child ($p < 0.001$). Patient comorbidities had a negative affect: 91% of those who were not successful had some type of co-morbidity. This proportion was significantly lower (51%) in those who reported success ($p = 0.02$). Specifically, a higher proportion of those who reported unsuccessful breastfeeding were asthmatic (46% vs. 6%, $p = 0.002$). Diabetes also trended toward significance in this direction. Breastfeeding success was not found to be associated with ASA score, or need for intraoperative sedative or analgesic medication ($p = 1$). However, there was a difference in anesthetic technique; a higher proportion of those who reported unsuccessful breast feeding had a combined spinal/epidural compared to those who reported successful breast feeding (27% vs. 1%, $p = 0.005$).

Surveyed patients were compared to non-surveyed patients ($n = 259$) for differences in demographics, pre and post -operative information. Aside from having a lower ASA score in the surveyed group, there were no discernible differences (not shown).

Discussion

Our analysis found no association between breastfeeding success and PONV or postoperative pain scores. We hypothesized that a better recovery profile would

Table 1 Breastfeeding success and antiemetic use, demographics, comorbidities, and delivery characteristics

Patient Characteristics	Unsuccessful Breastfeeding	Successful Breastfeeding	p value
Total Number of Patients	n = 11	n = 81	
Antiemetic Use			
PACU Antiemetics	2 (18.2%)	12 (14.8%)	0.67
48 Hour Antiemetics	4 (36.4%)	23 (28.4%)	0.73
Demographics			
Age (Years) - Median (IQR)	33 (28 - 34)	33 (28 - 36)	0.66
Height (cm) - Median (IQR)	160 (157 - 165)	162 (157 - 167)	0.44
Weight (kg) - Median (IQR)	93 (70- 100)	84.5 (74 - 94.5)	0.68
BMI (kg/m^2) - Median (IQR)	35.4 (27.1, 39.6)	32 (28.3 - 36)	0.53
Ethnicity (Caucasian vs. Non)	7 (63.6%)	53 (65.4%)	1
Parity (≥1)	4 (36.4%)	70 (86.4%)	<0.001
ASA Classification			
- ASA I	2 (18.2%)	32 (39.5%)	0.32
- ASA II	8 (72.7%)	45 (55.6%)	
- ASA III	1 (9.1%)	4 (4.9%)	
Gestational Age (Weeks) - Median (IQR)	39 (38 - 39)	39 (39 - 39.2)	0.07
Comorbidities			
Any Co-Morbidity	10 (90.9%)	41 (50.6%)	0.02
History of PONV	0 (0%)	13 (16.5%)	0.35
Diabetes	3 (27.3%)	6 (7.4%)	0.07
Asthma	5 (45.5%)	5 (6.2%)	0.002
Other Condition	4 (36.4%)	31 (38.3%)	1
Delivery Characteristics			
Indications for cesarean delivery			
Repeat Cesarean	4 (36.4%)	60 (75.0%)	0.01
Malpresentation	1 (9.1%)	10 (12.7%)	1
Macrosomia	2 (18.2%)	2 (2.5%)	0.07
Multiple gestation	1 (9.1%)	4 (5.0%)	0.48
Anesthetic technique			
- Spinal	8 (72.7%)	80 (98.8%)	0.005
- Combined Spinal Epidural	3 (27.3%)	1 (1.2%)	
Any Intraoperative Sedatives or Analgesics	2 (18.2%)	19 (23.5%)	1
Any Intraoperative Antiemetics	6 (54.6%)	50 (63.3%)	0.74

Table 2 Breastfeeding success and visual analog scale (VAS) pain scores

	Unsuccessful Breastfeeding	Successful Breastfeeding	P-value, Wilcox rank sum test
VAS 6 Hours	n = 10	n = 73	
Median (Q1/Q3)	1.5 (0/4)	3 (0/4)	0.56
Mean (Upper/Lower 95%)	2.0 (0.7-3.4)	2.73 (2.1-3.3)	
VAS 12 Hours	n = 9	n = 75	
Median (Q1/Q3)	1 (0/1)	2 (0/5)	0.39
Mean (Upper/Lower 95%)	1.6 (0-3.3)	2.6 (1.9-3.2)	
VAS 24 h	n = 10	n = 80	
Mean (Upper/Lower 95%)	4.5 (2/6)	3 (1/5)	0.31
Median (Q1/Q3)	4.1 (2.2-6.1)	3.2 (2.6-3.8)	

facilitate success at breastfeeding and that PONV and pain might make women more likely to give up trying to breastfeed. A previously published survey study demonstrated that mothers with increased pain after cesarean delivery had increased problems with breastfeeding (Karlstrom et al., 2007). We could find no data in the medical literature that correlated breastfeeding success with maternal PONV.

Our study found that mothers with previous children were more likely to be successful at breastfeeding, which is consistent with prior studies (Sutherland et al., 2012). It is interesting to note that mothers with asthma were much more likely to be unsuccessful at breastfeeding. It is unclear from our study if asthma causes a physical limitation that affects breastfeeding, or if asthma is a surrogate for demographic differences such as tobacco abuse or lower socioeconomic status. Lower socioeconomic status has been associated with lower breastfeeding rates (Brand et al., 2011). Future research should evaluate if improving breastfeeding rates in asthmatic mothers results in improved long-term outcomes for their children. A meta-analysis found that breastfeeding was associated with decreased incidence of asthma in children (Dogaru et al., 2014). Targeting breastfeeding resources toward first time mothers and asthmatic mothers may increase rates of breastfeeding success.

There are a limited number of studies that have looked at the effects of neuraxial anesthesia during childbirth on breastfeeding. Previous studies have suggested that epidural analgesia in labor is associated with lower breastfeeding rates (Baumgarner et al., 2003; Torvaldsen et al., 2006). However, a study by Halpern drew opposite conclusions demonstrating high breastfeeding rates in both patients who received or did receive labor epidural analgesia (Halpern et al., 1999). A systematic review found inconclusive evidence within the medical literature to determine the effect of epidural analgesia on breastfeeding (French et al., 2016).

A systematic review of breastfeeding worldwide reported a lower rate of breastfeeding in patients who had a cesarean versus a vaginal delivery (pooled odds ratio: 0.57 l 95% CI 0.50, 0.64, P, 0.00001). The rates of breastfeeding were also lower in patients who had a pre-labor (elective/scheduled) cesarean delivery versus an emergency, in-labor cesarean delivery (prelabor odds ratio: 0.83, 95% CI 0.80, 0.86, P, 0.00001, in labor odds ratio: 1.00, 95% CI 0.97, 1.04; $P = 0.86$) (Prior et al., 2012). The authors of this review speculated on several possible reasons for these findings. The first hours after delivery are important to establish breastfeeding between a mother and neonate. Postoperative evaluations and interventions may impede the creation of this bond between mother and child. Another idea is that there may be hormones released in labor that promote breastfeeding that are not released in prelabor cesarean delivery patients. However, these authors also observed that there were no differences at 6 months between vaginal delivery and cesarean delivery in the patients who had successful early breastfeeding (Thompson et al., 2010). Patients with greater blood loss due to postpartum hemorrhage were less likely to initiate and sustain full breastfeeding. There is speculation that less successful breastfeeding in these patients may be related to delays in initial contact/bonding between mother and child.

The World Health Organization reports that the exclusive breastfeeding rate at 6 months of life for newborns worldwide is 40%. (Global breastfeeding scorecard, 2017) In the United States, two thirds of mothers breastfed in the 1900s. Breastfeeding rates declined over the twentieth century reaching a nadir in 1972 with breastfeeding rates of 22%. Factors that are associated with the declining rates of breastfeeding include the increased use of breast milk substitutes, the need to return to work away from their babies, and lack of family support (Global breastfeeding scorecard, 2017; Raffle et al., 2011; Wolf, 2003). Breastfeeding rates have increased over the last few decades (Wolf, 2003).

Our high level of breastfeeding success may have little to do with the anesthetic management and may be more reflective of institutional policies that encourage breastfeeding. Our institution has worked toward earning a "Baby-Friendly" designation by instituting the AAP's *Ten Steps to Successful Breastfeeding* (So, 2012). Examples of these practices at our hospital include breastfeeding in the PACU after cesarean delivery, mothers and infants "room in" remaining together 24 h a day, pacifiers are not provided to the infants, postpartum lactation consultant services are available, and breastfeeding training is completed by all nursing staff. 32% of mothers at our institution exclusively breastfed during their hospital admission in 2012. Three years later, the exclusive breastfeeding rate increased to 56% of mothers in 2015. Implementation of these breastfeeding policies has allowed for consistently high rates of breastfeeding over time at other institutions (Philipp et al., 2003).

There are several limitations of this study. This is an historical cohort study and is thus subject to bias. Our breastfeeding analysis was performed in only 94 patients with completed survey data. Inclusion of more patients may have influenced our findings. Inclusion of more patients may have influenced our findings. We performed a sample size calculation that asked how many patients we would have needed in our study to obtain statistical significance with regard to breastfeeding, antiemetic use and pain scores. We calculated that we would have needed 3000 patients to detect a statistically significant difference in antiemetic use and breastfeeding success, and approximately 500-800 patients to detect a significant difference in pain score and breastfeeding success. We cannot rule out there being some association, however, these large required sample sizes suggest that any effect is probably small, given the large number of patients likely needed.

We used antiemetics as a well-established surrogate measure of PONV, however, it is possible that some patients may have had nausea but did not receive antiemetics (Myles & Wengritzky, 2012). Our definition of breastfeeding was subjective for each individual patient. We chose a subjective definition of breastfeeding success, as there is variability to what constitutes success between patients. Breastfeeding success could be defined as 1. successful breastfeed with formula supplementation (complementary feeding), 2. breastfeeding for 6 weeks until return to work, or 3. exclusive breastfeeding for 6 months. More objective measures (breastfeeding initiation, exclusive breastfeeding, breastfeeding at 6 months) may have provided more clinically meaningful information. Further investigation into the reasons as to why 29% of our patients did not intend to breastfeed may provide better insight into how to improve exclusive breastfeeding rates.

Conclusions
Breastfeeding success was not found to be associated with postoperative nausea and vomiting or postoperative pain. Efforts to improve PONV and pain after cesarean delivery may not be effective in increasing rates of breastfeeding success. To possibly improve breastfeeding rates, resources should be directed toward patients with no previous children and patients with asthma.

Abbreviations
AAP: American Academy of Pediatrics; PACU: Post anesthesia care unit; PONV: Postoperative nausea and vomiting; SQDUG: Surgical quality data use group; SQIP: Surgical quality improvement program; VAS: Visual Analog Scale

Acknowledgements
Not applicable

Funding
Funding for this project was provided by the Stony Brook Department of Anesthesiology.

Authors' contributions

RA (corresponding) was project coordinator, analyzed and interpreted the patient data and was in charge of the manuscript. JR was our statistician and created our database. SG, SR were the administrators of the database. RA, ES were involved in development of this project. EBG was involved in analysis and interpretation of patient data and manuscript preparation. All authors read and approved the final manuscript.

Competing interests

The authors declare that they have no competing interests.

References

Baumgarner DJ, Muehl P, Fischer M, Pribbenow B. Effect of labor epidural anesthesia on breast feeding of healthy full term newborns delivered vaginally. J Am Board Fam Pract. 2003;16:7–13.

Brand E, Kothari C, Stark MA. Factors related to breastfeeding discontinuation between hospital discharge and 2 weeks postpartum. J Perinat Educ. 2011; 20(1):36–44.

Dogaru CM, Nyffenegger D, Pescatore AM, Spycher BD, Kuehni CE. Breastfeeding and childhood asthma: systematic review and meta-analysis. Am J Epidemiol. 2014;179(10):1153–67.

French CA, Cong X, Chung KS. Labor epidural analgesia and breastfeeding: a systematic review. J Hum Lact. 2016;32(3):507–20.

Halpern SH, Levine T, Wilson DB, MacDonnell J, Katsiris SE, Leighton BL. Effect of labor analgesia of breastfeeding success. Birth. 1999;26(2):83–8.

Karlstrom A, Engstrom-Olofsson R, Norbergh KG, Sjoling M, Hildingsson I. Postoperative pain after cesarean birth affects breastfeeding and infant care. J Obstet Gynecol Neonatal Nurs. 2007;36(5):430–40.

Lin SY, Lee JT, Yang CC, Gau ML. Factors related to milk supply perception in women who underwent cesarean section. J Nurs Res. 2011;19(2):94–101.

Myles PS, Wengritzky R. Simplified postoperative nausea and vomiting impact scale for audit and post-discharge review. Br J Anaesth. 2012;108(3):423–9.

Osterman MJ, Martin JA. Trends in low-risk cesarean delivery in the United States, 1990-2013. National Vital Statistics Reports. 2014;63(6):1–16.

Philipp BL, Malone KL, Cimo S, Merewood A. Sustained breastfeeding rates at a US baby-friendly hospital. Pediatrics. 2003;112:e234–6.

Prior E, Santhakumaran S, Gale C, Philipps LH, Modi N, Hyde MJ. Breastfeeding after cesarean delivery: a systematic review and meta-analysis of world literature. Am J Clin Nutr. 2012;95(5):1113–35.

Raffle H, Ware LJ, Borchardt A, STrickland H. Factors that influence breastfeeding initiation and persistence in Ohio's Appalachian region. Athens: Boinovich School of Leadership and Public Affairs at Ohio University; 2011.

So B. Breastfeeding and the use of human milk. Pediatrics. 2012;129(3):e827–41.

Sutherland T, Pierce CB, Blomquist JL, Handa VL. Breastfeeding practices among first-time mothers and across multiple pregnancies. Matern Child Health J. 2012;16(8):1665–71.

Thompson JF, Heal LJ, Roberts CL, Ellwood DA. Women's breastfeeding experiences following a significant primary postpartum haemorrhage: a multicentre cohort study. Int Breastfeed J. 2010;5:5.

Torvaldsen S, Roberts CL, Simpson JM, Thompson JF, Ellwood DA. Intrapartum epidural analgesia and breastfeeding: a prospective cohort study. Int Breastfeed J. 2006;1:24.

Wallwiener S, Muller M, Doster A, Plewniok K, Wallwiener CW, Fluhr H, et al. Predictors of impaired breastfeeding initiation and maintenance in a diverse sample: what is important? Arch Gynecol Obstet. 2016;294(3):455–66.

WHO. Exclusive breastfeeding for six months best for babies everywhere. 2011 [Available from: http://www.who.int/mediacentre/news/statements/2011/breastfeeding_20110115/en/. Accessed 1 Oct 2017.

WHO. Global breastfeeding scorecard, 2017. Switzerland: Tracking Progress for Breastfeeding Policies and Programmes Geneve; 2017. [Available from: http://www.who.int/nutrition/publications/infantfeeding/global-bf-scorecard-2017.pdf?ua=1. Accessed 1 Oct 2017.

Wolf JH. Low breastfeeding rates and public health in the United States. Am J of Public Health. 2003;93(12):2000–10.

Intraoperative oxygenation in adult patients undergoing surgery (iOPS): a retrospective observational study across 29 UK hospitals

Clare M. Morkane[1†], Helen McKenna[1†], Andrew F. Cumpstey[2†], Alex H. Oldman[3], Michael P. W. Grocott[2], Daniel S. Martin[1*] and Pan London Perioperative Audit and Research Network (PLAN) South Coast Perioperative Audit and Research Collaboration (SPARC)

Abstract

Background: Considerable controversy remains about how much oxygen patients should receive during surgery. The 2016 World Health Organization (WHO) guidelines recommend that intubated patients receive a fractional inspired oxygen concentration (FIO_2) of 0.8 throughout abdominal surgery to reduce the risk of surgical site infection. However, this recommendation has been widely criticised by anaesthetists and evidence from other clinical contexts has suggested that giving a high concentration of oxygen might worsen patient outcomes. This retrospective multi-centre observational study aimed to ascertain intraoperative oxygen administration practice by anaesthetists across parts of the UK.

Methods: Patients undergoing general anaesthesia with an arterial catheter in situ across hospitals affiliated with two anaesthetic trainee audit networks (PLAN, SPARC) were eligible for inclusion unless undergoing cardiopulmonary bypass. Demographic and intraoperative oxygenation data, haemoglobin saturation and positive end-expiratory pressure were retrieved from anaesthetic charts and arterial blood gases (ABGs) over five consecutive weekdays in April and May 2017.

Results: Three hundred seventy-eight patients from 29 hospitals were included. Median age was 66 years, 205 (54.2%) were male and median ASA grade was 3. One hundred eight (28.6%) were emergency cases. An anticipated difficult airway or raised BMI was documented preoperatively in 31 (8.2%) and 45 (11.9%) respectively. Respiratory or cardiac comorbidity was documented in 103 (27%) and 83 (22%) respectively. SpO_2 < 96% was documented in 83 (22%) patients, with 7 (1.9%) patients desaturating < 88% at any point intraoperatively. The intraoperative FIO_2 ranged from 0.25 to 1.0, and median PaO_2/FIO_2 ratios for the first four arterial blood gases taken in each case were 24.6/0.5, 23.4/0.49, 25.7/0.46 and 25.4/0.47 respectively.

Conclusions: Intraoperative oxygenation currently varies widely. An intraoperative FIO_2 of 0.5 currently represents standard intraoperative practice in the UK, with surgical patients often experiencing moderate levels of hyperoxaemia. This differs from both WHO's recommendation of using an FIO_2 of 0.8 intraoperatively, and also, the value most previous interventional oxygen therapy trials have used to represent standard care (typically $FIO_2 = 0.3$). These findings should be used to aid the design of future intraoperative oxygen studies.

Keywords: Hyperoxia, Oxygen, Surgical procedures, Operative

* Correspondence: daniel.martin@ucl.ac.uk
†Clare M. Morkane, Helen McKenna and Andrew F. Cumpstey contributed equally to this work.
[1]Division of Surgery and Interventional Science (University College London) and Royal Free Perioperative Research Group, Department of Anaesthesia, Royal Free Hospital, 3rd Floor, Pond Street, London NW3 2QG, UK
Full list of author information is available at the end of the article

Background

Approximately 3 million patients undergo general anaesthesia in the UK each year and are routinely given supplemental oxygen as part of this procedure (Sury et al. 2014). This makes oxygen one of the most commonly used drugs during surgery, yet there still remains considerable uncertainty about how much oxygen patients should receive during the perioperative period. In November 2016, the World Health Organization (WHO) recommended that all intubated patients receive a fractional inspired oxygen concentration (FIO_2) of 0.8 throughout surgery and for up to 6 h in recovery, as this might reduce patients' risk of developing a surgical site infection (SSI) later (Allegranzi et al. 2016). However, this recommendation has already been widely criticised by anaesthetists (Ball et al. 2017; Myles and Kurz 2017), and a Cochrane systematic review and meta-analysis of 28 trials published in 2015 concluded that robust evidence is lacking for a beneficial effect of using a high FIO_2 to reduce SSIs (Wetterslev et al. 2015). In fact, this meta-analysis suggested using a high FIO_2 during surgery could increase the risk of adverse events, including mortality, after long-term findings of the PROXI study (the largest study included in this review) reported significantly higher 2-year mortality rate in patients with abdominal malignancy who received an FIO_2 of 0.8 (Wetterslev et al. 2015; Meyhoff et al. 2012).

WHO's recommendations would also appear to contradict the consensus opinion in other clinical contexts; concerns have been raised about potential harms associated with hyperoxaemia (defined by others as an arterial oxygen partial pressure (PaO_2) > 13.3 kPa or 100 mmHg (Damiani et al. 2014a)) after myocardial infarction, after cardiac arrest and also in critical illness (Farquhar et al. 2009; Damiani et al. Dell'Anna et al. 2014). Within 15–30 min of onset, FiO_2 0.8–1.0 has also been demonstrated to induce atelectasis (Edmark et al. 2003), systemic vasoconstriction (Reinhart et al. 1991), coronary vasoconstriction (McNulty et al. 2005) and (within hours) pulmonary inflammation as well (Davis et al. 1983). Furthermore, chemical free radicals generated from oxygen (known as reactive oxygen species, ROS) can also avidly oxidise proteins, lipids or DNA resulting in cellular oxidative stress—an integral part of the normal surgical stress response that may also be associated with the development of multiple post-operative complications (Kücükakin et al. 2009). A large meta-analysis of over 16,000 patients concluded that high-quality evidence now shows liberal oxygen therapy in acutely ill adults increases mortality without improving other patient-important outcomes, suggesting that supplemental oxygen administration might become unfavourable above an SpO_2 range of 94–98% (Chu et al. 2018).

Currently, there is limited data describing the intraoperative oxygen administration practices of UK anaesthetists. Given the current controversy surrounding WHO's recommendations for perioperative oxygen use, the aim of this multi-centre observational study was to characterise practice as regards the administration of oxygen to patients undergoing major surgery and to describe intraoperative arterial oxygenation during general anaesthesia.

Methods

A multi-centre retrospective observational study was conducted across 29 hospitals in London and parts of the South Coast of England affiliated with two trainee-led research networks: PLAN (Pan-London Perioperative Audit and Research Network—http://www.uk-plan.net) or SPARC (South Coast Perioperative Audit and Research Collaborative—http://wessex-sparc.com). The project was confirmed to be a clinical service evaluation by the Royal Free London and Southampton NHS Trust Clinical Governance departments, and research ethics committee approval and individual patient consent were not required. Appropriate approval was secured from the clinical governance department in each participating hospital.

Patients aged 18 years and over undergoing general anaesthesia for elective or emergency operations necessitating the insertion of an arterial cannula and subsequent arterial blood gas (ABG) monitoring were included. Patients receiving cardiopulmonary bypass were excluded (as during bypass, oxygen administration is often not controlled by the anaesthetist).

Data collection took place over five consecutive weekdays in April and May 2017; flexibility in the data collection window ensured maximum compliance locally. Anaesthetic trainees not involved in the clinical care of the patients collected data from the anaesthetic record. Patients were identified and assessed for inclusion daily from departmental operating lists. A retrospective review of anaesthetic charts and arterial blood gases was performed after the patients in question had been moved from theatre to the recovery area, ward or intensive care unit. Oxygenation data (including intraoperative SpO_2, FIO_2 and PaO_2 values), together with intraoperative positive end-expiratory pressure (PEEP) values and patient demographics, were collected using paper case report forms, held securely and treated as strictly confidential according to NHS policies.

Statistics were calculated using IBM SPSS Statistics, Version 24.0, Armonk, NY: IBM Corp. Data were examined for normality using the Shapiro-Wilk test. Unpaired data were compared using the Wilcoxon-Mann-Whitney U test and Kruskal-Wallis tests. Correlation was tested with Spearman's rank correlation coefficient. All tests were two-tailed, and significance was taken as $p < 0.05$. Continuous data were presented as median (IQR) and categorical data as number (percentage). Cumulative oxygen dose was determined in patients for whom more than one ABG was recorded, by calculating the area under the curve between the times of the first and final ABGs, in a plot of recorded PaO_2 as a function of time, with T0 equal to the time of the initial ABG.

Results

Data from 378 anaesthetic cases were contributed from 29 hospitals across London and Wessex. Results were reported from 17 (58.6%) district general hospitals (DGHs), 8 (27.6%) teaching hospitals and 4 (13.8%) speciality hospitals. Paper-based anaesthetic records were used in 334 (88.4%) cases, with electronic records contributed by three sites. The median patient age was 66 years

(IQR 52–74). Patient demographics and clinical details along with operation characteristics are shown in Table 1.

Surgical duration ranged from 1 to 13 h with a median of 4 h. Estimated blood loss was > 1000 ml in 31 (8.2%) patients. In total, 824 arterial blood gases were analysed. The number of ABGs recorded for each patient ranged from 1 to 13, with a median of 2. SpO_2 of < 96% was documented in 83 (22%) patients, with only 7 (1.9%) patients desaturating to < 88% at any point during the operation. Table 2 illustrates values for SpO_2, PaO_2 and haemoglobin concentration in the first five ABGs for each patient.

Table 1 Patient and operation characteristics

Variable		Patient/surgical characteristics number (%)
Gender	Male	205 (54.2%)
	Female	173 (45.8%)
ASA classification	1	17 (4.5%)
	2	158 (41.8%)
	3	153 (40.5%)
	4	34 (8.99%)
	5	5 (1.3%)
	Not recorded	11 (2.9%)
Documented respiratory disease	Asthma	37 (9.8%)
	COPD	31 (8.2%)
	Obstructive sleep apnoea	10 (2.6%)
	Other	25 (6.6%)
Documented cardiovascular disease	Hypertension	145 (38.4%)
	Ischaemic heart disease	49 (13%)
	Atrial fibrillation	31 (8.2%)
	Congestive cardiac failure	16 (4.2%)
	Valvular disease	18 (4.8%)
	Other	34 (9%)
National Confidential Enquiry into Patient Outcome and Death (NCEPOD) classification	Elective	270 (71.4%)
	Urgent/immediate/expedited	108 (28.6%)
Surgical specialty	Upper gastrointestinal/colorectal/general/breast	111 (29.4%)
	Urology/renal (including renal transplantation)	34 (9%)
	Vascular	37 (9.8%)
	Orthopaedics/spinal	29 (7.7%)
	Hepatopancreaticobiliary/liver transplant (including liver transplantation)	32 (8.5%)
	Ear nose and throat/maxillofacial	17 (4.5%)
	Neurosurgery	45 (11.9%)
	Gynaecology	23 (6.1%)
	Cardiothoracic	23 (6.1%)
	Plastics	2 (0.5%)
	Other	25 (6.6%)

Table 2 Oxygenation and haemoglobin values from the first five sequential arterial blood gas samples

ABG number	Median FIO_2 (IQR)	Median PaO_2 in kPa (IQR)	Median P:F ratio in kPa (IQR)	Median haemoglobin concentration g/l (IQR)
1 ($n = 378$)	0.5 (0.45–0.59)	24.5 (16.7–32.6)	51.2 (36.9–66.0)	113 (100–126)
2 ($n = 227$)	0.49 (0.4–0.54)	23.4 (17.4–29.5)	50.6 (38.1–62.9)	111 (100–124)
3 ($n = 116$)	0.46 (0.4–0.51)	25.7 (19.6–29.2)	54.5 (43.3–65.2)	108 (99–119)
4 ($n = 51$)	0.47 (0.4–0.5)	25.4 (20.7–30.8)	57.2 (43.9–71.1)	111 (93–153)
5 ($n = 24$)	0.49 (0.3–0.51)	26.3 (23.4–29.3)	58.6 (45.3–66.7)	99 (93–116)

The median PaO_2 and FIO_2 for all analysed ABGs combined were 24.7 kPa (IQR 17.9–30.8) and 0.50 kPa (IQR 0.41–0.55) respectively. There was no significant difference in the PaO_2 recorded across sequential ABGs ($p = 0.23$). Median FIO_2 was also consistent across sequential ABGs, although the variation about the median decreased by the fifth ABG (Fig. 1). Figure 1b demonstrates marked spread of data and a weak positive association between measured PaO_2 and FIO_2 ($r = 0.22$, $p \leq 0.001$). Supraphysiological values for PaO_2 (defined as > 13.3 kPa) were observed in 734 (89%) ABGs. Of the 769 ABGs for which the corresponding FIO_2 was recorded, an $FIO_2 \geq 0.8$ was administered on 32 (4.2%) occasions. Of these 32 occasions, 20 (62.5%) were at the time of taking the baseline arterial gas, closest to induction of anaesthesia.

The median cumulative oxygen dose, calculated for those patients for whom at least two ABGs were documented ($n = 223$), was 3824 kPa min (IQR 2121–6923) over a median time of 159 min (IQR 91–291). The administration of 13.3 kPa O_2 over the same time period would have resulted in a median cumulative oxygen dose of 2088 kPa. Representative traces of the cumulative oxygen dose administered to four individual patients are illustrated in Fig. 2.

Positive end-expiratory pressure (PEEP) was recorded in 287 (75.9%) of cases, and the median PEEP administered was 5 cmH_2O (range 0–12). A PEEP of 4, 5 or 6 cmH_2O was administered in 207 (72.1%) of cases where PEEP was recorded. A change in the level of PEEP administered was documented during only 28 cases.

Discussion

These results demonstrate that the amount of oxygen anaesthetists administer to adult patients undergoing major surgery in the UK currently varies widely—the recorded FIO_2 ranged from 0.25 to 1.0 throughout surgery. In many patients, FIO_2 was nearer 0.5 for the duration of surgery, resulting in PaO_2 values of approximately 25 kPa throughout.

An FIO_2 of 0.5 is much higher than "standard" therapy used for control groups (where FIO_2 is typically 0.3) in previous studies of "high" versus "standard" oxygen therapy (Wetterslev et al. 2015) and also considerably less than the WHO now recommends (Allegranzi et al. 2016). Interestingly, the findings from this UK-based sample exactly match values recently reported as representing current practice in the Cleveland Clinic, USA (Kurz et al. 2018). These results are also similar to the LAS VEGAS study (a prospective cross-sectional study of 9808 patients from 29 different countries) where half of all patients received an FIO_2 between 0.4 and 0.6 and one third between 0.6 and

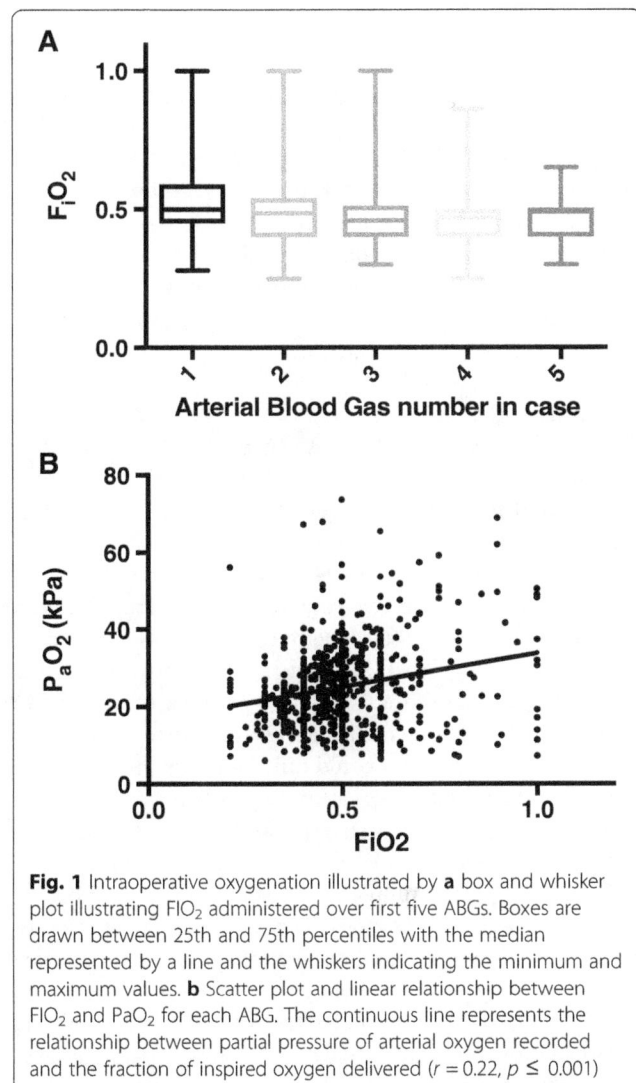

Fig. 1 Intraoperative oxygenation illustrated by **a** box and whisker plot illustrating FIO_2 administered over first five ABGs. Boxes are drawn between 25th and 75th percentiles with the median represented by a line and the whiskers indicating the minimum and maximum values. **b** Scatter plot and linear relationship between FIO_2 and PaO_2 for each ABG. The continuous line represents the relationship between partial pressure of arterial oxygen recorded and the fraction of inspired oxygen delivered ($r = 0.22$, $p \leq 0.001$)

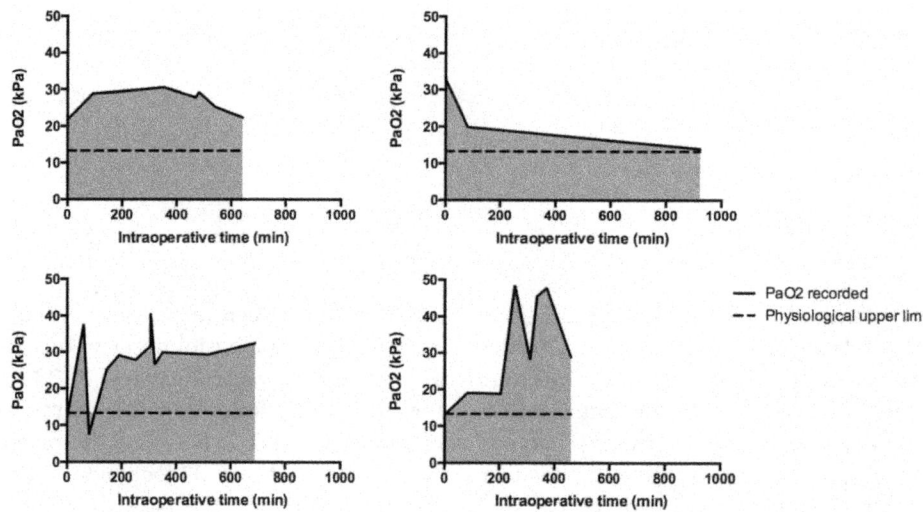

Fig. 2 Sample traces demonstrating of cumulative oxygen dose for four individual patients. The solid line represents the actual PaO₂ recorded in successive blood gases, whilst the dashed line represents the physiological upper limit (13.3 kPa). Area under the curve (shaded) was calculated between the times of the first and final ABGs

0.8 Rogerson et al. (2017). LAS VEGAS also reported a median PEEP of 5 cmH₂O (the value in > 50% cases where PEEP was recorded in this study) suggesting this also represents the current "standard" of practice Rogerson et al. (2017).

In many other clinical contexts, including on the critical care unit, PaO₂ values around 25 kPa would likely be classed as moderate hyperoxia rather than normoxia (Damiani et al. 2014a). However, median intraoperative PaO₂ values of approximately 25 kPa are consistent with an earlier single UK centre pilot study carried out by our group, reporting a mean PaO₂ of 24.4 kPa in 75 surgical patients over a 6-week period (Martin and Grocott 2015), and observational data also suggests that current practice still favours hyperoxaemia in critically ill patients (de Jonge et al. 2008; Eastwood et al. 2012).

Intraoperative hyperoxaemia may be a consequence of several factors. Firstly, up to now, evidence associating hyperoxia under anaesthesia with harm has been relatively limited. However, high intraoperative FIO₂ has been retrospectively associated in a dose-dependent manner with increased post-operative respiratory complications and with increased mortality (Staehr-Rye et al. 2017); the PROXI study demonstrated a higher 2-year mortality in patients with abdominal malignancy who received an FIO₂ of 0.8; and similarly, in 2018, a trial of over 5000 patients reported that using an FIO₂ of 0.8 intraoperatively instead of 0.3 did not alter SSI rates but did double 30-day mortality rates (*p* = 0.08) (Kurz et al. 2018). Secondly, continuous monitoring of arterial oxygenation during general anaesthesia occurs mainly via pulse oximetry with a scale that stops at 100%. New technology may

allow non-invasive measurement of surrogate markers of PaO₂ in the future (e.g. the oxygen reserve index (Applegate et al. 2016)), but the use of these devices is currently limited. The duration of oxygen exposure may also possibly affect the outcomes, yet this has often not been considered or reported in clinical trials previously. The method of determining cumulative oxygen dose demonstrated here could represent a more relevant measure for use in future outcome studies.

Strengths and limitations

This study characterises how anaesthetists in the UK currently use oxygen during a mixed selection of major surgery and in a large number of different hospitals. The biggest limitation to these findings is that corresponding clinical outcomes could not be collected. This should be a focus of future prospective research studies, and although this study was never designed to collect outcome data itself, our findings that FIO₂ of 0.5 currently represents "standard care" (and not 0.3 as used by most trials to date) should be considered in the design of future trials. Area under the curve analysis could only be performed between times of arterial blood gas sampling, which could not be specified due to the retrospective and observational study design, and consequently, our data may represent underestimates of total cumulative oxygen doses as FIO₂ is often increased at the start and end of anaesthesia to prepare for intubation and extubation. Because of the way most recruiting hospitals routinely document anaesthesia, the majority of data were collected from paper anaesthetic records. Previous studies have suggested a paper anaesthetic chart is not always the most accurate record of intraoperative events (Devitt et al. 1999); however, in our study, findings from centres using paper charts were still very similar to those using electronic recording systems. In order to record PaO_2 values, we included patients undergoing procedures necessitating arterial line insertion; implying our findings might only be applicable to those in whom invasive monitoring was deemed necessary by the anaesthetist, either due to patient or operative factors. However, despite all of these limitations, our findings corroborated reports of current practice in other countries exactly (Kurz et al. 2018).

Conclusions

Anaesthetists are currently faced with an international recommendation on the intraoperative administration of oxygen that conflicts with the majority of evidence from other clinical contexts. It is perhaps not surprising therefore that the amount of oxygen administered to patients undergoing general anaesthesia in the UK varies widely. The administration of an FIO_2 of 0.5 appears to be the current standard of care for UK-based anaesthetists, which is often associated with moderate levels of hyperoxaemia intraoperatively. These findings are very similar to the reports from other countries and need to be considered in the design of any future studies investigating the potential impact intraoperative oxygen therapy may have on surgical patients' outcomes.

Abbreviations
ABG: Arterial blood gas; DGH: District general hospital; F_iO_2: Fractional inspired oxygen concentration; IQR: Interquartile range; PaO_2: Arterial oxygen partial pressure; PEEP: Positive end-expiratory pressure; PLAN: Pan-London Perioperative Audit and Research Network; ROS: Reactive oxygen species; SPARC: South Coast Perioperative Audit and Research Collaborative; SpO_2: Peripheral oxygen saturation; SSI: Surgical site infection; WHO: World Health Organization

Acknowledgements
PLAN:
Louise Carter, Cyrus Razavi, Ryan Howle, Alex Eeles, Kate C. Tatham, Victoria Winter, Lena Al-Shammari, Leda Lignos, Gagandeep Dhotar, Emma Karsten, Justine Lowe, Noel Young, Lindsey Iles, Colin Coulter, Michael Shaw, Liam Gleeson, Liana Zucco, Charlie Cox, Amanda Bruce, John N Cronin, James Arlidge, Rachel Krol, Rasha Abouelmagd, Phil Dart, Mohamed Ahmed, Kathy Shammas, Carly Webb, Luke Foster, Rafi Kanji, Darragh Hodnett, Lusha Suntharanathan, Amy Sangam, Zain Malik, Eleanor Jeffreys, Jonathan Williamson, Marika Chandler, Nick Dennison, Jan Schumacher, Kariem El-Boghdadly, Peter Odor, Helen Laycock, Sibtain Anwar, Harriet Wordsworth, Alex Wickham, Shaima Elnour, Edward Burdett, Sioned Phillips, Matt Oliver, Carolyn Johnston, Mitul Patel, Kate Grailey, Queenie Lo, Benjamin Frost, James O'Carroll, Hew D Torrance, Vimal Grover, Chris Whiten, Justine Lowe, Matthew C. Dickinson, Vanessa Cowie, Richard George, Julian Giles, Otto Mohr, Ahmer Mosharaf, Jon Brammall.
SPARC:
Jamie Plumb, Alexander I. R. Jackson, Erica Jolly, Huw Wilkins, Hannah Wong, Suzanne Shuttleworth, Nick Hayward, J. Joseph Kinsella, Emma Killick, Tom Daubeny, Philip McGlone, Sophie Yelland, Kushmandinie Goonetilleke, Victoria Tuckey, Alan Radford, Rebecca Fry, Jessie Rose, Mukunder Patel, Hugh Cutler, Kate Blethyn, Jeremy Whittles, Paul Stevens, Rebecca Sands, Matt Taylor, Fiona Linton, Tom Blincoe, Lucy Chumas, Sarah Bates, Heidi Lightfoot, Olivia Shields, Francesca Riccio.

Authors' contributions
CMM, HM and AFC contributed to the study conception and design, data collection, data analysis and writing of the manuscript. AO contributed to the study design and data collection. DSM and MPWG contributed to the study conception and design and writing and editing of the manuscript. All authors read and approved the final manuscript.

Competing interests
Professor Michael P. W. Grocott (MPWG) serves on the medical advisory board of Sphere Medical Ltd. and is a director of Oxygen Control Systems Ltd. He has received honoraria for speaking for and/or travel expenses from BOC Medical (Linde Group), Edwards Lifesciences and Cortex GmBH. MPWG leads the Xtreme Everest Oxygen Research Consortium and the Fit-4-Surgery research collaboration. Some of this work was undertaken at University Southampton NHS Foundation Trust–University of Southampton NIHR Biomedical Research Centre. MPWG serves as the UK NIHR CRN national specialty group lead for Anaesthesia Perioperative Medicine and Pain and is an elected council member of the Royal College of Anaesthetists, an elected board member of the Faculty of Intensive Care Medicine and president of the Critical Care Medicine Section of the Royal Society of Medicine.
Daniel Martin has received consultancy fees from Siemens Healthcare and Masimo and lecture honoraria from Edwards Lifesciences and Deltex Medical. He is also a Director of Oxygen Control Ltd.
Dr. Andrew Cumpstey is currently funded through the NIHR as an Academic Clinical Fellow. The other authors declare that they have no competing interests.

Author details
[1]Division of Surgery and Interventional Science (University College London) and Royal Free Perioperative Research Group, Department of Anaesthesia, Royal Free Hospital, 3rd Floor, Pond Street, London NW3 2QG, UK. [2]University of Southampton/University Hospital Southampton and NIHR Biomedical Research Centre, Tremona Rd, Southampton SO16 6YD, UK. [3]University Hospital Southampton, Tremona Rd, Southampton SO16 6YD, UK.

References
Allegranzi B, Zayed B, Bischoff P, Kubilay NZ, de JS, de VF, et al. New WHO recommendations on intraoperative and postoperative measures for surgical site infection prevention: an evidence-based global perspective. Lancet Infect Dis. 2016;16(12):e288–303.

Applegate RL, Dorotta IL, Wells B, Juma D, Applegate PM. The relationship between oxygen reserve index and arterial partial pressure of oxygen during surgery. Anesth Analg. 2016;123(3):626–33.

Ball L, Lumb AB, Pelosi P. Intraoperative fraction of inspired oxygen: bringing back the focus on patient outcome. BJA Br J Anaesth. 2017;119(1):16–8.

Chu DK, Kim LH-Y, Young PJ, Zamiri N, Almenawer SA, Jaeschke R, et al. Mortality and morbidity in acutely ill adults treated with liberal versus conservative oxygen therapy (IOTA): a systematic review and meta-analysis. Lancet. 2018; 391(10131):1693–705.

Damiani E, Adrario E, Girardis M, Romano R, Pelaia P, Singer M, et al. Arterial hyperoxia and mortality in critically ill patients: a systematic review and meta-analysis. Crit Care. 2014;18(16):711.

Davis WB, Rennard SI, Bitterman PB, Crystal RG. Pulmonary oxygen toxicity. N Engl J Med. 1983;309(15):878–83.

de Jonge E, Peelen L, Keijzers PJ, Joore H, de Lange D, van der Voort PH, et al. Association between administered oxygen, arterial partial oxygen pressure and mortality in mechanically ventilated intensive care unit patients. Crit Care. 2008;12(6):R156.

Dell'Anna AM, Lamanna I, Vincent J-L, Taccone FS. How much oxygen in adult cardiac arrest? Crit Care. 2014;18:555.

Devitt JH, Rapanos T, Kurrek M, Cohen MM, Shaw M. The anesthetic record: accuracy and completeness. Can J Anaesth J Can Anesth. 1999;46(2):122–8.

Eastwood G, Bellomo R, Bailey M, Taori G, Pilcher D, Young P, et al. Arterial oxygen tension and mortality in mechanically ventilated patients. Intensive Care Med. 2012;38(1):91–8.

Edmark L, Kostova-Aherdan K, Enlund M, Hedenstierna G. Optimal oxygen concentration during induction of general anesthesia. Anesthesiol J Am Soc Anesthesiol. 2003;98(1):28–33.

Farquhar H, Weatherall M, Wijesinghe M, Perrin K, Ranchord A, Simmonds M, et al. Systematic review of studies of the effect of hyperoxia on coronary blood flow. Am Heart J. 2009;158(3):371–7.

Kücükakin B, Gögenur I, Reiter RJ, Rosenberg J. Oxidative stress in relation to surgery: is there a role for the antioxidant melatonin? J Surg Res. 2009;152(2): 338–47.

Kurz A, Kopyeva T, Suliman I, Podolyak A, You J, Lewis B, et al. Supplemental oxygen and surgical-site infections: an alternating intervention controlled trial. Br J Anaesth. 2018;120(1):117–26.

Martin DS, Grocott MPW. Oxygen therapy and anaesthesia: too much of a good thing? Anaesthesia. 2015;70(5):522–7.

McNulty PH, King N, Scott S, Hartman G, McCann J, Kozak M, et al. Effects of supplemental oxygen administration on coronary blood flow in patients undergoing cardiac catheterization. Am J Physiol - Heart Circ Physiol. 2005; 288(3):H1057–62.

Meyhoff CS, Jorgensen LN, Wetterslev J, Christensen KB, Rasmussen LS, PROXI Trial Group. Increased long-term mortality after a high perioperative inspiratory oxygen fraction during abdominal surgery: follow-up of a randomized clinical trial. Anesth Analg 2012;115(4):849–854.

Myles PS, Kurz A. Supplemental oxygen and surgical site infection: getting to the truth. BJA Br J Anaesth. 2017;119(1):13–5.

Reinhart K, Bloos F, König F, Bredle D, Hannemann L. Reversible decrease of oxygen consumption by hyperoxia. Chest. 1991;99(3):690–4.

Rogerson D, Williams JP, Yates S, Rogers E. Epidemiology, practice of ventilation and outcome for patients at increased risk of postoperative pulmonary complications. Eur J Anaesthesiol. 2017;34(8):492–507.

Staehr-Rye AK, Meyhoff CS, Scheffenbichler FT, MF MV, Gätke MR, et al. High intraoperative inspiratory oxygen fraction and risk of major respiratory complications. BJA Br J Anaesth. 2017;119(1):140–9.

Sury MRJ, Palmer JHMG, Cook TM, Pandit JJ, Mahajan RP. The state of UK anaesthesia: a survey of National Health Service activity in 2013. BJA Br J Anaesth. 2014;113(4):575–84.

Wetterslev J, Meyhoff CS, Jørgensen LN, Gluud C, Lindschou J, Rasmussen LS. The effects of high perioperative inspiratory oxygen fraction for adult surgical patients. Cochrane Database Syst Rev. 2015;6(6). https://doi.org/10.1002/14651858.CD008884.pub2.

The sensitivity of the human thirst response to changes in plasma osmolality

Fintan Hughes[*] 🆔, Monty Mythen and Hugh Montgomery

Abstract

Background: Dehydration is highly prevalent and is associated with adverse cardiovascular and renal events. Clinical assessment of dehydration lacks sensitivity. Perhaps a patient's thirst can provide an accurate guide to fluid therapy. This systematic review examines the sensitivity of thirst in responding to changes in plasma osmolality in participants of any age with no condition directly effecting their sense of thirst.

Methods: Medline and EMBASE were searched up to June 2017. Inclusion criteria were all studies reporting the plasma osmolality threshold for the sensation of thirst.

Results: A total of 12 trials were included that assessed thirst intensity on a visual analogue scale, as a function of plasma osmolality (pOsm), and employed linear regression to define the thirst threshold. This included 167 participants, both healthy controls and those with a range of pathologies, with a mean age of 41 (20–78) years. The value ±95% CI for the pOsm threshold for thirst sensation was found to be 285.23 ± 1.29 mOsm/kg. Above this threshold, thirst intensity as a function of pOsm had a mean ± SEM slope of 0.54 ± 0.07 cm/mOsm/kg. The mean ± 95% CI vasopressin release threshold was very similar to that of thirst, being 284.3 ± 0.71 mOsm/kg. Heterogeneity across studies can be accounted for by subtle variation in experimental protocol and data handling.

Conclusion: The thresholds for thirst activation and vasopressin release lie in the middle of the normal range of plasma osmolality. Thirst increases linearly as pOsm rises. Thus, osmotically balanced fluid administered as per a patient's sensation of thirst should result in a plasma osmolality within the normal range. This work received no funding.

Keywords: Dehydration, Osmoregulation, Thirst

Background

Dehydration is prevalent amongst hospital inpatients. Amongst those aged > 65 years old admitted to UK hospitals, 37% had a plasma osmolality > 300 mOsm/kg on admission, and 62% of these where still afflicted 48 h later (Siervo et al., 2014). While 62% of Scottish stroke patients had a ratio of serum urea: creatinine concentration > 80 mmol/L:μmol/L at some point during hospital admission (Rowat et al., 2012). Over 70% of intensive care unit patients report at least moderately distressing thirst (Puntillo et al., 2010). Dehydration is also highly prevalent outside hospitals; in UK residential homes,

measurements of plasma osmolality suggest 46% of residents to be dehydrated (El-Sharkawy et al., 2015).

Such dehydration is not benign: its presence is associated with an increased risk of myocardial infarction (Kloner, 2006), renal calculi (Feehally & Khosravi, 2015), venous thromboembolic disease (Saad et al., 2016) and acute kidney injury (Kanagasundaram, 2015). Meanwhile, dehydration increases pain perception (Farrell et al., 2006) and the associated risk of delirium is comparable with that related to opiate administration (Boettger et al., 2015). As a consequence, dehydration is associated with increased length of hospital stay and greater healthcare costs (Pash et al., 2014; Frangeskou et al., 2015), and preventing dehydration has become a focus of concern for England's Care Quality Commission (Comission NuTCQ, 2011), patient associations (Association HP, 2010), The British

* Correspondence: fint@nhugh.es
Institute for Sport, Exercise and Health, University College London, 170 Tottenham Court Road, London W1T 7HA, UK

Parliamentary Ombudsman (Parliamentary OH, 2011) and independent inquiries (RF, 2013).

Clinical features of dehydration only appear when fluid losses exceed at least 4–5% of total body water (Mackenzie et al., 1989; Gross et al., 1992) and even then may be variably present or poorly detected. Clinical features of total body water loss include reduced skin turgor, lack of sweat, sunken eyes, and dry mucous membranes, and reflect a reduction in cellular and interstitial water content. Reductions in intravascular volume may be associated with delayed capillary refill time, hypotension (or a postural drop in blood pressure) and tachycardia. However, clinicians are poor at diagnosing dehydration overall when osmolality is used as a gold standard. Diagnosis of dehydration based solely on these signs is unreliable and generally of very low sensitivity (between 0 and 44%) (Fortes et al., n.d.) and poor specificity (Thomas et al., 2004).

Nor can urine or serum osmolality be readily and routinely used to guide hour-by-hour fluid administration. Indeed, no single gold standard test yet exists which can routinely determine hydration status in the clinical environment (Armstrong, 2007). Such factors might account for the huge variation in fluid administration seen in clinical care. By way of example, the volume of fluid administered in the perioperative period was found to vary sixfold between individual doctors at two US institutions irrespective of the patients' condition (Lilot et al., 2015). Fluid overload can lead to organ dysfunction through the development of tissue oedema. Wound healing can be impaired, and gut function likewise negatively impacted. Oedema increases the diffusion distance of oxygen from capillary to cell, but can also raise the hydrostatic pressure within capsulated organs (such as the kidney) and thus impair tissue perfusion. Pulmonary oedema can also cause a reduction in systemic oxygenation, and increase in end-diastolic pressure can impair subendocardial myocardial perfusion and thus ventricular contractility (Holte et al., 2002).

Physiologically, plasma osmolality (pOsm) is maintained between 275 and 295 mOsm/kg by the combination of thirst sensation and arginine vasopressin release (AVP), stimulated by activation of central osmoreceptors lying outside the blood brain barrier (Baylis & Thompson, 1988). Thirst stimulation will drive fluid consumption to increase total body water, while AVP inserts aquaporins in the collecting duct to promote free-water reabsorption at the nephron via the V2 receptor to prevent further losses from the intravascular space, as well as acting as a potent vasoconstrictor through the V1 receptor (Table 1).

Additionally, plasma volume reductions are sensed both directly and indirectly by baroreceptors primarily located in the pulmonary and renal arteries and the atria. Volume depletion also stimulates renin release and thence increased circulating angiotensin II

levels which are tightly coupled to increasing thirst (Johnson et al., 1981).

These processes interact; haemodynamic controls amplify the osmotic thirst response. Baroreceptor-signalling mechanisms alter the threshold and sensitivity of both thirst and AVP release to changes in pOsm (Kimura et al., 1976). In hypovolaemic states, the pOsm thresholds for thirst and AVP release are reduced, while the slope of their response to pOsm is increased (Andersson & Rundgren, 1982). This interaction can be explained by the shared vagal and glossopharyngeal pathway from the atria to the supraoptic and paraventricular nuclei of the hypothalamus (Johnson, 2007), which coordinate thirst and AVP release. The osmotic thirst mechanism detects small variations in hydration, while hypovolaemic thirst is specific for large falls in plasma volume of over 8–10% (Kimura et al., 1976).

Given the integrative nature of these homeostatic mechanisms, could a patient's own subjective sense of thirst be a better guide to the need for further hydration than our current clinical assessment? The degree to which clinicians include assessment of thirst when considering fluid prescription is not known. Anecdotal evidence suggests that some more experienced clinicians may do so. However, the value of this may be influenced by the degree to which thirst reflects a dehydration-related rise in serum osmolality. Perhaps thirst is one of the few sensitive symptoms of underlying reductions in total body water, and should prompt further clinical and biochemical investigation. If so, this might guide fluid administration in hospitalised patients, fluid being delivered until thirst is no longer present. However, before such practice can be recommended, it is essential to quantify the diagnostic accuracy of thirst so as not to pose a risk of iatrogenic dehydration or fluid overload. To explore the feasibility of this approach, we performed a systematic review to determine the value of plasma osmolality associated with developing a sense of thirst, how this relates to age and gender, and those factors which might influence thirst in hospitalised patients (Fig. 1).

Methods

Medline and EMBASE were searched (up to June 1, 2017) for human trials in all languages for the combined terms 'thirst' AND 'osmolality' AND 'threshold', the bibliographies of extracted papers were also searched for relevant articles.

Included studies were those that reported the plasma osmolality threshold, in dehydrated subjects, for the sensation of thirst, as measured on a visual analogue scale. Full journal publication was required. Participants were of any age, with no condition directly effecting their sense of thirst. The types of interventions included were

Table 1 Summary of included trials investigating the threshold of AVP release and thirst stimulation in response to increasing plasma osmolality

Author (year) (citation)	Age mean	Subject condition	Sample size	Dehydration mechanism	Thirst threshold mean (±SD) mOsm/kg	Relevant findings
(Thompson, Bland et al. 1986)	24.3	Healthy	10	5% NaCl @ 0.06 ml/kg/min for 2 h	281.1 ± 3.2	High individual repeatability of threshold results. Lower threshold found, stimulating thirst before significant dehydration occurs.
(Phillips, Bretherton et al. 1991)	25 69.8	Healthy Young Healthy Elderly	7 7	5% NaCl @ 0.06 ml/kg/min for 2 h	261.0 ± 18.5 276.0 ± 13.2	Elderly show reduced thirst
(Davies, O'Neill et al. 1995)	26.8 70.5	Healthy Young Healthy Elderly	10 10	5% NaCl @ 0.1 ml/kg/min for 2 h	287.5 ± 12.6 292.4 ± 8.5	Thirst threshold is not elevated in healthy elderly, but inter-subject variation is greater. Linear response of thirst to pOsm identified.
(Thompson and Baylis 1987)	29.2 28.6	Healthy Controls Diabetes insipidus	15 14	5% NaCl @ 0.06 ml/kg/min for 2 h	286.3 ± 3.9 286.3 ± 3.9	Diabetes insipidus does not alter thirst or AVP response to pOsm
(Thompson, Davis et al. 1988)	30 29.1	Healthy Controls Type 1 Diabetes	7 7	5% NaCl @ 0.1 ml/kg/min for 2 h vs: Glucose raised from 4 to 20 mmol/l over 2 h	284.7 ± 1.6 287.0 ± 6.9	Oral fluid intake rapidly abolished thirst independent of pOsm. Type 1 Diabetes does not alter thirst and AVP response.
(Thompson, Edwards et al. 1991)	29.6	Healthy controls	7	5% NaCl @ 0.05 ml/kg/min for 2 h	286.5 ± 3.2	No significant difference between thirst and AVP thresholds.
(Thompson, Selby et al. 1991)	34.1	Healthy	16	5% NaCl @ 0.06 ml/kg/min for 2 h	286.3 ± 4.2	Very high 6 month repeatability of AVP and thirst threshold seen within individuals
(Argent, Burrell et al. 1991)	41.1 41.4	Healthy Chronic Kidney Disease	7 8	5% NaCl @ 0.06 ml/kg/min for 2 h	279.4 ± 5.8 281.8 ± 6.8	Threshold of AVP & Thirst are very close in both subject groups
(Phillips, Butler et al. 1994)	41.5	Healthy	8	5% NaCl @ 0.06 ml/kg/min for 2 h vs. 20% Mannitol @ 0.07 ml/ kg/min for 2 h	291.0 ± 5.8	5% saline is a more powerful osmotic stimulant than mannitol. The threshold for mannitol is similar but the slope lower
(Martinez-Vea, Garcia et al. 1992)	43.1 55.0	Healthy Controls Chronic Kidney Disease	6 5	5% NaCl @ 0.06 ml/kg/min for 2 h	289.8 ± 8.3 288.9 ± 19.0	High degree of sensitivity and repeatability in individual responses of thirst to osmolality. Thirst unaffected by chronic kidney disease, but dialysis causes a variation.
(Smith, Moore et al. 2004)	51.8	Healthy Controls	8	5% NaCl @ 0.05 ml/kg/min for 2 h	285.9 ± 2.8	Oral fluid intake abolishes osmotically stimulated thirst. Some individuals can lack thirst response.
(McKenna, Morris et al. 1999)	69.8 70.5	Healthy Controls Type 2 Diabetes	7 7	8 h water deprivation	285.5 ± 2.5 283.9 ± 2.0	Osmoregulation of thirst and AVP are normal in Type 2 Diabetes.

any which simulated or induced dehydration by increasing plasma osmolality.

Trials included were required to assess thirst intensity as a function of plasma osmolality, and employ linear regression to define the threshold value of pOsm for the sensation of thirst. This allows for both averaging of the thirst response across a range of dehydration severity and identifies the threshold more precisely than a subject reporting their onset of thirst.

Tabulated data were extracted from the included trials directly into spreadsheets to become the input for our statistical analysis. The primary variable sought was the pOsm threshold for thirst. Secondary variables, analysed where available, included pOsm threshold for the release of arginine vasopressin (AVP), the rates at which thirst score and AVP concentration varied with increasing pOsm, and linear correlation coefficients of both the thirst and AVP response to pOsm. Each value extracted was accompanied by a measure of variation, being either standard deviation, standard error or 95% confidence intervals. Data relating to the rate of increase in thirst were normalised to account for differences in size of the visual analogue thirst scales between the studies.

The factors affecting the sensitivity of thirst are poorly understood and no fixed effects can be assumed for the individuals in these studies. As the cohorts studied are not identical, some measurement errors exist and the results are intended to be generalised, a DerSimonian and

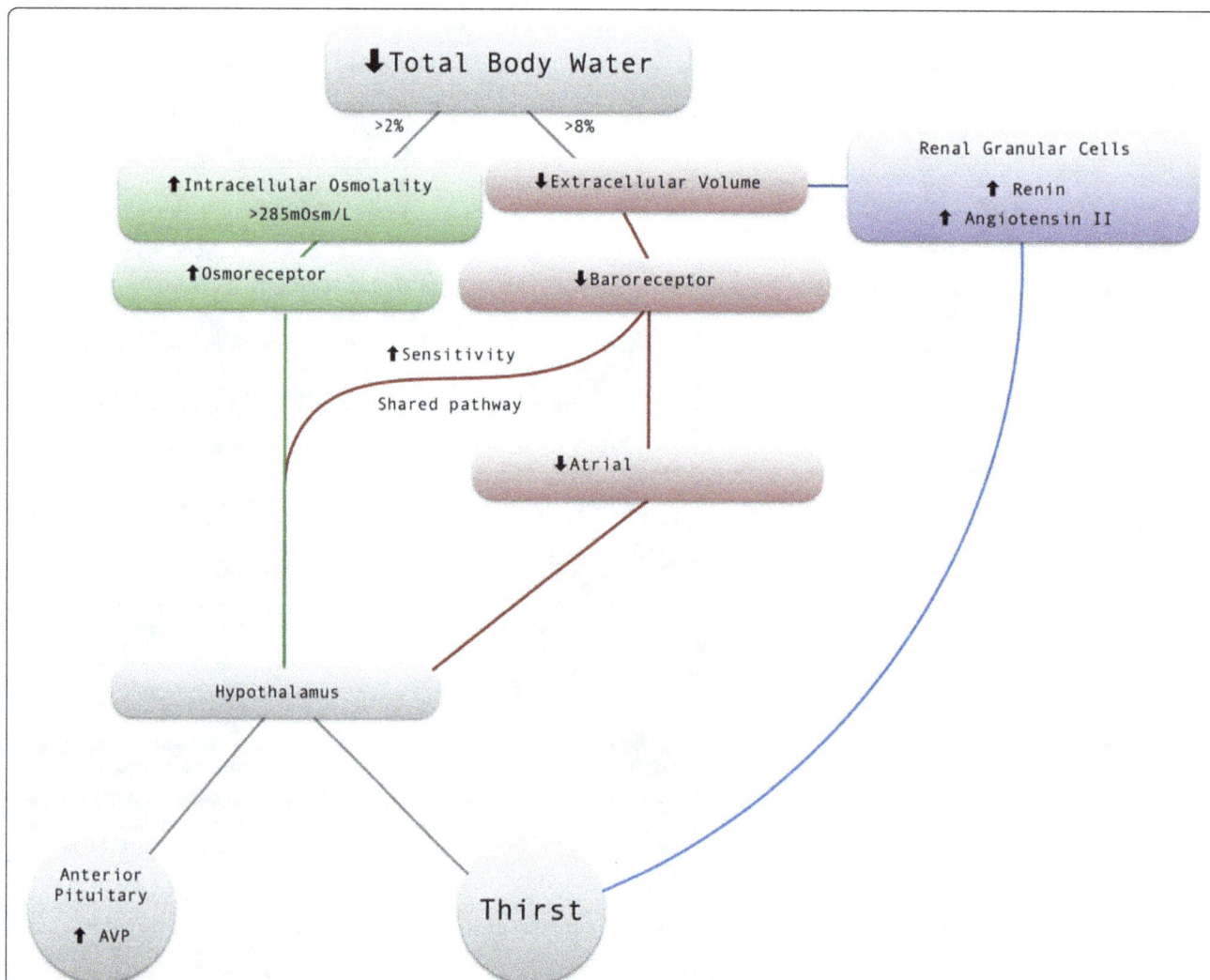

Fig. 1 The pathways initiated by total body water deficit leading to the stimulation of the thirst response. Whilst osmoreceptor stimulation is one of three mechanisms which influence the thirst response, it the most sensitive of these, signalling to the hypothalamus after a 2% reduction in total body water. The convergence of baroreceptor and osmoreceptors onto a shared pathway allows for integration of these distinct physiological parameters, such that thirst increases exponentially with large reductions in extracellular volume

Laird random effects model was employed with the R metafor package (Figure 3), which also provided an inconsistency metric for heterogeneity.

Whilst the synthesis of regression slopes is the topic of much discussion, this complexity arises from the combination of dissimilar studies and resulting nonequivalence of metrics (Becker & Wu, 2007). In the case of each of the studies included in this analysis, however, which employ a univariate approach, the two parameters, pOsm and thirst intensity or AVP concentration were measured in a comparable manner. As such it is appropriate to synthesise regression slopes using an arithmetic mean.

Papers varied in their reporting of either standard error of the mean, standard deviation or 95% confidence intervals; these were converted into variances and combined by Satterthwaite approximation (Satterthwaite,

1946), due to the non-equal variances within each patient cohort, to produce a composite variance for each secondary parameter.

Studies were subjectively assessed for sources of bias, with respect to selection of participants, performance bias, detection bias, and attrition bias.

Additional analysis was performed on the thirst thresholds reported in the subgroup of female trials. A paired t test was used to assess the mean difference between follicular and luteal phases within the menstrual cycle across four studies. These paired values were also combined to give a mean value for the female thirst threshold.

Results

One-hundred seventeen studies identified by our search strategy were screened and assessed, with 22 deemed eligible. Two studies were excluded that reported thirst threshold based on a single data point, not through least squared regression. A further study which did not include distribution data for each outcome was also excluded.

In women, there is known variation in thirst between different hormonal states. Seven studies investigating the effects of hormonal variation on thirst were excluded from the analysis and reviewed separately. The values reported in these trials are for specific cohorts of subjects across a range of hormonal states, which are either pharmacologically or pathologically induced, or related to the physiological variations at discrete time points in pregnancy and the menstrual cycle. Thus, the distribution of hormonal states in the pooled cohort from these studies is not representative of the normal population.

In the primary analysis, a total of 12 trials were included. Cohorts of patients with a significant disturbance in fluid balance (e.g., dialysis causing > 5% weight gain, compulsive water drinking, syndrome of inappropriate antidiuretic hormone secretion and those following hyperosmotic non-ketotic coma) were excluded from the analysis (Fig. 2).

Study characteristics

Included studies involved 167 participants with a mean age of 41, ranging from 20 to 78 years. These included both healthy controls and those with a range of pathologies: diabetes insipidus, diabetes mellitus type 1 and 2, and chronic kidney disease.

During the period prior to each trial, the intake of participants was standardised in different ways, ranging from 12 h of fasting with free water intake, to avoidance of caffeine on the morning of the trial. One trial imposed a standard protocol for fluid consumption in the 12 h prior to the experiment.

In all but one trial, which employed water deprivation, subjects rested in a recumbent or supine position for 15 to 60 min before intravenous cannulae were placed into each antecubital fossa.

One cannula was used for the infusion with blood samples drawn from the opposite arm. In all but one trial, pOsm was determined by freezing point depression.

All studies of high enough quality to include in our analysis followed the same general experimental design; defining thirst score as a function of plasma osmolality, they studied each participant's data over the course of a progressive rise in plasma osmolality. Seven trials administered a peripheral intravenous infusion of hypertonic saline at a rate of 0.06 ml/kg/min over 2 h (Thompson et al., 1986; Phillips et al., 1991; Thompson & Baylis, 1987; Thompson et al., 1991; Argent et al., 1991; Phillips et al., 1994; Martinez-Vea et al., 1992), with four others using

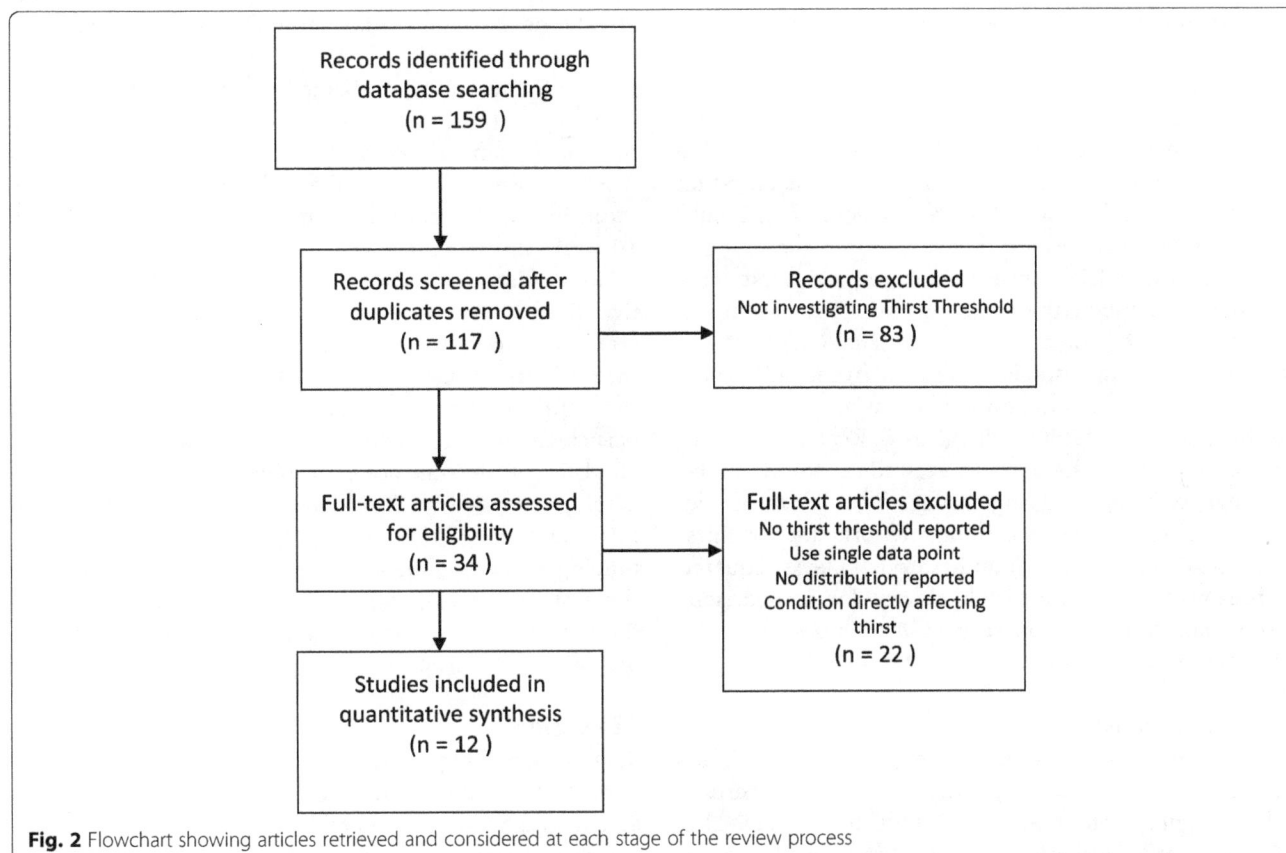

Fig. 2 Flowchart showing articles retrieved and considered at each stage of the review process

rates of 0.1 (Davies et al., 1995; Thompson et al., 1988) and 0.05 ml/kg/min (Thompson et al., 1991; Smith et al., 2004). One trial compared saline infusion to a 2 h 20% mannitol infusion at 0.07 ml/kg/min (Phillips et al., 1994), and another compared hypertonic saline to a steady infusion of hypertonic D-glucose, at a rate adjusted to each participant, sufficient to raise plasma glucose from 4 to 5 mmol/L to 20 mmol/L over 2 h (Thompson et al., 1988), another enforced 8 h of fluid restriction as a method of dehydration (McKenna et al., 1999).

These protocols led to an increase in pOsm of approximately 20 mOsm/kg, from starting values of between 276 and 290 mOsm/kg.

Trial participants reported thirst intensity (using a visual analogue scale, ranging from 100 mm long to 180 mm long) over the course of the dehydration challenge. Participants would mark the intensity of their subjective sense of thirst on these scales, and the distance from the zero point defined the degree of thirst intensity. None of the scales were graduated, but some included text at the extremes of the scale, indicating 'not thirsty' or 'very thirsty'. Linear regression analysis was applied to a series of subjective thirst scores taken throughout the course of the dehydration challenge, plotted against measurements of plasma osmolality. These linear regression models were then used by each study to determine primary outcome, the minimum value of plasma osmolality required for the sensation of thirst. This was achieved by calculating the abscissal intercept, which is the value of plasma osmolality above which thirst starts to increase. Secondary outcomes reported in several studies were the pOsm threshold for AVP release, the rate of increase of both thirst and AVP concentration with pOsm and the correlation coefficients of each subject to the linear regression model.

Four of these trials investigating female thirst were conducted in much the same way as those in males, reporting thirst scores on a visual analogue scale to changes in plasma osmolality due to hypertonic saline infusion or fluid restriction (Evbuomwan et al., 2001; Stachenfeld et al., 1999; Stachenfeld & Keefe, 2002; Calzone et al., 2001). The other three studies, whilst similar in design, only reported single values for thirst threshold; whilst this technique consistently reports higher thirst thresholds than those found through least squared regression, these data are still relevant for comparisons within each trial (Davison et al., 1988; Thompson et al., 1988; Spruce et al., 1985).

Data analysis results

Data on the thirst threshold were available in all included trials. The value ±95% C.I. for the pOsm threshold for thirst sensation was found to be 285.23 ± 1.29 mOsm/kg ($n = 167$). There was evidence of significant heterogeneity between studies ($I^2 = 0.73$, $\tau = 4.53$). None of the secondary outcome measures were present in all studies. Above this threshold, thirst intensity as a function of pOsm was found to have a mean ± SEM slope of 0.54 ± 0.07 cm/mOsm/kg ($n = 143$). The mean correlation coefficient of each individual linear regression was 0.91 ($n = 120$), indicating that above the threshold for sensation, the increase in thirst with pOsm is linear.

Eight studies also examined the threshold of AVP release in response to changes in pOsm. The mean ± 95% C.I. AVP release threshold was very similar to that of thirst, being 284.3 ± 0.71 mOsm/kg ($n = 150$). Above this threshold, AVP release was also linear, as shown by a mean regression coefficient of 0.91 ($n = 57$), and had a mean ± SEM slope of 0.35 ± 0.09 pmol/mOsm ($n = 72$) (Fig. 3).

Female thirst data

The pooled data from four studies (Stachenfeld et al., 1999; Calzone et al., 2001; Thompson et al., 1988; Spruce et al., 1985) in women demonstrated the mean reduction in thirst threshold in the luteal phase to be 3.1 mOsm/kg ($p < 0.001$). Averaging the control values for both follicular and luteal phases returns a threshold of 282.7 mOsm/kg ($n = 26$).

Combined administration of oestrogen and progesterone produced a threshold 4 mOsm/kg lower than administration of oestrogen alone (Stachenfeld & Keefe, 2002), and 2–4 mOsm/kg lower than that of progesterone alone (Stachenfeld et al., 1999; Calzone et al., 2001). Female thirst is further affected by pregnancy, one study showing that thirst threshold consistently falls from a pre-conception value of 285.5 to 281.5, 277.5, and 275.5 mOsm/kg across the gestation period, before returning to the starting value (Davison et al., 1988) by 10 weeks postpartum.

No bias likely to have significantly affected the cumulative results was identified. Only 3 of the 12 studies employed randomisation to the selection of participant or their allocation into groups. In the other studies, allocation into experimental or control arm was determined by participant factors (either age or pathology). Double blinded control infusions of physiological saline were employed in two studies, which caused no alteration in thirst sensation. Trials were supported either by national funding bodies or medical research charities, except for three studies which did not report the source of their funding. In no case was bias considered a likely contributing factor to heterogeneity in reported thirst threshold.

Discussion

Sources of heterogeneity

Whilst the heterogeneity seen in our primary outcome across studies was considerable, it is not indicative of the degree of thirst threshold variation within the population.

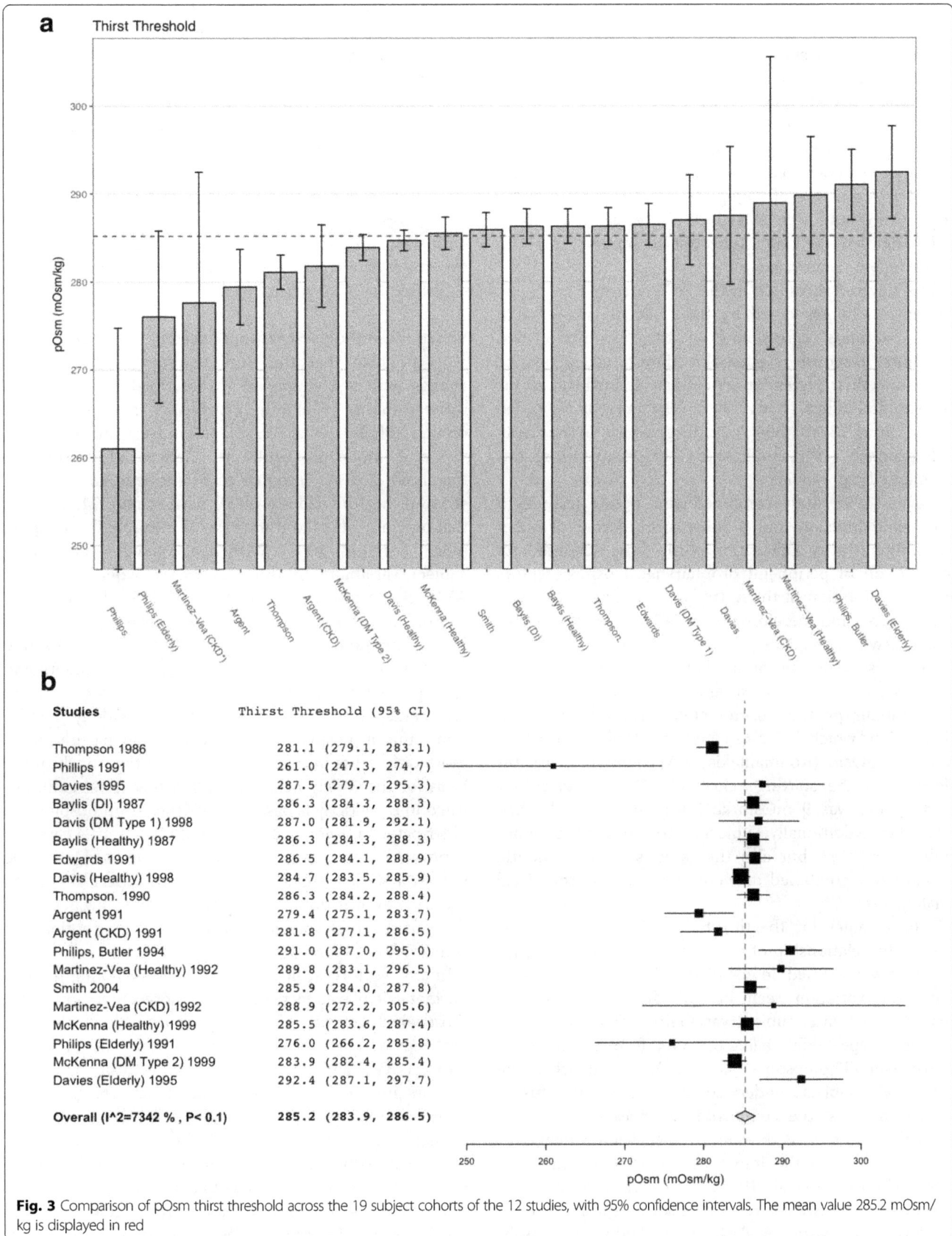

Fig. 3 Comparison of pOsm thirst threshold across the 19 subject cohorts of the 12 studies, with 95% confidence intervals. The mean value 285.2 mOsm/kg is displayed in red

Instead, subtle variation in experimental protocol and data handling can account for much of the heterogeneity.

Both studies of chronic kidney disease report adjusted pOsm values to facilitate comparison between controls and subjects; in the case of Argent (Argent et al., 1991), these were corrected to a urea concentration of 0, which will give an artificially low thirst threshold; conversely Martinez-vea corrected pOsm upwards to a standardised blood urea nitrogen of 10 mg/100 ml, accounting for the higher threshold seen (Martinez-Vea et al., 1992). Notably, this was the only study not to impose limits on subjects' pre-trial intake.

The elevated threshold in the 1994 trial by Philips and Butler can be explained by their use of two-segment piecewise linear regression. From their assumption that the thirst response is parabolic, they forced a turning point into their regression model and defined this as the threshold (Phillips et al., 1994). The experiment raised pOsm from 287 to 304 mOsm/kg, which by necessity will produce a threshold within this range, using this segmented regression.

Davies' 1995 study combined data points from both the saline infusion and a subsequent period of water drinking into their calculation of the thirst threshold. As stimulation of peripheral oropharyngeal osmoreceptors leads to inhibition of thirst, this method produces lower thirst scores and therefore reports a higher threshold for thirst (Davies et al., 1995).

The most significant outlier is Philips' 1991 study. This study is unique in its measurement of pOsm, determined by a vapour pressure osmometer, based on dew point depression, which has a tendency to produce lower results for pOsm (Koumantakis & Wyndham, 1989). Indeed, even the starting values of pOsm reported for participants was 9 mOsm/kg lower in this study than any other. Additionally, subjects were asked to score not only their thirst, but also the dryness of their mouth, which likely combined to increase ratings on the visual analogue scale.

Whilst values for the threshold fall within a narrow range, the relationship of thirst intensity to rising osmolality shows marked inter-individual variation. Importantly the variation seen in this threshold is mainly derived from inter-subject variability, with a very high degree of repeatability being observed for each individual participant (Thompson et al., 1986). Indeed, when the same eight subjects underwent a repeat saline infusion after 6 months, the composite variances in values for both thirst and AVP thresholds of each individual subject compared to the initial values, were found to be 0.6% (Thompson et al., 1991). It thus appears that each person's thirst response remains a consistent indicator of his level of dehydration. Perhaps this 'individual threshold' is associated with 'healthy hydration' for that

subject, and the stimulation of thirst and AVP release act to return a subject to this set point of hydration.

There exists some disagreement in the literature regarding whether AVP release shares the same response to pOsm as the thirst. Our analysis demonstrates a 0.9 mOsm/kg difference between these two thresholds. This result is consistent with the findings of Thompson et al.'s 1986 study of healthy men, which concluded that AVP release and thirst sensation have a shared threshold (Thompson et al., 1986). However, such a result conflicts with data reported by others, Robertson suggesting that the thirst threshold was consistently higher than the threshold for AVP release (Robertson, 1984).

Variations in the thirst response seen in the elderly

It is possible that the thirst and/or AVP thresholds change with age. Philips et al. described a reduction in thirst response in elderly men despite normal AVP secretion (Phillips et al., 1991). In contrast, however, Davies et al. found no significant difference in the slope or threshold of thirst response to pOsm between young (< 40) and 'healthy' elderly (> 70) participants. They found that age only affected thirst response to rapidly changing pOsm (Arnaud, 2003). With age, the inter- and intra-subject variability of thirst increases, whereas that of AVP release does not (Phillips et al., 1991; Davies et al., 1995). This variability is seen in response to differences in experimental conditions, such as altered rate of saline infusion; it is possible that the subjects undergoing healthy ageing, described in Davies et al.'s work, are not representative of the cross section of the elderly population found in hospital, many of whom may have multiple morbidities. It is important to recognise that much of the basis for the widely held assumption that thirst is diminished in the elderly is based on evidence from hospitalised older patients (Kenney & Chiu, 2001). Yet, in the carefully controlled experimental conditions utilised in the reviewed studies, thirst sensing did not appear altered by age. However, it does appear that elderly subjects do not drink as much as younger subjects upon dehydration and similar AVP responses (Phillips et al., 1984).

In any work regarding thirst, it is worth noting the important role played by peripheral osmoreceptors, primarily those which generate afferent signals from the oropharyngeal region. These produce a marked and sudden inhibition of AVP and thirst in response to drinking, which appears greater than can be ascribed to any change in systemic osmolality and which antecedes such osmolality changes (Figaro & Mack, 1997). As such, access to oral fluids may reduce the thirst score associated with any rise in plasma osmolality, and may thus increase experimental thirst threshold values and thirst-osmolar gradient. Most notably, those studies reporting a reduction of thirst sensing in the elderly have examined this question in relation to oral fluid intake (Mack et al., 1994; Miescher & Fortney, 1989; Phillips et al., 1984; Takamata et al., 1999). It remains to be seen whether this finding is consistent in the case of intravenous rather than oral rehydration, although it is possible that oropharyngeal suppression of osmotic thirst is greater in the elderly. If so, thirst will remain a good guide to intravenous fluid management of dehydration in both the young and old. The thirst of elderly subjects' is less sensitive to isolated experimental variations in plasma volume (Stachenfeld et al., 1997). However, given the interdependence of osmotic and haemodynamic thirst mechanisms, future studies should focus on the combined hypertonic-hypovolaemic dehydration typical in clinical practice.

Variations in the thirst response seen in women

Over the course of the menstrual cycle, there is marked variation in the levels of circulating oestrogen and progesterone. Whist the follicular phase is dominated by an oestrogen spike at day 12, the luteal phase sees high levels of both oestrogen and progesterone peaking at day 22. These hormones are known to influence the thirst response by several possible mechanisms of actions. AVP's effect at the kidneys is modulated by oestrogen, whilst α and β oestrogen receptors are found in AVP neurons of the hypothalamus, and along both osmoreceptor and baroreceptor pathways, controlling AVP release (Sladek & Somponpun, 2008).

Whilst the combination of oestrogen and progesterone produce a threshold-lowering effect, neither hormone in isolation is responsible for this effect. Combined administration of oestrogen and progesterone produced a greater reduction in threshold than either hormone in isolation.

Application to a hospitalised population

'Thirst threshold' appears remarkably consistent in the healthy, suggesting that patient thirst may be a useful guide to fluid administration in such individuals. However, this may not be so in hospitalised patients: haemodialysis (Martinez-Vea et al., 1992) and opioid administration, for instance, might perhaps both be associated with increases in thirst (Stotts et al., 2015). Morphine use was associated with a dry mouth in 47% of intensive care patients, with 3% of fentanyl users afflicted (Wiffen et al., 2014). Whilst causation was unproven in this study, high doses of morphine may stimulate drinking whilst low doses may inhibit thirst (Vokes, 1987). The specific nature of thirst response to opioids is thus hypothesised to depend on dose administered and the receptor being targeted, with μ_2, δ_1, and κ receptors modulating angiotensin II-induced thirst (Wilson et al., 1999). Likewise, insulin and epinephrine appear to stimulate thirst, whilst norepinephrine, haloperidol, and glucocorticoids may be inhibitory (Vokes, 1987). Thirst is shown to increase the intensity of contemporaneous pain

whilst no changes were seen in thirst rating in response to pain (Farrell et al., 2006). Whether such influences are of clinical relevance is not known.

Interestingly, diabetes mellitus, a condition often associated with disturbances in thirst, was found to have no influence on thirst threshold (McKenna et al., 1999). The administration of a glucose infusion, raising blood glucose levels to 20 mmol/L did not influence either thirst or AVP levels. This suggests that the polydipsia experienced in uncontrolled diabetes is a consequence of hypovolaemia induced by polyuria, rather than disturbances in plasma osmolality (Thompson et al., 1988).

Conclusion

Thirst and AVP respond to increases is plasma osmolality in unison, acting as the primary homeostatic mechanism of body water regulation. Across a range of physiological states including young healthy males, in patients with chronic kidney failure, and in subjects over the age of 70 and participants with both types 1 & type 2 diabetes, values for the pOsm threshold of thirst response fell within a narrow range.

Our analysis has demonstrated that across a diverse population of participants the thresholds for thirst activation and AVP release are exactly in the middle of the normal range of plasma osmolality. Both rise linearly with pOsm, intensifying the mechanisms acting to reduce pOsm, either by stimulating water consumption or stimulating water retention at the nephron. It can be assumed that the presence of the symptom of thirst likely indicates a hyperosmotic state. Thus, clinicians might use the symptom of thirst to screen for the need for further assessment of hydration status. This clinical examination can be facilitated by requesting a measurement of plasma osmolality, or alternatively through simple calculations from the patient's existing biochemistry data. The best formula for doing do being: plasma osmolarity (in mmol/L) = $1.86 \times (Na^+ + K^+) + 1.15 \times$ [glucose] + [urea] + 14 (Hooper et al., 2015).

Whilst the exact levels of plasma osmolality at which thirst can be sensed vary between individuals, intra-individual measures are highly consistent and reproducible. Thirst may be a more sensitive indicator of dehydration than a clinician's assessment of physical signs. As such, our patient's feedback as to their sense of thirst could hold the essential information needed to accurately manage their fluid administration for both pre- and post- operative optimisation.

These existing trials are limited in their scope, in that they artificially induced a hyperosmolar state in small and restrictive cohorts. The time consuming and invasive nature of the experimental designs used limit the cohort size to an extent. The volume expansion caused by the administration of fluids may also interfere with the sensation of thirst as baroreceptors stimulate atrial natriuretic peptide release, inhibiting thirst. The lack of hypovolaemia accompanying the hyperosmolar plasma excludes a true investigation of the thirst response which increases exponentially as plasma volume falls. The model of thirst examined by these studies remains representative of mild to moderate degrees of dehydration, more relevant to perioperative optimisation. These studies remain of value in their assessment of a fundamental physiological parameter, but further investigations in surgical patients throughout the perioperative period would be of value. Our analysis of these trials was limited by their age, and the associated difficulty in attaining the raw data. We rely on the data analysis of each individual author and our analysis inherits a degree of heterogeneity as a result. Our review is further limited in that it does not include hospitalised patients.

Fluid management is an area that still requires significant improvements, yet the thirst response has been overlooked as an area of research over the last decade. A full population based model of thirst is still lacking, and we would advocate further research in this area. Firstly, the true prevalence of elevated plasma osmolarity might be systematically sought in patient electronic records. Secondly, the ability of a variety of clinicians to identify varying degrees of dehydration should be assessed across a range of severities. All such findings might be related to the quantified thirst intensity as perceived by patients. This may be facilitated by the prospective inclusion of thirst intensity into clinical research databases as a patient reported outcome measure. Factors influencing that thirst response (such as opioid analgaesic use, anticholinergic drug effects, obtundation, use of dry inhaled gases) might also be systematically sought. The full description of those factors that affect thirst in the hospitalised patient, by way of large-scale observation studies would allow for the design of individualised thirst-based fluid administration systems, specific to a patient's pathology and medications. Furthermore, explicit investigation of whether thirst might be used to guide or trigger the administration of intravenous fluid boluses in the clinical setting is warranted. Clinical trials might asses the ability of healthy volunteers and of patients to better guide their intravenous fluid therapy.

Abbreviations
AVP: Arginine vasopressin; pOsm: Plasma osmolality; SEM: Standard error in the mean

Acknowledgements
There are no acknowledgements to be made.

Funding
This work received no funding.

Author's contributions
FH performed the literature searches, wrote the primary manuscript, and incorporated the regular inputs from the other authors. FH also performed the statistical analysis and prepared the final manuscript. HM identified the need for such a work and provided guidance on the scope of the review and the framework for its initial conception. HM also drafted the regular alterations and gave critical comments. HM also performed a significant redrafting of the manuscript to reduce its length and read and approved final draft. MM identified the need for such a work. Provided additional sources to include in the review, and guided its development, ensuring that all aspects of the topic were addressed. MM also drafted the alterations and gave critical comments and read and approved final draft. All authors read and approved the final manuscript.

Competing interests
FH declares that he/she has no competing interests. HM and MM are named co-inventors on a patent relating to a device to allow patient-controlled fluid delivery. MM is a paid consultant for Edwards Lifesciences and Deltex. MM is also University Chair endowed by Smiths Medical.

References
Andersson B, Rundgren M. Thirst and its disorders. Annu Rev Med. 1982;33:231–9.

Argent NB, Burrell LM, Goodship TH, Wilkinson R, Baylis PH. Osmoregulation of thirst and vasopressin release in severe chronic renal failure. Kidney Int. 1991; 39:295–300.

Armstrong LE. Assessing hydration status: the elusive gold standard. J Am Coll Nutr. 2007;26:575S–84S.

Arnaud MJ. Mild dehydration: a risk factor of constipation? Eur J Clin Nutr. 2003; 57(Suppl 2):S88–95.

Association HP: Listen to patients, speak up for change. 2010.

Baylis PH, Thompson CJ. Osmoregulation of vasopressin secretion and thirst in health and disease. Clin Endocrinol. 1988;29:549–76.

Becker BJ, Wu M-J. The synthesis of regression slopes in meta-analysis; 2007. p. 414–29.

Boettger S, Jenewein J, Breitbart W. Delirium and severe illness: etiologies, severity of delirium and phenomenological differences. Palliat Support Care. 2015;13:1087–92.

Calzone WL, Silva C, Keefe DL, Stachenfeld NS. Progesterone does not alter osmotic regulation of AVP. Am J Physiol Regul Integr Comp Physiol. 2001; 281:R2011–20.

Comission NuTCQ. Dignity and nutrition inspection program: national overview. Commission CQ. 2011;

Davies I, O'Neill PA, McLean KA, Catania J, Bennett D. Age-associated alterations in thirst and arginine vasopressin in response to a water or sodium load. Age Ageing. 1995;24:151–9.

Davison JM, Shiells EA, Philips PR, Lindheimer MD. Serial evaluation of vasopressin release and thirst in human pregnancy. Role of human chorionic gonadotrophin in the osmoregulatory changes of gestation. J Clin Invest. 1988;81:798–806.

El-Sharkawy AM, Watson P, Neal KR, Ljungqvist O, Maughan RJ, Sahota O, Lobo DN. Hydration and outcome in older patients admitted to hospital (the HOOP prospective cohort study). Age Ageing. 2015;44:943–7.

Evbuomwan IO, Davison JM, Baylis PH, Murdoch AP. Altered osmotic thresholds for arginine vasopressin secretion and thirst during superovulation and in the ovarian hyperstimulation syndrome (OHSS): relevance to the pathophysiology of OHSS. Fertil Steril. 2001;75:933–41.

Farrell MJ, Egan GF, Zamarripa F, Shade R, Blair-West J, Fox P, Denton DA. Unique, common, and interacting cortical correlates of thirst and pain. Proc Natl Acad Sci U S A. 2006;103:2416–21.

Feehally J, Khosravi M. Effects of acute and chronic hypohydration on kidney health and function. Nutr Rev. 2015;73(Suppl 2):110–9.

Figaro MK, Mack GW. Regulation of fluid intake in dehydrated humans: role of oropharyngeal stimulation. Am J Phys. 1997;272:R1740–6.

Fortes MB, Owen JA, Raymond-Barker P, Bishop C, Elghenzai S, Oliver SJ, Walsh NP. Is this elderly patient dehydrated? Diagnostic accuracy of hydration assessment using physical signs, urine, and saliva markers. J Am Med Dir Assoc. 2015;16:221–8.

Frangeskou M, Lopez-Valcarcel B, Serra-Majem L. Dehydration in the elderly: a review focused on economic burden. J Nutr Health Aging. 2015;19:619–27.

Gross CR, Lindquist RD, Woolley AC, Granieri R, Allard K, Webster B. Clinical indicators of dehydration severity in elderly patients. J Emerg Med. 1992; 10:267–74.

Holte K, Sharrock NE, Kehlet H. Pathophysiology and clinical implications of perioperative fluid excess. Br J Anaesth. 2002;89:622–32.

Hooper L, Abdelhamid A, Ali A, Bunn DK, Jennings A, John WG, Kerry S, Lindner G, Pfortmueller CA, Sjostrand F, et al. Diagnostic accuracy of calculated serum osmolarity to predict dehydration in older people: adding value to pathology laboratory reports. BMJ Open. 2015;5:e008846.

Johnson AK. The sensory psychobiology of thirst and salt appetite. Med Sci Sports Exerc. 2007;39:1388–400.

Johnson AK, Mann JF, Rascher W, Johnson JK, Ganten D. Plasma angiotensin II concentrations and experimentally induced thirst. Am J Phys. 1981;240:R229–34.

Kanagasundaram NS. Pathophysiology of ischaemic acute kidney injury. Ann Clin Biochem. 2015;52:193–205.

Kenney WL, Chiu P. Influence of age on thirst and fluid intake. Med Sci Sports Exerc. 2001;33:1524–32.

Kimura T, Minai K, Matsui K, Mouri T, Sato T. Effect of various states of hydration on plasma ADH and renin in man. J Clin Endocrinol Metab. 1976;42:79–87.

Kloner RA. Natural and unnatural triggers of myocardial infarction. Prog Cardiovasc Dis. 2006;48:285–300.

Koumantakis G, Wyndham LE. An evaluation of osmolality measurement by freezing point depression using micro-amounts of sample. J Automat Chem. 1989;11:80–3.

Lilot M, Ehrenfeld JM, Lee C, Harrington B, Cannesson M, Rinehart J. Variability in practice and factors predictive of total crystalloid administration during abdominal surgery: retrospective two-centre analysis. Br J Anaesth. 2015;114:767–76.

Mack GW, Weseman CA, Langhans GW, Scherzer H, Gillen CM, Nadel ER. Body fluid balance in dehydrated healthy older men: thirst and renal osmoregulation. J Appl Physiol (1985). 1994;76:1615–23.

Mackenzie A, Barnes G, Shann F. Clinical signs of dehydration in children. Lancet. 1989;2:605–7.

Martinez-Vea A, Garcia C, Gaya J, Rivera F, Oliver JA. Abnormalities of thirst regulation in patients with chronic renal failure on hemodialysis. Am J Nephrol. 1992;12:73–9.

McKenna K, Morris AD, Azam H, Newton RW, Baylis PH, Thompson CJ. Exaggerated vasopressin secretion and attenuated osmoregulated thirst in human survivors of hyperosmolar coma. Diabetologia. 1999;42:534–8.

Miescher E, Fortney SM. Responses to dehydration and rehydration during heat exposure in young and older men. Am J Phys. 1989;257:R1050–6.

Parliamentary OH: Care and compassion?: report of the Healeth service ombudsman on ten investigations into NHS Care of Older People. 2011.

Pash E, Parikh N, Hashemi L. Economic burden associated with hospital postadmission dehydration. JPEN J Parenter Enteral Nutr. 2014;38:58S–64S.

Phillips EM, Butler T, Baylis PH. Osmoregulation of vasopressin and thirst: comparison of 20% mannitol with 5% saline as osmotic stimulants in healthy man. Clin Endocrinol. 1994;41:207–12.

Phillips PA, Bretherton M, Johnston CI, Gray L. Reduced osmotic thirst in healthy elderly men. Am J Phys. 1991;261:R166–71.

Phillips PA, Rolls BJ, Ledingham JG, Forsling ML, Morton JJ, Crowe MJ, Wollner L. Reduced thirst after water deprivation in healthy elderly men. N Engl J Med. 1984;311:753–9.

Phillips PA, Rolls BJ, Ledingham JG, Morton JJ. Body fluid changes, thirst and drinking in man during free access to water. Physiol Behav. 1984;33:357–63.

Puntillo KA, Arai S, Cohen NH, Gropper MA, Neuhaus J, Paul SM, Miaskowski C. Symptoms experienced by intensive care unit patients at high risk of dying. Crit Care Med. 2010;38:2155–60.

QC RF: Mid Staffordshire NHS foundation trust public inquiry. 2013.

Robertson GL. Abnormalities of thirst regulation. Kidney Int. 1984;25:460–9.

Rowat A, Graham C, Dennis M. Dehydration in hospital-admitted stroke patients: detection, frequency, and association. Stroke. 2012;43:857–9.

Saad E, Ron H, Gleb S, Benjamin B, Yona N. Dehydration as a possible cause of monthly variation in the incidence of venous Thromboembolism. Clin Appl Thromb Hemost. 2016;22:569–74.

Satterthwaite FE. An approximate distribution of estimates of variance components. Biom Bull. 1946;2:110–4.

Siervo M, Bunn D, Prado CM, Hooper L. Accuracy of prediction equations for serum osmolarity in frail older people with and without diabetes. Am J Clin Nutr. 2014;100:867–76.

Sladek CD, Somponpun SJ. Estrogen receptors: their roles in regulation of vasopressin release for maintenance of fluid and electrolyte homeostasis. Front Neuroendocrinol. 2008;29:114–27.

Smith D, Moore K, Tormey W, Baylis PH, Thompson CJ. Downward resetting of the osmotic threshold for thirst in patients with SIADH. Am J Physiol Endocrinol Metab. 2004;287:E1019–23.

Spruce BA, Baylis PH, Burd J, Watson MJ. Variation in osmoregulation of arginine vasopressin during the human menstrual cycle. Clin Endocrinol. 1985;22:37–42.

Stachenfeld NS, DiPietro L, Nadel ER, Mack GW. Mechanism of attenuated thirst in aging: role of central volume receptors. Am J Phys Regul Integr Comp Phys. 1997;272:R148–57.

Stachenfeld NS, Keefe DL. Estrogen effects on osmotic regulation of AVP and fluid balance. Am J Physiol Endocrinol Metab. 2002;283:E711–21.

Stachenfeld NS, Silva C, Keefe DL, Kokoszka CA, Nadel ER. Effects of oral contraceptives on body fluid regulation. J Appl Physiol (1985). 1999;87:1016–25.

Stotts NA, Arai SR, Cooper BA, Nelson JE, Puntillo KA. Predictors of thirst in intensive care unit patients. J Pain Symptom Manag. 2015;49:530–8.

Takamata A, Ito T, Yaegashi K, Takamiya H, Maegawa Y, Itoh T, Greenleaf JE, Morimoto T. Effect of an exercise-heat acclimation program on body fluid regulatory responses to dehydration in older men. Am J Phys. 1999;277: R1041–50.

Thomas DR, Tariq SH, Makhdomm S, Haddad R, Moinuddin A. Physician misdiagnosis of dehydration in older adults. J Am Med Dir Assoc. 2004;5:S30–4.

Thompson CJ, Baylis PH. Thirst in diabetes insipidus: clinical relevance of quantitative assessment. Q J Med. 1987;65:853–62.

Thompson CJ, Bland J, Burd J, Baylis PH. The osmotic thresholds for thirst and vasopressin release are similar in healthy man. Clin Sci (Lond). 1986;71:651–6.

Thompson CJ, Burd JM, Baylis PH. Osmoregulation of vasopressin secretion and thirst in cyclical oedema. Clin Endocrinol. 1988;28:629–35.

Thompson CJ, Davis SN, Butler PC, Charlton JA, Baylis PH. Osmoregulation of thirst and vasopressin secretion in insulin-dependent diabetes mellitus. Clin Sci (Lond). 1988;74:599–606.

Thompson CJ, Edwards CR, Baylis PH. Osmotic and non-osmotic regulation of thirst and vasopressin secretion in patients with compulsive water drinking. Clin Endocrinol. 1991;35:221–8.

Thompson CJ, Selby P, Baylis PH. Reproducibility of osmotic and nonosmotic tests of vasopressin secretion in men. Am J Phys. 1991;260:R533–9.

Vokes T. Water homeostasis. Annu Rev Nutr. 1987;7:383–406.

Wiffen PJ, Derry S, Moore RA. Impact of morphine, fentanyl, oxycodone or codeine on patient consciousness, appetite and thirst when used to treat cancer pain. Cochrane Database Syst Rev. 2014:CD011056.

Wilson J, Woods I, Fawcett J, Whall R, Dibb W, Morris C, McManus E. Reducing the risk of major elective surgery: randomised controlled trial of preoperative optimisation of oxygen delivery. BMJ. 1999;318:1099–103.

Patient-reported outcomes 6 months after enhanced recovery after colorectal surgery

Thomas Deiss[1]* (iD), Lee-lynn Chen[2], Ankit Sarin[3] and Ramana K. Naidu[4]

Abstract

Background: Enhanced recovery after surgery (ERAS) programs have been established as perioperative strategies associated with improved outcomes. However, intermediate and long-term patient-reported outcome data for patients undergoing ERAS interventions remain limited. We utilized an automated telephone survey 6 months post-colorectal surgery from patients who participated in an ERAS program to determine 6-month patient-reported outcomes and associated predictive factors.

Methods: We conducted a prospective observational study, using an automated telephone survey and researcher-administered telephone questionnaire 6 months after patients underwent abdominal colorectal surgery. Six-month significant outcomes were defined by persistent pain, hospital readmission, and patient satisfaction. Patients reporting these outcome variables were compared with patients who met none of these criteria. Additionally, analysis was performed to determine differences between patients that did and did not respond to the 6-month survey. A chi-square test was used to determine any relationship for categorical variables, a two independent sample t test for length of procedure/stay, and a Wilcoxon-Mann-Whitney test for pain scores.

Results: One hundred fifty-four of 324 patients contacted 6 months after surgery completed the automated telephone survey (47.53%). There was no statistical difference between patient populations completing and not completing the survey. Hospital 6-month readmission was associated with patients with a diagnosis of cancer ($P = .049$) and with a longer mean length of index procedure (282 vs. 206 minutes, $P = .006$). Median 6-month pain scores were higher for patients that underwent an open procedure compared to laparoscopic ($Z = -2.06$, $P = .04$).

Conclusions: Long-term benefits of an ERAS program were mostly confirmed. Longer procedure time and patients with cancer correlated with an increased likelihood of hospital 6-month readmission, suggesting that perioperative outcomes in complex cancer patients need to be evaluated over a longer time frame. In addition, invasiveness of procedure continues to have a significant effect on pain scores even 6 months later.

Keywords: Enhanced recovery after surgery, Colorectal surgery, Postoperative pain, Long-term outcomes, Hospital readmission

Background

Enhanced recovery after surgery (ERAS) programs are becoming an essential component of any perioperative management paradigm. They have been shown to be effective at improving early postoperative outcomes in several settings (Lau and Chamberlain 2017; Visioni et al. 2017; Ni et al. 2015) and especially in colorectal surgery (Sarin et al. 2016a). However, information on recovery after discharge in this group of patients is limited (Jakobsson et al. 2014),

and this information is becoming increasingly important as convalescence from surgery shifts to the outpatient setting in the era of shortening postoperative length of stays. Current postoperative data focuses on physiological parameters, which are key in the early postoperative period, but are neither available nor reflective of recovery in the post discharge longer term period when patients are under less surveillance by healthcare providers. Therefore, there is merit in obtaining and analyzing patient-reported outcomes during this period.

Previous studies (Kehlet et al. 2006a) have shown that acute postoperative pain is followed by persistent pain in

* Correspondence: thomas.deiss@ucsf.edu
[1]Department of Biochemistry & Biophysics, University of California San Francisco, 505 Parnassus Ave., San Francisco, CA 94143, USA
Full list of author information is available at the end of the article

10–50% of individuals after common operations. Chronic postoperative pain can range from 15 to 30% after major and minor abdominal and pelvic operations, 6–36% following inguinal hernia, 3–56% following gall bladder surgery, (Perkins and Kehlet 2000), and 17% incidence for colorectal operations (Joris et al. 2015). In addition to pain, other factors such as fatigue, muscle weakness, and gastrointestinal dysfunction, which can persist for several weeks, contribute to the dissatisfaction felt by patients. Our study attempted to identify the percentage of patients that have a less than satisfactory 6-month outcome following colorectal surgery within an enhanced recovery program and to analyze the cause of these outcomes using patient-reported data.

Methods

After obtaining Institutional Review Board approval, we conducted a prospective observational study of patients that underwent abdominal colorectal surgery at a single tertiary medical center from February 2015 to June 2016. All adult patients ($n = 324$) that were part of the

ERAS program for colorectal surgery within this period were included in the study. As part of standard care in the ERAS program, patients receive automated telephone calls (CipherHealth LLC, New York, NY) 6 months after discharge following surgery. The automated telephone call script was designed to ask questions about persistent pain, readmissions, and satisfaction with their stay at the medical center (Fig. 1). These data were collected monthly and sent to our research team. For the first 2 months of data collection, a researcher called patients that had completed the automated telephone call to validate their survey responses. The period of validation ended when no difference between the automated telephone call and research-administered questionnaire results were found. After the initial period of validation, a researcher called all patients that reported a significant outcome in the automated telephone call and administered a telephone questionnaire (Fig. 2). Significant outcomes were defined by any of the following: (1) pain associated with the surgery 6 months after discharge, (2) any hospital readmissions between discharge and 6 months, regardless of cause, and (3) patients reporting "somewhat

Fig. 1 Script for automated telephone call

Questionnaire:

1.) Are you currently having pain related to your colorectal surgery on __/__/__?
      YES   NO
(If no skip to question 4)
2.) Can you please rate your pain on a scale from 1-9, with 1 being a little and 9 being the worst pain?
  1   2   3   4   5   6   7   8   9

3.) Where, specifically, are you experiencing pain?

_____

3.) Are you taking prescription medications to manage your pain?
      YES   NO
If yes, what medications are you currently taking?

_____

4.) Have you been re-admitted to the hospital since your discharge on __/__/__?
      YES   NO
If yes,
Why were you admitted to the hospital?_____

_____

When was this hospital admission? _____

How long were you in the hospital?_____

7.) Were you satisfied with your stay at UCSF Medical Center on __/__/__ to __/__/__?

a. COMPLETELY SATISFIED   b. SOMEWHAT SATISFIED c. NOT SATISFIED

(If b or c) Can you briefly describe to me what we could have done differently to improve your experience?

_____

_____

If applicable (reported pain, poor outcome, dissatisfaction):

You reported (stated issue/concerns) during this survey. Have you brought up this issue with your surgical team or primary medical doctor and is it currently being addressed?
      YES   NO

If no, why not? _____

Fig. 2 Research telephone questionnaire

satisfied" or "not satisfied" with their stay at the medical center. The researcher-administered telephone questionnaire confirmed data collected from the automated telephone call and also collected additional information. The additional information collected by the researcher-administered telephone questionnaire included, when applicable, the site of the patient's pain, what specific medications were being taken for pain, when they were readmitted to a hospital, why they were readmitted to a hospital, the length of their hospital readmission, and/or what could have been done

differently to improve their experience during their initial stay. Researcher-administered telephone questionnaires were done within 2 weeks of receiving the monthly data and up to three attempts were made to contact each patient. The Institutional Review Board granted a waiver of informed consent for patients in which only information from the medical record and automated telephone calls was obtained. For patients that completed the researcher-administered telephone questionnaire, verbal consent was first obtained for the collection of the questionnaire data.

Baseline patient and surgical data was retrieved from electronic medical records for all patients that received an automated telephone call 6 months post-colorectal surgery. Patient data included age, gender, diagnoses (cancer/non-cancer), and ASA rating. Surgical data included use of an epidural, type of procedure (open vs. minimally invasive), preoperative and postoperative pain scores, length of procedure, and length of hospital stay. Preoperative pain scores were collected in the pre-operative holding room when patients were checked in before surgery, and average postoperative pain scores were collected while patients were in the post-anesthesia care unit after surgery.

Significant outcomes were based off the six-month automated telephone call and researcher-administered telephone questionnaire. Patients reporting any of the significant outcomes were compared with patients that did not report any significant outcomes.

Data were analyzed using STATA software (Version 12.1, StataCorp LLC, College Station, TX). Statistical analysis was performed to determine any relationship between surgical or patient data and the significant outcomes. P values were obtained from the chi-square test to determine any relationship between the categorical variables (age, gender, diagnoses, ASA rating, type of procedure, epidural use) and each significant outcome. P values were obtained from the two independent sample t test to determine the relationship between length of procedure and length of stay to each significant outcome. A Wilcoxon-Mann-Whitney test was used to determine any relationship between preoperative and postoperative pain (1–10 scale used for both) and any significant outcome. Analysis was also performed to determine if there was a statistically significant difference between the surgical and patient data of those who completed the automated 6-month survey and those that did not, using the same statistical tests described above (Table 1).

Results

During the 17-month study period from February 2015 to June 2016, 324 patients received automated telephone calls 6 months after discharge following colorectal surgery. One hundred fifty-four of 324 (48%) patients completed the automated telephone survey and 39 of 324 (12%) patients completed the researcher-administered telephone questionnaire. Of the patients that completed the 6-month automated telephone call, 61 of 154 (40%) reported a significant outcome (Fig. 3). Twenty-seven of those 61 patients (44%) completed a researcher-administered telephone questionnaire, while the remaining 34 patients (56%) could not be reached in the follow-up call and/or all relevant data was collected from the automated telephone questionnaire and electronic medical records at UC San Francisco Medical Center. One patient that was contacted by a researcher refused participation in the telephone questionnaire,

Table 1 Difference between the patient population that completed the automated 6-month telephone survey and the population that did not complete the survey

	Completed 6-month call ($N = 154$)	Unsuccessful 6-month call ($N = 170$)	P value
Age	55 ± 14	53 ± 15	0.246
Male sex	81 (53)	80 (47)	0.319
Dx of cancer	75 (49)	73 (43)	0.299
Open procedure	64 (42)	73 (43)	0.801
Median length of stay (hours)	126	126	0.839
Median length of Procedure (min)	187	197	0.572
Median ASA rating	2	2	0.579
Pre-op pain	29 (19)	40 (24)	0.302
Post-op pain	73 (47)	81 (48)	0.948
Epidural use	90 (58)	108 (64)	0.348

and none of that patient's data was included in the study. There were no statistical differences between those completing and not completing the telephone survey when examining age, gender, cancer diagnosis, and variables related to the patient's procedure (Table 1).

Thirty of 154 (19%) patients reported persistent surgical pain, 31 of 154 (20%) patients reported a hospital readmission, and 21 of 154 (14%) patients reported less than complete satisfaction with their stay (Fig. 4).

Of the 30 patients reporting persistent surgical pain, 19 (63%) reported taking medication for their pain, 10 of which were using opioids to manage their pain. Median 6-month pain scores were significantly higher for patients that underwent an open procedure compared to minimally invasive

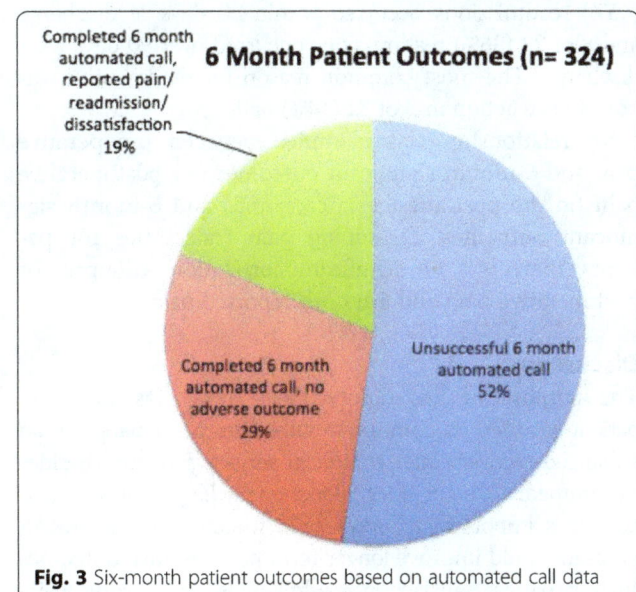

Fig. 3 Six-month patient outcomes based on automated call data

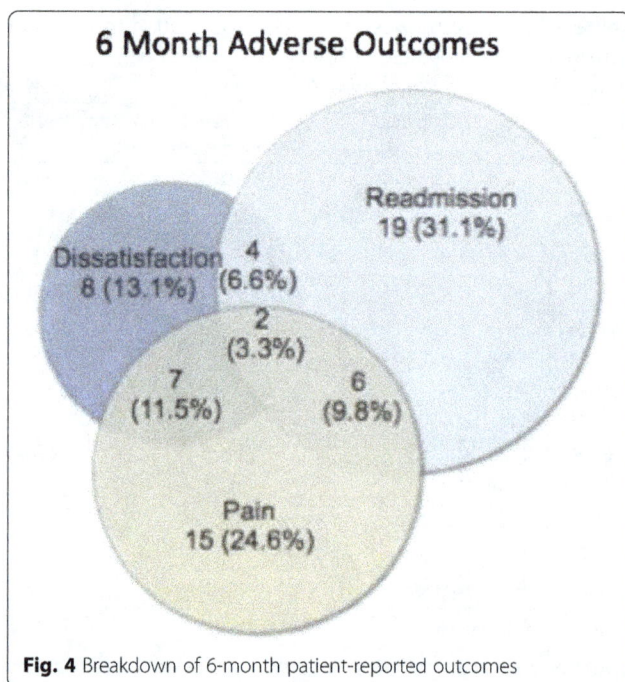

Fig. 4 Breakdown of 6-month patient-reported outcomes

Table 2 Characteristics of patients with and without a hospital readmission within 6 months of discharge

	Hospital readmission within 6 months of discharge (N = 31)	No hospital readmission within 6 months of discharge (N = 123)	P value
Age	57 ± 16	54 ± 14	0.290
Male sex	21 (68)	60 (49)	0.059
Dx of cancer	20 (65)	55 (45)	0.049
Open procedure	12 (39)	52 (42)	0.719
Length of stay (hours)	202 ± 118	184 ± 170	0.839
Length of procedure (min)	282 ± 167	206 ± 126	0.006
Median ASA rating	2	2	0.127
Pre-op pain	7 (23)	22 (18)	0.550
Post-op pain	14 (48)	61 (50)	0.836
Epidural use	19 (61)	71 (58)	0.719
Dissatisfaction with stay	6 (19)	15 (12)	0.299
6 month pain	8 (26)	22 (18)	0.320

($Z = -2.06$, $P = 0.04$). All patients reporting persistent pain confirmed that the site of pain was surgical and not a chronic or non-surgical pain.

Of the patients reporting less than complete satisfaction with their hospital stay, postoperative pain (9 of 21, 43%) and postoperative complications (8 of 21, 38%) were the most common reasons.

Hospital readmission was associated with a diagnosis of cancer ($P = .049$) and with longer mean length of procedure (282 vs. 206 min, $P = .006$) (Table 2). Of the patients with hospital readmissions, readmission data was only available for 22 of 31 (71%) patients. Of those patients, 10 of 22 (45%) readmissions occurred within 30 days of discharge and 8 of 22 (36%) readmissions occurred over 90 days after discharge. The most common reason for readmission was bowel obstruction in 3 of 22 (14%) patients.

No relationship was identified between preoperative pain and 6-month significant outcomes nor postoperative pain (in the post-anesthesia care unit) and 6-month significant outcomes. Examining pain trajectories for patients, there was no significant correlation with pre- or postoperative pain and 6-month reported pain.

Discussion

The purpose of this observational study was to assess patient-reported outcomes 6 months after participation in an enhanced recovery after colorectal surgery program. Besides the immediate benefits of reduction in length of stay and cost, it is important to understand whether such an ERAS program could improve longer-term postoperative outcomes such as patient satisfaction, readmissions, and chronic pain.

Hospitals typically use surveys from vendors such as Press Ganey to collect patient satisfaction data after an inpatient stay (between 48 h and 6 weeks after discharge). With our initial rollout of ERAS for the colorectal service line, we observed improved patient outcomes while maintaining our Press Ganey scores (Sarin et al. 2016b). However, most studies and registries have concentrated on 30-day outcomes.

By using a similar automated phone call system to screen for patient-reported post-operative pain, readmission, and/ or satisfaction, we were able to focus on 6-month outcomes without requiring significant additional resources.

The survey response rate of 48% compares favorably with results reported in the literature (Kehlet et al. 2006b). Since there was no statistical difference between the responders and non-responders to the survey (based on age, gender, cancer diagnosis, and variables related to the patient's procedure), it was assumed that the reported outcomes for responders would represent those of non-responders. Similar survey techniques can be considered in the future.

Though the majority of patients were satisfied with their surgical experience, those who were dissatisfied either suffered from persistent post-surgical pain or another complication related to their surgery. These longer term patient-reported outcomes are often underappreciated by the perioperative team. Our study suggests that perioperative complications and persistent pain can be a source of patient dissatisfaction long after the index surgery when they may no longer be under the care of their surgeon.

The development of chronic persistent post-surgical pain (PPSP) is an area of growing interest. It is estimated that the incidence of PPSP after abdominal surgery is anywhere from 10 to 50% depending on the type of surgery (cholecystectomy, herniorrhaphy, laparotomy) and surveying methods (Kehlet et al. 2006b; Laufenberg-Feldmann et al. 2016). One of the main objectives of this study was to determine the prevalence of PPSP in patients after colorectal surgery and understand the role of the ERAS program in affecting this pain. This study showed a PPSP rate of 19%, of which 63% of patients were taking pain medications to address this pain. Of note, only 33% of patients were using opioids to manage this pain, which we hypothesize is directly related to their participation in an ERAS program focused on multimodal analgesia and patient education on attenuating opioid consumption postoperatively. With the current American opioid epidemic, this is a reassuring outcome.

Readmission rates at 30 days were 10%, which is similar to previously published data. The majority of readmissions were related to infection, obstruction, or nausea/vomiting. Not all data regarding readmissions were available, because patients might have been admitted to other institutions. Readmission rate at 6 months was 20%, which was twice the readmission rate at 30 days. Readmissions were associated with a diagnosis of cancer and with longer surgical procedure times, suggesting that patients with more complex operations or underlying malignancy were driving longer term readmissions, rather than postoperative care.

Limitations

This is an observational study and is dependent on telephone responses; therefore, it is inherently susceptible to selection bias. Detailed readmission data was only available for patients admitted to our institution, although the telephone surveys did capture all readmissions (subject to recall bias) as these were reported by patients themselves. The vendor through which the automated telephone surveys were administered only offered a 9-point scale for pain scores, rather than the standard 11-point numerical rating scale (NRS), which may have introduced slight differences in pain score results.

Conclusion

Nineteen percent of patients after colorectal surgery within an ERAS program went on to develop persistent post-surgical pain. However, only two out of three used any analgesic medications, and only one out of three used opioids to mitigate this pain, suggesting that a focus on multimodal non-opioid analgesia in the ERAS program may be of benefit beyond just the immediate postoperative period. Pain and postoperative complications account for the majority of dissatisfaction in patients 6 months following colorectal surgery. Readmissions occur as often in the period from 1 to 6 months following surgery as they do in the first month, and this is related to more complex surgical procedures and a diagnosis of cancer.

Abbreviations
ASA: American Society of Anesthesiologists; ERAS: Enhanced recovery after surgery; PSPP: Persistent post-surgical pain

Acknowledgements
Ramana K. Naidu has received speaker's honoraria from Halyard Health, Abbott, and Sonosite in the past year. This project did not have involvement from any of these entities.

Authors' contributions
TD conceived the study, participated in its design and coordination, performed the statistical analysis, and helped to draft the manuscript. L-LC conceived the study, participated in its design and coordination, and helped to draft the manuscript. AS conceived the study, participated in its design and coordination, and helped to draft the manuscript. RKN conceived the study, participated in its design and coordination, and helped to draft the manuscript. All authors read and approved the final manuscript.

Competing interests
The authors declare that they have no competing interests.

Author details
[1]Department of Biochemistry & Biophysics, University of California San Francisco, 505 Parnassus Ave., San Francisco, CA 94143, USA. [2]Department of Anesthesia & Perioperative Medicine, University of California San Francisco, 1825 4th St., San Francisco, CA 94158, USA. [3]Department of Surgery, University of California San Francisco, 1825 4th St., San Francisco, CA 94158, USA. [4]California Orthopedics and Spine, Director of Pain Management at Marin General Hospital, 18 Bon Air Road, Larkspur, CA 94939, USA.

References
Jakobsson J, Idvall E, Wann-Hansson C. Patient-reported recovery after enhanced colorectal cancer surgery: a longitudinal six-month follow-up study. Int J Color Dis. 2014;29(8):989–98. https://doi.org/10.1007/s00384-014-1939-2. Epub 2014 Jul 4

Joris J, Georges M, Medjahed K, et al. Prevalence, characteristics and risk factors of chronic postsurgical pain after laparoscopic colorectal surgery. Eur J Anaesthesiol. 2015;32:712–7.

Kehlet H, Jensen TS, Woolf C. Persistent postsurgical pain: risk factors and prevention. Lancet. 2006a;367:1618–25.

Kehlet H, Jensen TS, Woolf C. Persistent postsurgical pain: risk factors and prevention. Lancet. 2006b;367:1618–25.

Lau CS, Chamberlain RS. Enhanced recovery after surgery programs improve patient outcomes and recovery: a meta-analysis. World J Surg. 2017;41(4): 899–913. https://doi.org/10.1007/s00268-016-3807-4.

Laufenberg-Feldmann, et al. BMC Anesthesiology. 2016;16:91. https://doi.org/10.1186/s12871-016-0261-7.

Ni TG, Yang HT, Zhang H, Meng HP, Li B Enhanced recovery after surgery programs in patients undergoing hepatectomy: a meta-analysis. World J Gastroenterol 2015;21(30):9209–16. https://doi.org/10.3748/wjg.v21.i30.9209.

Perkins FM, Kehlet H. Chronic pain as an outcome of surgery. Anesthesiology. 2000;93:1123–33.

Sarin A, Litonius ES, Naidu R, Yost CS, Varma MG, Chen LL. Successful implementation of an enhanced recovery after surgery program shortens length of stay and improves postoperative pain, and bowel and bladder function after colorectal surgery. BMC Anesthesiol. 2016a;16(1):55. https://doi.org/10.1186/s12871-016-0223-0.

Sarin A, Litonius ES, Naidu R, Yost CS, Varma MG, Chen LL. Successful implementation of an enhanced recovery after surgery program shortens length of stay and improves postoperative pain, and bowel and bladder function after colorectal surgery. BMC Anesthesiol. 2016b;16(1):55. https://doi.org/10.1186/s12871-016-0223-0.

Visioni A, Shah R, Gabriel E, Attwood K, Kukar M, Nurkin S. Enhanced recovery after surgery for noncolorectal surgery? A systematic review and meta-analysis of major abdominal surgery. Ann Surg. 2017 Apr 21; https://doi.org/10.1097/SLA.0000000000002267.

A systematic review and meta-analysis of perioperative oral decontamination in patients undergoing major elective surgery

Philip Spreadborough[1], Sarah Lort[1], Sandro Pasquali[2], Matthew Popplewell[1], Andrew Owen[3], Irene Kreis[4], Olga Tucker[2,5], Ravinder S Vohra[1,6*] and on behalf of the Preventing Postoperative Pneumonia Study Group and the West Midlands Research Collaborative

Abstract

Background: Oral antiseptics reduce nosocomial infections and ventilator-associated pneumonia in critically ill medical and surgical patients intubated for prolonged periods. However, the role of oral antiseptics given before and after planned surgery is not clear. The aim of this systematic review and meta-analysis is to determine the effect of oral antiseptics (chlorhexidine or povidone–iodine) when administered before and after major elective surgery.

Methods: Searches were conducted of the MEDLINE, EMBASE and Cochrane databases. The analysis was performed using the random-effects method and the risk ratio (RR) with 95 % confidence interval (CI).

Results: Of 1114 unique identified articles, perioperative chlorhexidine was administered to patients undergoing elective surgery in four studies. This identified 2265 patients undergoing elective cardiac surgery, of whom 1093 (48.3 %) received perioperative chlorhexidine. Postoperative pneumonia and nosocomial infections were observed in 5.3 and 20.2 % who received chlorhexidine compared to 10.4 and 31.3 % who received a control preparation, respectively. Oral perioperative chlorhexidine significantly reduced the risk of postoperative pneumonia (RR = 0.52; 95 % CI 0.39–0.71; $p < 0.01$) and overall nosocomial infections (RR = 0.65; 95 % CI 0.52–0.81; $p < 0.01$), with no effect on in-hospital mortality (RR = 1.01; 95 % CI 0.49–2.09; $p = 0.98$).

Conclusions: Perioperative oral chlorhexidine significantly decreases the incidence of nosocomial infection and postoperative pneumonia in patients undergoing elective cardiac surgery. There are no randomised controlled studies of this simple and cheap intervention in patients undergoing elective non-cardiac surgery.

Trial Registration: This systematic review was registered with the International prospective register of systematic reviews (PROSPERO). The registration number is CRD42015016063.

Keywords: Anti-infective agents, Chlorhexidine, Perioperative care, Pneumonia

Background

An estimated 234 million patients undergo major surgery worldwide every year. Nosocomial infections, particularly postoperative pneumonia, following surgery are common, affecting 1.5–57 % of patients depending on the type and extent of surgery (Weiser et al. 2008; Hemmes et al. 2014; Niggebrugge et al. 1999; Treschan et al. 2012; Seiler et al. 2009; Hulscher et al. 2002). Following major elective abdominal surgery, postoperative pneumonia results in six to nine extra hospital days and costs the healthcare system an additional $30,000 per patient (Khuri et al. 2005). Even after risk adjustment, it is associated with a 66 % lower survival at 5 years following surgery (Khuri et al. 2005). In those who do survive, the limited available evidence suggests a detrimental effect on early and late health-related quality of life (Thompson et al. 2006).

* Correspondence: ravinder.vohra@nuh.nhs.uk
Olga Tucker and Ravinder S Vohra are Joint or Co-senior authors.
[1]West Midlands Research Collaborative, University of Birmingham, Edgbaston, Birmingham B15 2TH, UK
[6]Nottingham Oesophagi-Gastric unit, Nottingham University Hospitals NHS Trust, Queens Medical Centre, Nottingham NG7 2UH, UK
Full list of author information is available at the end of the article

The definition of postoperative pneumonia used in the majority of studies is based on clinical, radiological and microbiological criteria defined by the Center of Disease Control and Prevention (CDC) for nosocomial pneumonia between the 2nd and 30th postoperative days (Garner et al. 1988). One of the primary causes of postoperative pneumonia is aspiration of oral and pharyngeal secretions at the time of intubation before surgery. Continued micro-aspiration of secretions due to small folds in the endotracheal tube cuff with prolonged ventilation (days to weeks) contributes to ventilator-associated pneumonia (VAP) (du Moulin et al. 1982; Cook et al. 1998; American Thoracic Society 2005). Oral antiseptics such as chlorhexidine gluconate or povidone–iodine have been shown to reduce the oral bacterial load in patients mechanically ventilated for 3 days or more. Chlorhexidine gluconate is a broad-spectrum antimicrobial, effective against gram-positive and gram-negative bacteria, anaerobes and fungi within 20 s (Horner et al. 2012; Fitzgerald et al. 1989). Three recent systematic reviews demonstrate reduction in VAP by 20 % with regular oral chlorhexidine application after intubation in critically ill patients mechanically ventilated for 3 days or more, with conflicting effects on early mortality (Labeau et al. 2011; Klompas et al. 2014; Price et al. 2014). Recent recommendations support daily chlorhexidine mouth care to prevent VAP in the intensive care setting (Scottish Intensive Care Society Audit Group 2008). However, the majority of elective surgical patients are extubated immediately following surgery in the operating room. These recommendations of daily chlorhexidine mouth care do not apply to this group, and pre-anaesthesia oral decontamination or prophylaxis with oral antiseptics is currently not part of the routine care. The aim of this systematic review and meta-analysis is to determine the effect of oral decontamination using antiseptics (chlorhexidine or povidone–iodine) before and after major elective surgery on infective complications and postoperative mortality.

Methods

Study selection

The meta-analysis was performed following the Preferred Reporting Items for Systematic Reviews and Meta-Analyses (PRISMA) guidelines (Moher et al. 2009). A systematic review was conducted by searching the MEDLINE, EMBASE and Cochrane databases. The full search criteria used are included at Appendix A. They contain search terms used relating to "surgery" and any combination of "chlorhexidine", "iodine", "povidone" with terms relating to "mouth", "oral" and "decontamination". This was limited to a 20-year period between October 1994 and 2014 and English language publications.

All trial designs and interventions (mouthwash, nasal, gel) were included. Studies in patients under 18 years and including dental, oral or maxillofacial surgery were excluded.

Data extraction and synthesis

Two investigators independently reviewed the search results. A third investigator resolved any disagreements. Two additional investigators assessed all included papers. The perioperative period was defined as any time period before and after the operation. Risk of bias was assessed using the Cochrane Collaboration checklist and the Jadad score (Jadad et al. 1996).

Main outcomes and measures

Outcomes assessed were postoperative pneumonia and overall nosocomial infections, mortality, and intervention-related adverse events. Postoperative pneumonia was defined as nosocomial pneumonia between the 2nd and 30th postoperative days based on the CDC criteria (Garner et al. 1988). Nosocomial infections were defined as surgical site infections and any other infections including postoperative pneumonia, urinary tract infections and bacteraemia between the 2nd and 30th postoperative days (Garner et al. 1988). The additional following information was sought from all the included papers: study design, eligibility criteria, randomization method, allocation method, risk category, strength of solutions used, treatment regime and number of randomised patients.

Statistical analysis

A meta-analysis methodology was applied to determine the effect of a perioperative oral antiseptic on the incidence of postoperative pneumonia, nosocomial infections and mortality following surgery (Higgins and Green 2011). Data were analysed on an intention-to-treat principle. When this information was not available, per-protocol data were used. The outcome measures were the risk ratio (RR), with 95 % confidence interval (CI), weighted by the inverse of their variances. In this meta-analysis, mouthwash is considered the "experimental" treatment with RR reported as mouth wash-to-placebo/observation ratios.

We assessed heterogeneity using chi^2-based Cochran's Q test and I^2 statistic tests. Inconsistency across studies was considered low, moderate and high for I^2 statistic values lower than 25 %, between 25 and 50 % and greater than 50 %, respectively. Heterogeneity was significant when the I^2 statistic was greater than 50 %, the Cochran's Q test p value was smaller than 0.1 or both. A random-effects model was used to calculate the overall effect.

Results

One thousand six hundred seventy-six articles were identified (Fig. 1). Five hundred sixty-two duplicates and a

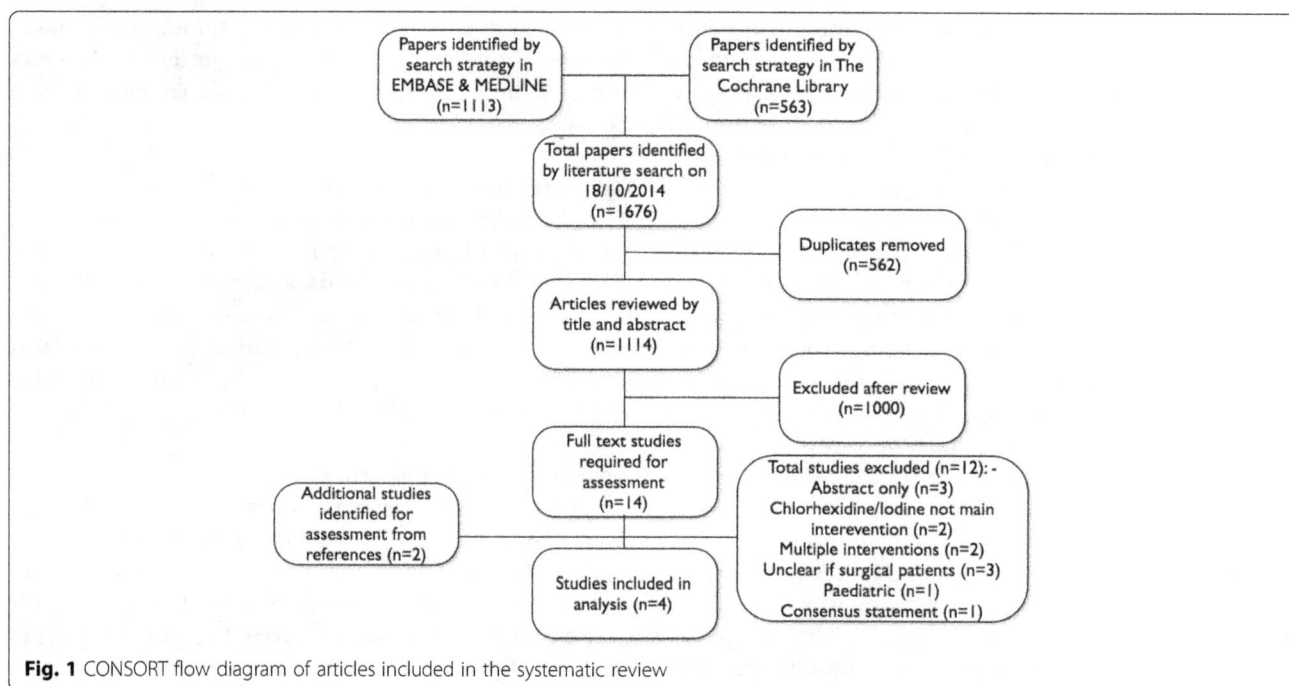

Fig. 1 CONSORT flow diagram of articles included in the systematic review

further 1100 were excluded after abstract review. Full text was not available for 3 of the 14 remaining abstracts. Four of the 11 publications met the criteria after full manuscript review. These studies included 2205 participants of whom 1093 received perioperative chlorhexidine mouthwash or gel. None of the studies reported iodine use. All four studies, three randomised controlled and one quasi-experimental, included patients having elective cardiac surgery only. Table 1 summarises the sample sizes, population, intervention regime and outcomes of the eligible studies. Additional preparations were administered in two studies with nasal chlorhexidine gel in one, and dental brushing in another. All four studies included a placebo (mouthwash, gel or nasal ointment).

All four studies reported postoperative pneumonia rates and mortality, while three reported nosocomial infection rates (Segers et al. 2006; DeRiso et al. 1996; Nicolosi et al. 2014). Three studies used intention-to-treat analysis (DeRiso et al. 1996; Nicolosi et al. 2014; Houston et al. 2002), and one a *per-protocol* analysis (Segers et al. 2006). The risk of bias and Jadad scores are summarised in Table 2. The chlorhexidine regime used varied. All four studies included preoperative chlorhexidine. Three studies continued the intervention postoperatively with varying

Table 1 Summary of sample sizes, population, regime, and outcomes

Author	Location	Patients (chlorhexidine vs. control)	Population	Chlorhexidine strength	Regime	Overall nosocomial infection	Postoperative pneumonia	Mortality
De Riso 1996	USA	353 (173 vs. 180)	Cardiac	0.12 %	Preop (no time scale given) and postop (discharge from ITU or death). Mean = 8.2 days	8/173 (4.6 %) 24/180 (13.3 %)	5/173 (2.9 %) 17/180 (9.4 %)	3/173 (1.7 %) 10/180 (5.6 %)
Houston et al 2002	USA	561 (270 vs. 291)	Cardiac	0.12 %	Preop (no time scale given) and postop (10 days or extubation, tracheostomy, development of POP or death)	–	4/270 (1.5 %) 9/291 (3.1 %)	6/270 (2.2 %) 3/291 (1 %)
Nicolosi et al 2014	Argentina	300 (150 vs. 150)	Cardiac	0.12 %	Preop (3 days)	46/150 (30.7 %) 69/150 (46 %)	4/150 (2.7 %) 13/150 (8.7 %)	8/150 (5.3 %) 7/150 (4.7 %)
Segers et al. 2006	USA	991 (500 vs. 491)	Cardiac	0.12 %	Preop (mean = 1.9 days) and postop (no time scale given)	116/500 (23.2 %) 164/491 (33.4 %)	45/500 (9 %) 74/491 (15.1 %)	8/500 (1.6 %) 6/491 (1.2 %)

Table 2 Risk of bias in studies

Study	Random sequence generation	Allocation concealment	Blinding	Incomplete data outcome addressed
Nicolosi et al. 2014	N/A	N/A	N/A	N/A
Segers et al. 2006	Low risk	Low risk	Low risk	Low risk
Houston et al. 2002	High risk	Unclear	Unclear	Low risk
DeRiso et al. 1996	Low risk	Low risk	Low risk	Low risk

N/A not applicable

duration and preparations (Segers et al. 2006; DeRiso et al. 1996; Houston et al. 2002). Only one study reported duration and dosing (Nicolosi et al. 2014).

Postoperative pneumonia

Three of the four studies used the CDC definition (American Thoracic Society 2005; Segers et al. 2006; DeRiso et al. 1996; Houston et al. 2002; Rotstein et al. 2008). Timing of the diagnosis was variable and not reported in one study (Segers et al. 2006; DeRiso et al. 1996; Nicolosi et al. 2014; Houston et al. 2002). Fifty-eight (5.3 %) patients in the chlorhexidine group developed postoperative pneumonia compared with 113 (10.2 %) patients in the control group (RR = 0.52; 95 % CI 0.39–0.71; $p < 0.01$). There was no statistical significant between study heterogeneity ($p = 0.45$; $I^2 = 0$ %). This produced a number needed to treat of 14 (Fig. 2).

Nosocomial infections

Of the three studies that reported nosocomial infection rates, 170 (20.7 %) patients in the chlorhexidine group, compared with 265 (31.3 %) in the control arm, developed a nosocomial infection (RR = 0.65; 95 % CI 0.52–0.81; $p < 0.01$). There was no statistical significant between study heterogeneity ($p = 0.23$; $I^2 = 32$ %). This produced a number needed to treat of 9 (Fig. 3).

Mortality

All four studies reported in-hospital mortality (Fig. 4) with 25 (2.3 %) deaths in the chlorhexidine group compared with 26 (2.3 %) in the control arm (RR = 1.01; 95 % CI 0.49–2.09; $p = 0.98$). There was no statistical significant between study heterogeneity ($p = 0.19$; $I^2 = 37$ %).

Adverse events

Temporary teeth discolouration was reported in a study, in 1 of 500 patients (0.2 %) who received chlorhexidine.

Discussion

Routine administration of oral chlorhexidine preparations before and after oral surgery reduces local and systemic infective complications (Berchier et al. 2010; Supranoto S et al. 2015; Lambert et al. 1997). This is the first systematic review to determine the effectiveness of perioperative oral antiseptic use in patients undergoing major elective surgery. When administered both before and after elective cardiac surgery, oral antiseptic use with chlorhexidine significantly reduces the incidence of postoperative pneumonia and nosocomial infections with no effect on early mortality. The previous meta-analyses and current National Institute for Health and Care Excellence (NICE) and CDC guidelines focus on critically ill patients including emergency and elective surgical patients mechanically ventilated for 3 days or more (National Institute for Health and Care Excellence 2014; Tablan et al. 2004). The meta-analysis by Labeau et al. demonstrated a significant reduction in VAP (RR 0.67; 95 % CI 0.50–0.88; $p < 0.01$) with oral chlorhexidine or povidone–iodine use (Labeau et al. 2011). The effect was highest with chlorhexidine (RR 0.72; 95 % CI 0.55–0.94; $p = 0.02$). A subgroup analysis of two studies suggested patients undergoing cardiac surgery

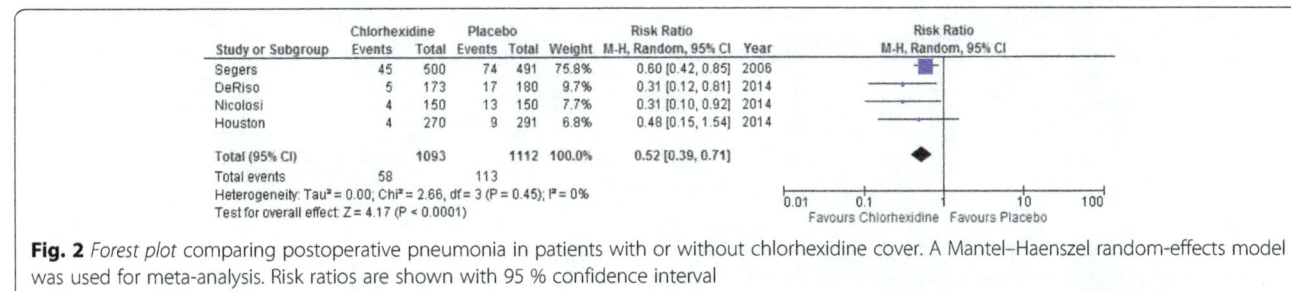

Fig. 2 *Forest plot* comparing postoperative pneumonia in patients with or without chlorhexidine cover. A Mantel–Haenszel random-effects model was used for meta-analysis. Risk ratios are shown with 95 % confidence interval

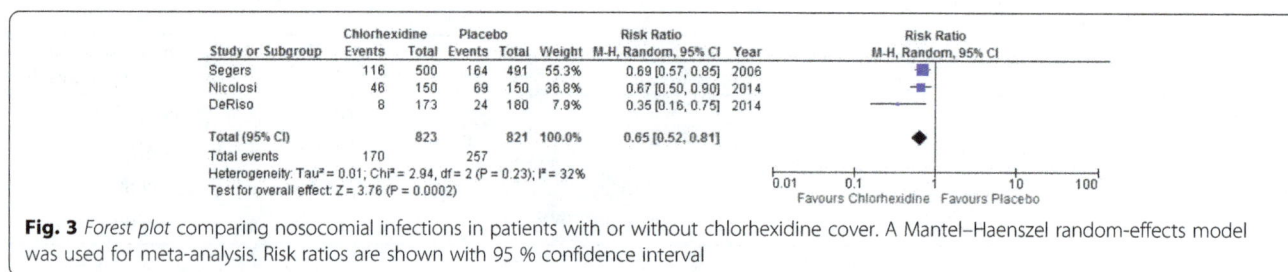

Study or Subgroup	Chlorhexidine Events	Total	Placebo Events	Total	Weight	Risk Ratio M-H, Random, 95% CI	Year
Segers	116	500	164	491	55.3%	0.69 [0.57, 0.85]	2006
Nicolosi	46	150	69	150	36.8%	0.67 [0.50, 0.90]	2014
DeRiso	8	173	24	180	7.9%	0.35 [0.16, 0.75]	2014
Total (95% CI)		823		821	100.0%	0.65 [0.52, 0.81]	
Total events	170		257				

Heterogeneity: Tau² = 0.01; Chi² = 2.94, df = 2 (P = 0.23); I² = 32%
Test for overall effect: Z = 3.76 (P = 0.0002)

Fig. 3 *Forest plot* comparing nosocomial infections in patients with or without chlorhexidine cover. A Mantel–Haenszel random-effects model was used for meta-analysis. Risk ratios are shown with 95 % confidence interval

might have the greatest benefit from oral antiseptic use (RR 0.41; 95 % CI 0.17–0.98; $p = 0.05$) (Labeau et al. 2011).

This systematic review aimed to identify studies investigating the effectiveness of oral antiseptic use before and after major elective surgery. No studies were identified that included patients undergoing elective non-cardiac surgery or who were administered oral povidone–iodine.

Even though the number of studies performed is small, a clear benefit was demonstrated in the reduction of the incidence of postoperative pneumonia and nosocomial infection with perioperative oral chlorhexidine. Perioperative oral chlorhexidine would need to be administered to 14 patients to prevent one episode of postoperative pneumonia and 9 patients to prevent one episode of nosocomial infection. These small numbers needed to treat further supports the effectiveness of the intervention.

Other approaches, including selective decontamination of the digestive tract with antibiotics, reduce the incidence of postoperative pneumonia and nosocomial infection; however, uptake of this technique is limited by concerns of emerging antibiotic resistance (Silvestri and van Saene 2010; Nathens and Marshall 1999; Silvestri and van Saene 2012; Bastin and Ryanna 2009). These approaches were not considered in this systematic review. As the four studies identified included cardiac patients only the findings may not be generalisable to non-cardiac surgical cohorts.

Currently, oral chlorhexidine preparations are used to control dental plaque, treat gingivitis and given routinely before and after oral surgery to reduce local and systemic infective complications (Berchier et al. 2010; Supranoto et al. 2015; Lambert et al. 1997). Outside

this setting, oral chlorhexidine preparations are not routinely administered in the perioperative setting. A recent international consensus statement from over 1000 anaesthetists, intensive care specialists, surgeons, and epidemiologists identified oral chlorhexidine preparations as an inexpensive intervention that may reduce perioperative mortality across surgical disciplines (Landoni et al. 2012). The expert panel commented that the lack of availability of effectiveness studies evaluating the use of perioperative chlorhexidine preparations has in part prevented its widespread adoption (Landoni et al. 2012; Rello et al. 2007).

Oral chlorhexidine is recommended in patients who remain intubated for prolonged periods as it is proven to reduce the incidence of VAP. Perioperative oral chlorhexidine reduces the incidence of postoperative pneumonia and nosocomial infections following elective cardiac surgery. No studies have been performed to evaluate the effectiveness of perioperative oral chlorhexidine on nosocomial infections and postoperative pneumonia after elective non-cardiac surgery. We suggest that a pragmatic, multi-centre and large clinical trial is needed to demonstrate the effectiveness of this simple, well-tolerated, and cheap intervention before and after elective major non-cardiac surgery before it will be accepted and introduced into complex perioperative clinical care pathways.

Conclusions

Perioperative oral chlorhexidine significantly decreases the incidence of nosocomial infection and postoperative

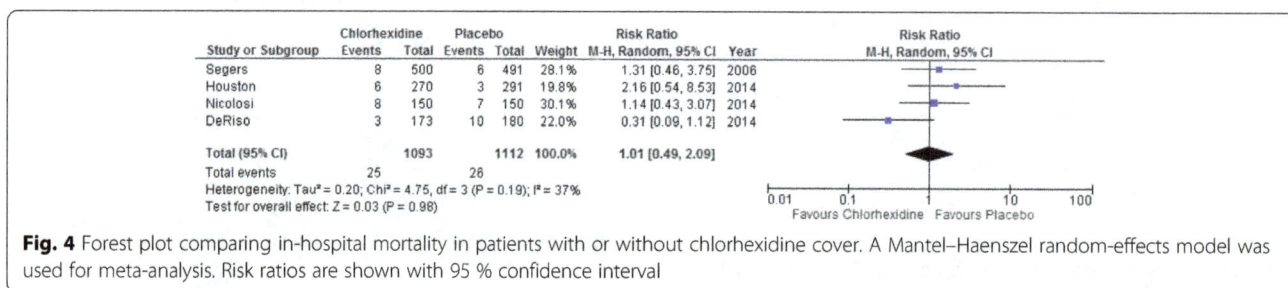

Study or Subgroup	Chlorhexidine Events	Total	Placebo Events	Total	Weight	Risk Ratio M-H, Random, 95% CI	Year
Segers	8	500	6	491	28.1%	1.31 [0.46, 3.75]	2006
Houston	6	270	3	291	19.8%	2.16 [0.54, 8.53]	2014
Nicolosi	8	150	7	150	30.1%	1.14 [0.43, 3.07]	2014
DeRiso	3	173	10	180	22.0%	0.31 [0.09, 1.12]	2014
Total (95% CI)		1093		1112	100.0%	1.01 [0.49, 2.09]	
Total events	25		26				

Heterogeneity: Tau² = 0.20; Chi² = 4.75, df = 3 (P = 0.19); I² = 37%
Test for overall effect: Z = 0.03 (P = 0.98)

Fig. 4 Forest plot comparing in-hospital mortality in patients with or without chlorhexidine cover. A Mantel–Haenszel random-effects model was used for meta-analysis. Risk ratios are shown with 95 % confidence interval

pneumonia in patients undergoing elective cardiac surgery. There are no randomised controlled studies of this simple and cheap intervention in patients undergoing elective non-cardiac surgery. Given the low number needed to treat to prevent either event, we suggest that this intervention may benefit patients undergoing major elective non-cardiac surgery, but additional research is required prior to its routine adoption in perioperative care pathways.

Abbreviations

CDC: Center of Disease Control and Prevention; CI: confidence interval; I^2: percentage variation across studies attributed to heterogeneity; NICE: National Institute for Health and Care Excellence; PRISMA: Preferred Reporting Items for Systematic Reviews and Meta-Analyses; RR: risk ratio; VAP: ventilator-associated pneumonia.

Competing interests

The authors declare that they have no competing interests.

Authors' contributions

RSV, AO and OT contributed to the conception of the review. PS, SL, MP and RSV performed the systematic review. SP, SL, PS and RSV participated in the statistical analysis. IK provided educational supervision on behalf of the RCS. RSV acts as the guarantor. All authors read and approved the manuscript.

Acknowledgements

We thank Professor Dion Morton for his advice and comments on the manuscript.

Funding

This work was supported by an educational grant from the Royal College of Surgeons of England, London, UK.
AO is a clinical research training fellow, funded by the Medical Research Council (MRC).

Author details

[1]West Midlands Research Collaborative, University of Birmingham, Edgbaston, Birmingham B15 2TH, UK. [2]Department of Upper Gastro-Intestinal Surgery, Queen Elizabeth Hospital, Birmingham, UK. [3]School of Immunity and Infection, University of Birmingham, Birmingham, UK. [4]Clinical Effectiveness Unit, Royal College of Surgeons England, London, UK. [5]Academic Department of Surgery, University of Birmingham, 4th Floor, (Old) Queen Elizabeth Hospital, Edgbaston, Birmingham B15 2TH, UK. [6]Nottingham Oesophagi-Gastric unit, Nottingham University Hospitals NHS Trust, Queens Medical Centre, Nottingham NG7 2UH, UK.

References

Weiser TG, Regenbogen SE, Thompson KD, Haynes AB, Lipsitz SR, Berry WR, et al. An estimation of the global volume of surgery: a modelling strategy based on available data. Lancet. 2008;372:139–44.

Hemmes SN, Gama de Abreu M, Pelosi P, Schultz MJ, PROVE Network Investigators for the Clinical Trial Network of the European Society of Anaesthesiology. High versus low positive end-expiratory pressure during general anaesthesia for open abdominal surgery (PROVHILO trial): a multicentre randomised controlled trial. Lancet. 2014;384:495–503.

Niggebrugge AH, Trimbos JB, Hermans J, Steup WH, Van De Velde CJ. Influence of abdominal-wound closure technique on complications after surgery: a randomised study. Lancet. 1999;353:1563–7.

Treschan TA, Kaisers W, Schaefer MS, Bastin B, Schmalz U, Wania V, et al. Ventilation with low tidal volumes during upper abdominal surgery does not improve postoperative lung function. Br J Anaesth. 2012;109:263–71.

Seiler CM, Deckert A, Diener MK, Knaebel HP, Weigand MA, Victor N, et al. Midline versus transverse incision in major abdominal surgery: a randomized, double-blind equivalence trial (POVATI: ISRCTN60734227). Ann Surg. 2009;249:913–20.

Hulscher JB, van Sandick JW, de Boer AG, Wijnhoven BP, Tijssen JG, Fockens P, et al. Extended transthoracic resection compared with limited transhiatal resection for adenocarcinoma of the esophagus. N Engl J Med. 2002;347:1662–9.

Khuri SF, Henderson WG, DePalma RG, Mosca C, Healey NA, Kumbhani DJ. Participants in the VANSQIP: determinants of long-term survival after major surgery and the adverse effect of postoperative complications. Ann Surg. 2005;242:326–41. discussion 341–323.

Thompson DA, Makary MA, Dorman T, Pronovost PJ. Clinical and economic outcomes of hospital acquired pneumonia in intra-abdominal surgery patients. Ann Surg. 2006;243:547–52.

Garner JS, Jarvis WR, Emori TG, Horan TC, Hughes JM. CDC definitions for nosocomial infections, 1988. Am J Infect Control. 1988;16:128–40.

du Moulin GC, Paterson DG, Hedley-Whyte J, Lisbon A. Aspiration of gastric bacteria in antacid-treated patients: a frequent cause of postoperative colonisation of the airway. Lancet. 1982;1:242–5.

Cook D, De Jonghe B, Brochard L, Brun-Buisson C. Influence of airway management on ventilator-associated pneumonia: evidence from randomized trials. JAMA. 1998;279:781–7.

American Thoracic Society, Infectious Diseases Society of America. Guidelines for the management of adults with hospital-acquired, ventilator-associated, and healthcare-associated pneumonia. Am J Respir Crit Care Med. 2005;171:388–416.

Horner C, Mawer D, Wilcox M. Reduced susceptibility to chlorhexidine in staphylococci: is it increasing and does it matter? J Antimicrob Chemother. 2012;67:2547–59.

Fitzgerald KA, Davies A, Russell AD. Uptake of 14C-chlorhexidine diacetate to Escherichia coli and Pseudomonas aeruginosa and its release by azolectin. FEMS Microbiol Lett. 1989;51:327–32.

Labeau SO, Van de Vyver K, Brusselaers N, Vogelaers D, Blot SI. Prevention of ventilator-associated pneumonia with oral antiseptics: a systematic review and meta-analysis. Lancet Infect Dis. 2011;11:845–54.

Klompas M, Speck K, Howell MD, Greene LR, Berenholtz SM. Reappraisal of routine oral care with chlorhexidine gluconate for patients receiving mechanical ventilation: systematic review and meta-analysis. JAMA Intern Med. 2014;174:751–61.

Price R, MacLennan G, Glen J, Su DC. Selective digestive or oropharyngeal decontamination and topical oropharyngeal chlorhexidine for prevention of death in general intensive care: systematic review and network meta-analysis. BMJ. 2014;348:g2197.

Scottish Intensive Care Society Audit Group: VAP prevention bundle: guidance for implementation. National Health Services Scotland 2008.

Moher D, Liberati A, Tetzlaff J, Altman DG, Group P. Preferred Reporting Items for Systematic Reviews and Meta-Analyses: the PRISMA statement. BMJ. 2009;339:b2535.

Jadad AR, Moore RA, Carroll D, Jenkinson C, Reynolds DJ, Gavaghan DJ, et al. Assessing the quality of reports of randomized clinical trials: is blinding necessary? Control Clin Trials. 1996;17:1–12.

Higgins JPT, Green S (editors): Cochrane handbook for systematic reviews of interventions version 5.1.0. March 2011 edition: The Cochrane Collaboration; 2011. Available from www.cochranehandbook.org.

Segers P, Speekenbrink RG, Ubbink DT, Ogtrop ML, Mol BA. Prevention of nosocomial infection in cardiac surgery by decontamination of the nasopharynx and oropharynx with chlorhexidine gluconate: a randomized controlled trial. JAMA. 2006;296:2460–6.

DeRiso AJ, Ladowski JS, Dillon TA, Justice JW, Peterson AC. Chlorhexidine gluconate 0.12 % oral rinse reduces the incidence of total nosocomial respiratory infection and nonprophylactic systemic antibiotic use in patients undergoing heart surgery. Chest. 1996;109:1556–61.

Nicolosi LN, del Carmen Rubio M, Martinez CD, Gonzalez NN, Cruz ME. Effect of oral hygiene and 0.12 % chlorhexidine gluconate oral rinse in preventing ventilator-associated pneumonia after cardiovascular surgery. Respir Care. 2014;59:504–9.

Houston S, Hougland P, Anderson JJ, LaRocco M, Kennedy V, Gentry LO. Effectiveness of 0.12 % chlorhexidine gluconate oral rinse in reducing prevalence of nosocomial pneumonia in patients undergoing heart surgery. Am J Crit Care. 2002;11:567–70.

Rotstein C, Evans G, Born A, Grossman R, Light RB, Magder S, et al. Clinical practice guidelines for hospital-acquired pneumonia and ventilator-associated pneumonia in adults. Can J Infect Dis Med Microbiol. 2008;19:19–53.

Berchier CE, Slot DE, Van der Weijden GA. The efficacy of 0.12 % chlorhexidine mouthrinse compared with 0.2 % on plaque accumulation and periodontal parameters: a systematic review. J Clin Periodontol. 2010;37:829–39.

Supranoto S, Slot D, Addy M, Van der Weijden G: The effect of chlorhexidine dentifrice or gel versus chlorhexidine mouthwash on plaque, gingivitis, bleeding and tooth discoloration: a systematic review. Int J Dent Hyg 2015;13(2):83-92.

Lambert PM, Morris HF, Ochi S. The influence of 0.12 % chlorhexidine digluconate rinses on the incidence of infectious complications and implant success. J Oral Maxillofac Surg. 1997;55:25–30.

National Institute for Health and Care Excellence. Technical patient safety solutions for ventilator-associated pneumonia in adults. London: London: National Institute for Health and Care Excellence; 2014.

Tablan OC, Anderson LJ, Besser R, Bridges C, Hajjeh R. CDC, Healthcare Infection Control Practices Advisory C: Guidelines for preventing health-care-associated pneumonia, 2003: recommendations of CDC and the Healthcare Infection Control Practices Advisory Committee. MMWR Recomm Rep. 2004;53:1–36.

Silvestri L, van Saene HK. Selective digestive decontamination to prevent pneumonia after esophageal surgery. Ann Thorac Cardiovasc Surg. 2010;16:220–1. author reply 221.

Nathens AB, Marshall JC. Selective decontamination of the digestive tract in surgical patients: a systematic review of the evidence. Arch Surg. 1999;134:170–6.

Silvestri L, van Saene HK. Selective decontamination of the digestive tract: an update of the evidence. HSR Proc Intensive Care Cardiovasc Anesth. 2012;4:21–9.

Bastin AJ, Ryanna KB. Use of selective decontamination of the digestive tract in United Kingdom intensive care units. Anaesthesia. 2009;64:46–9.

Landoni G, Rodseth RN, Santini F, Ponschab M, Ruggeri L, Szekely A, et al. Randomized evidence for reduction of perioperative mortality. J Cardiothorac Vasc Anesth. 2012;26:764–72.

Rello J, Koulenti D, Blot S, Sierra R, Diaz E, De Waele JJ, et al. Oral care practices in intensive care units: a survey of 59 European ICUs. Intensive Care Med. 2007;33:1066–70.

17

Effects of different colloid infusions on ROTEM and Multiplate during elective brain tumour neurosurgery

N. Li[1], S. Statkevicius[2], B. Asgeirsson[2] and U. Schött[2*]

Abstract

Background: The European Medicines Agency does not recommend the use of hydroxyethyl starch-based volume replacement solutions in critically ill patients due to an increased risk of renal failure. However, this recommendation is questionable for its perioperative use. Several recent randomised controlled studies do not indicate a risk for renal failure—not even after high-risk surgery. Human albumin is used in our neurointensive care unit as a part of the "Lund concept" of brain injury resuscitation, and albumin has been introduced in elective neurosurgery instead of starch. The aim of our prospective unblinded observational cohort study was to compare the degree of dilutive coagulopathy after albumin and starch intra-operative fluid therapy.

Methods: Thirty-nine patients undergoing elective brain tumour surgery with craniotomy received either 130/0.42 hydroxyethyl starch or 5 % albumin infusions. The first 18 patients received starch, whereas the rest received albumin. Rotational thromboelastometry with ROTEM and platelet aggregometry with Multiplate were performed before surgery, after the first and second consecutive colloid infusions (250/500 ml albumin or 500/1000 ml starch) and at the end of surgery.

Results: Both intra- and inter-group comparisons showed more deranged ROTEM parameters after the higher doses of starch. Multiplate detected changes only in the albumin group after 500-ml infusion. Blood los did not differ between groups, nor did haemoglobin preoperatively or at end of surgery. Lower volumes of albumin were required to maintain stable intra-operative haemodynamic parameters; 250/500 ml albumin corresponded to 500/1000 ml starch.

Conclusions: Hydroxyethyl starch affected coagulation at lower volumes, with a more prominent effect on clot structure at the end of surgery, corroborating previous research. Only albumin decreased platelet aggregation, and 5 % albumin had a more potential volume effect than 130/0.42 hydroxyethyl starch.

Keywords: Thromboelastography, Platelet aggregation, Albumin, Hydroxyethyl starch, Neurosurgery

Background

In brain tumour neurosurgery, intra- and post-operative bleeding in brain tumour resection can be linked to the vascularity of the tumours, tumour size and localization (Goh et al. 1997). Most of the losses will be surgical, and as the field is open, direct haemostasis with cautery or topical coagulants is more relevant. Post-operative hematomas are rare but may be more related to a coagulopathy than a surgical bleed. During surgery, different fluids are used to replace blood loss and maintain arterial pressure, including crystalloids and blood products, and during the last few decades, synthetic colloids as well. However, all of these fluids are associated with adverse effects, and an ideal fluid for haemodynamic stabilisation and resuscitation has yet to be found.

Hydroxyethyl starches (HESs) are synthetic colloids with different molecular weights and substitutions that are used for their plasma-expanding effects. In recent years, several studies have highlighted the adverse effects of this colloid, particularly the risk of acute renal failure (Zarychanski et al. 2013), allergic skin manifestations

* Correspondence: ulf.schott@skane.se
[2]Department of Anaesthesia and Intensive Care, Lund University and Skane University Hospital, Lund S-22185, Sweden
Full list of author information is available at the end of the article

and hypocoagulability following infusion. HES has been shown to impair clot strength, platelet function and increase fibrinolysis to an extent that cannot be explained by haemodilution alone (Levi & Jonge 2007). HES infusions decrease plasma levels of fibrinogen and several coagulation factors, leading to weaker and smaller clots (Fenger-Eriksen et al. 2009). It can also decrease circulating levels of von Willebrand's factor (F), thus impairing platelet function (de Jonge et al. 2001).

In Europe, market authorisations for HES have been suspended due to these findings (Agency EM. PRAC recommends suspending marketing authorisations for infusion solutions containing hydroxyethyl starch: European Medicines Agency & [cited 2013 Jun 14]). However, the clinical perioperative implications of these findings are still uncertain for stable patients undergoing elective surgery (Moral et al. 2013). Human albumin (HA) is an alternative fluid that has recently been replacing HES in neurosurgery at Lund University Hospital. Albumin is used by us in accordance with the "Lund concept" of brain injury resuscitation (Grande 2011), and for us, it was natural to replace HES with HA. However, in large meta-analyses on the effectiveness of HA on patient mortality and morbidity, no significant benefits have been shown when comparing HA to synthetic colloids or crystalloids (Perel et al. 2013; Roberts et al. 2011). HA may have lesser impact on coagulation compared to synthetic colloids (Niemi et al. 2006), which is a desirable quality for perioperative use. The coagulopathy caused by HA also seems to be easily reversed by fibrinogen and FXIII concentrate (Winstedt et al. 2013), making it a potentially better fluid for patients that might already suffer from a coagulopathy or risk of developing one.

Routine clinical laboratory analyses of coagulation, such as activated partial thromboplastin time (aPTT) and prothrombin time (PT), are plasma-based and might not correctly predict a clinical coagulopathy. Whole blood viscoelastic methods, such as thromboelastometry (e.g. ROTEM®) and whole blood-aggregometry (e.g. Multiplate®), have gained recognition as alternative methods. Thromboelastometry is able to assess global haemostatic functions, and platelet aggregometry assesses platelet function in response to different reagents. These systems have already been introduced clinically as point-of-care methods for quickly determining bleeding risk and helping to guide transfusions (Shore-Lesserson et al. 1999). They have also been used to study haemostasis in different critical care situations, such as trauma (Solomon et al. 2011) and sepsis (Brenner et al. 2012). ROTEM is known to detect colloid-induced coagulopathy (Fenger-Eriksen et al. 2009), even at low levels of dilution (Tynngård et al. 2014).

The purpose of this study was to compare the effects on coagulation of 5 % HA and HES 130/0.42 in elective brain tumour neurosurgical patients. Our aim was to investigate whether HA had a more favourable effect on coagulation and platelet function, assessed by a viscoelastic method and a platelet aggregometry method (ROTEM and Multiplate, respectively). Our hypothesis was that HA infusions would induce less hypocoagulability than HES, as seen on ROTEM and Multiplate.

Methods

This study was performed as a prospective unblinded observational cohort study with two colloid fluid regimens. During 2013 and 2014, our fluid regimen for haemodynamic stabilisation and initial blood-loss substitution during elective brain tumour resection was changed from HES to 5 % HA. We had studied 18 consecutive patients with HES according to a protocol, and our initial aim was to include more patients with HES and the combined testing with ROTEM and Multiplate when the department replaced HES with HA.

We therefore decided to continue the protocol with HA and compare its effects on ROTEM and Multiplate with the data from the previous HES-patients. According to a power analysis from an in vitro study (Winstedt et al. 2013), >15 patients in each group would give a statistical power of 0.8 at a significance level of $p < 0.05$, defined by detected differences in FIBTEM-MCF (see below), as this is the best predictive ROTEM parameter for dilutive coagulopathy, correlating with fibrinogen; the first coagulation factor to reach critical low levels during haemodilution (Winstedt et al. 2013).

General ethical approval was obtained from the Regional Ethical Review Board (Lund, Protocol DNR 2012/482) for monitoring neurosurgery patients with ROTEM and Multiplate. Signed consent was received from all patients in the two test groups. All patients were over 18 years.

No patients with a known haemostatic disturbance, anticoagulants, antiplatelet drugs (also including aspirin/nonsteroidal anti-inflammatory drugs), abnormal preoperative coagulation analysis (aPTT/PT, platelet count), known renal impairment or increased plasma-creatinine level were included.

Anaesthesia was induced and maintained with propofol (Diprivan®; AstraZeneca, Sweden) and remifentanil (Ultiva®, GlaxoSmithKline, Sweden). Intubation was facilitated with rocuronium (Esmeron®; MSD, USA) (0.5–0.8 mg/kg), and ventilation was maintained with positive pressure ventilation in a circle system. Minute ventilation was adjusted to maintain normocapnia (PaCO2 of 4.5–5.5 kPa).

After induction, a radial arterial catheter was inserted for continuous measurement of blood pressure and for collection of blood samples, and a bladder catheter was inserted for hourly measurement of diuresis.

All patients received thromboprophylaxis with mechanical calf compression (Kendall SCD™ Express Sleeves; Covidien, USA) during surgery and postoperatively for 24 h.

Normothermia during the surgery was maintained with a Bair Hugger™ (3 M, St. Paul, USA) and oesophageal temperature monitoring.

During this study, there was no intervention on our part in the transfusion/infusion protocols. The crystalloid/colloid infusions and transfusion of blood components were solely determined by the anaesthetist in charge, based on a standard protocol from the anaesthesia department (see below) and were not affected by the study protocol or the ROTEM/Multiplate test results.

Standard Lund departmental protocol for perioperative fluids during neurosurgery: After the induction of anaesthesia, a basal infusion of 1.5–2.0 ml/kg/h of saline (NaCl 0.9 %; B. Braun Medical AB) was started. Initial bleeding up to 200–300 ml was substituted with saline (2–3 ml per 1 ml of bleeding). The HES group received hydroxyethyl starch 130/0.42 in sodium chloride for maintaining mean arterial pressure of >60–65 mm Hg, systolic blood pressure >90 mmHg, pulse pressure variation (PPV) <12 mmHg and replacing bleeding of >200–300 ml (see above) (1–2 ml HES per 1 ml of bleeding) (HES; Venofundin® 60 mg/ml hydroxyethyl starch; MW 130 kDa; substitution 0.42; B. Braun Medical AG, Germany). HES was thus also used to compensate for the haemodynamic effects of anaesthesia. HES was restricted to 1000 ml by the departmental protocol. The HA group was given 5 % human albumin (Albumin; CSL Behring, Germany) at 1–2 ml HA per 1 ml of bleeding of >200–300 ml (see above). HA was also used to compensate for the haemodynamic effects of anaesthesia as for HES. Albumin was restricted to 500 ml by the departmental protocol.

According to departmental protocol, packed red blood cells (PRBCs) are to be administered when the concentration of haemoglobin reaches <95–100 gram/L, and blood loss of more than 30 % of the calculated blood volume is substituted with PRBCs, fresh-frozen plasma (FFP) and platelet concentrates (PC).

Arterial blood was sampled from radial arterial catheters with a continuous sodium chloride flush system with no heparin. The blood samples were collected in 2.7-ml citrated plastic vacuum tubes (3.2 % citrate; BD Vacutainer systems, UK) for ROTEM and in 3.0-ml hirudin tubes (Dynabyte GmbH, Germany) for Multiplate analysis. Blood sampling was performed before surgical incision, after every colloid unit (i.e. after every 250 ml HA or 500 ml HES infusion) and at the end of surgery; altogether, three or four samples were collected per patient. Blood loss during surgery was evaluated from suction reservoir and swabs.

Arterial blood gases with haemoglobin, electrolyte, lactate and glucose levels were analysed before the beginning of surgery and during surgery every 1–2 h (Radiometer ABL800 FLEX; Radiometer, Denmark).

Rotational thromboelastometry (ROTEM®; TEM Innovations GmbH, Germany) measures the coagulation initiation, amplification and propagation kinetics of whole blood. It uses a cup with a rotating pin, whose movement is impeded as blood coagulates inside the cup. The impedance reflects clot firmness and is plotted graphically against time. Analysis was carried out within 1 h from blood sampling, during which time the samples were kept at 37 °C. The following two assays were run on each sample: EXTEM and FIBTEM. EXTEM measures coagulation activated by tissue factor (extrinsic pathway), while the FIBTEM assay includes a platelet inhibitor (cytochalasin D), thus measuring only fibrinogen activity. For EXTEM, the following parameters are assessed for each analysis (normal range within brackets): clotting time/CT (42–74 s), clot formation time/CFT (46–148 s), alpha-angle/AA (63–81°) and maximum clot firmness/MCF (63–81 mm). For FIBTEM, only MCF (9–25 mm) was analysed. The normal ranges used were established in a multi-centre study (Lang et al. 2005).

Multiple electrode aggregometry (Multiplate®; Roche Diagnostics, Basel, Switzerland) measures platelet aggregation in whole blood using electrical resistance between two electrodes. As aggregation occurs, the increasing impedance is plotted against time, and the area under the curve (AUC) is a measure of platelet function. The blood samples were kept at room temperature for 30–40 min before analysis, which was done at 37 °C. The following two test assays were performed for each sample: platelet aggregation in response to adenosine diphosphate (ADP-test, AUC reference range 57–113) and thrombin receptor-activating peptide (TRAP-test, AUC reference range 84–128). For statistical analysis of the data, both inter- and intra-group comparisons were made. Normal distribution was not assumed (non-parametric data). Samples after first colloid infusion, after second colloid infusion and at the end of surgery were tested against the preoperative sample using the Wilcoxon signed-rank test for paired samples. All ROTEM and Multiplate values in one test group were also compared to the corresponding values in the other test group, using the Mann-Whitney U test for unpaired samples. The level of significance was set to $p < 0.017$ after correction in accordance to Bonferroni, in order to decrease the risk of type I errors due to multiple comparisons. Results are presented as boxplots showing median and interquartile range, with min-max whiskers and + signs identifying mean values.

Results

In total, 18 patients were included in the HES group and 21 patients in the HA group during a 5-month period. The demographic, bleeding and transfusion/infusion data for these patients are shown in Table 1. Six patients received erythrocyte transfusions, one patient received platelet transfusions and one patient received plasma transfusions intra-operatively. There were no differences in median haemoglobin concentration at the end of surgery between the groups (Table 1). The decrease in haemoglobin preoperative-postoperative was the same in both groups.

Intra-group comparisons

Results from each sampling occasion were compared to the preoperative results. In the HA group, the most significant differences were detected after the second HA infusion, as well as at the end of surgery (Tables 2 and 3 and Figs. 1, 2 and 3). After 250 ml HA, ROTEM only showed a significant decrease in FIBTEM-MCF. After 500 ml HA, CFT, AA and EXTEM-MCF also differed as compared to pre-surgery levels. At the end of surgery, changes were detected in all ROTEM parameters except for CT. Multiplate detected changes in the ADP parameter only after 500 ml HA. No other significant changes could be shown in ADP or TRAP parameters. In the HES group, significant differences could be detected already after the first infusion (Table 2 and 3 and Figs. 1, 2 and 3). After 500 ml HES, CFT was markedly prolonged, as seen in Fig. 1. AA and EXTEM-MCF both decreased (Fig. 2 (AA not shown)). Only after 1000 ml HES was CT prolonged (Tables 2 and 3 and Fig. 1). Additionally, changes could be seen in the CFT, AA and FIBTEM-MCF parameters after 1000 ml

HES, as well as after surgery (Tables 2 and 3). Multiplate did not detect any significant differences within the HES group (Fig. 3).

Inter-group comparisons

When comparing the two test groups against each other, each parameter was compared to the corresponding one in the other test group. Most of the changes occurred after the first dose of colloid. Before the start of surgery, only the CT parameter differed between the groups ($p = 0.0001$), with a lower median CT in the HES group. After the first colloid infusion, CT was still significantly shorter in the HES group ($p = 0.0014$), while CFT was longer ($p = 0.0002$). EXTEM-MCF were lower ($p = 0.001$ and $p = 0.0107$, respectively) in the HES group as compared to the HA group. After the second dose of colloid infusion, no further changes between the groups were detected. At the end of surgery, the following two parameters differed between the groups: CT ($p = 0.0068$) and FIBTEM-MCF ($p = 0.0117$), which registered significantly lower values in the HES test group. For Multiplate analysis, no parameters were found to be different between the two test groups.

There were no differences in the median arterial blood gas parameters nor were there any differences in median systolic, diastolic or mean arterial blood pressures, heart rate or pulse pressure variation (only measured during anaesthesia, with muscle relaxation and tidal volumes of >10 ml/kg body weight and no arrhytmias) or in intra- and post-operative median hourly diuresis between the groups. Post-operatively, there was no increase in plasma creatinine in either group (controlled 3–8 weeks postoperatively).

Table 1 Demographic and bleeding data for patients receiving 5 % human albumin (HA) or hydroxyethyl starch 130/0.4 (HES) during elective neurosurgery up to the end of surgery (eos)

	HES ($n = 18$)	HA ($n = 21$)
Gender (male/female)	10/8	7/14
Median age (min-max)	51(21–86)	54(20–73)
Blood loss (n)	100–499 ml (7)	100–499 ml (8)
	500–999 ml (4)	500–999 ml (3)
	1000–1999 ml (5)	1000–1999 ml (4)
	≥2000 ml (1)	≥2000 ml (0)
Total colloid volume received (n)	500 ml (5)	250 ml (10)
	1000 ml (13)	500 ml (11)
Total NaCl volume received (n)	2000 ml (15)	2000 ml (16)
	2500 ml (2)	2500 ml (5)
	3000 ml (2)	
Median preoperative Hb (min-max)	128 g/L (99–148)	127 (97–144)
Median eos Hb (min-max)	116 g/L (96–122)	113 (94–144)

Table 2 ROTEM and Multiplate parameters (median values, first and third quartiles within brackets) of patients receiving hydroxyethyl starch 130/0.4 (HES) during brain tumour neurosurgery ($n = 18$), blood samples taken at different times during surgery

	Pre-surgery	After 500 ml HES	After 1000 ml HES	End of surgery
CT (s)	48 (45–53)	52 (47–57)	58 (54–63)	47 (44–56)
CFT (s)	96 (84–131)	137 (115–145)	144 (134–148)	130 (110–144)
AA (°)	72 (67–73)	64 (62–65)	63 (61–65)	65 (62–68)
MCF (mm)	59 (57–63)	55 (52–58)	57 (50–58)	56 (51–62)
FIBTEM-MCF (mm)	14 (11–17)	12 (8–18)	9 (6–12)	11 (8–13)
Multiplate-ADP(AUC)	77 (51–89)	69 (58–101)	66 (53–79)	80 (53–102)
Multiplate-TRAP(AUC)	135 (120–171)	139 (123–169)	140 (128–152)	158 (128–177)

Discussion

Our results indicate that the two types of colloid infusions induce coagulation defects in elective brain tumour neurosurgical patients, most notably seen with ROTEM parameters and after HES infusion. There are dose-response effects with both HA and HES. At the end of surgery, the HES group had more deranged ROTEM values than the HA group, but had been infused at a much higher volume ratio to assessed bleeding. Multiplate showed only one significant intra-group deterioration in the ADP parameter, detected after 500 ml HA, as compared to pre-surgery, and normalised already at the end of surgery. No significant Multiplate changes could be seen in the HES group.

Using viscoelastic or aggregometric techniques as point-of-care methods for assessing perioperative bleeding risks is a desirable option, since they provide faster results than traditional laboratory-based tests. ROTEM has already been used for this purpose and is able to detect colloid-induced coagulopathies (Fenger-Eriksen et al. 2009; Hartog et al. 2011); Multiplate has not been studied as thoroughly in this aspect. One study used Multiplate to detect impaired platelet function after 60 % colloid dilution in vitro (Kind et al. 2013), but the clinical implications are uncertain as this represents an extreme dilution seldom observed in clinical practice. In our study with colloid dilutions of 10–20 %, Multiplate indicated a statistically significant lowered

ADP aggregation as compared to the preoperative result only after 500 ml HA. However, at all sampling points, median levels were within normal ranges for both the ADP and TRAP reagents for both fluids. It is possible that Multiplate is not sensitive enough to detect changes in platelet function at low degrees of colloid dilution in vivo. Multiplate is also affected by platelet count, especially at levels beneath 100×10^9/L (Hanke et al. 2010).

Only one of our patients had a low borderline platelet count due to radiation therapy prior to surgery, and received one unit of platelet transfusion at the beginning of the surgery due to increased wound bleeding, and additionally, 250 ml HA and three units of platelets intra-operatively. This patient's Multiplate values for TRAP/ADP were 67/30 preoperatively, 59/18 after 250 ml HA and 128/34 at the end of surgery (after the three units of platelet transfusions; patient's data is not included in the Multiplate data statistical evaluation). This might indicate a colloid-induced effect on a low-platelet function/count that is restored after additional platelet transfusions.

In this study, blood samples were taken before the start of surgery to determine a baseline value. Some of these preoperative values fell outside of the normal ROTEM ranges, possibly induced by the tumour itself or stress due to anaesthesia (Hahnenkamp et al. 2002). After the first volume of colloid infusion, there were significant changes in several ROTEM parameters in the

Table 3 The p values when comparing ROTEM and Multiplate parameters of brain tumour neurosurgery patients after colloid infusions before surgery. Results after each colloid infusion (250 ml for HA and 500 ml for HES) as well as at the end of surgery were compared to pre-operative results using Wilcoxon's signed ranked test

	CT (s)	CFT (s)	AA (°)	EXTEM-MCF (mm)	FIBTEM-MCF (mm)	Multiplate ADP(AUC)	Multiplate TRAP(AUC)
HA 250 ml	ns	ns	ns	ns	0.0015 (**)	ns	ns
HA 500 ml	ns	0.0098 (**)	0.0156 (*)	0.0039 (**)	0.0039 (**)	0.0020 (*)	ns
HA end of surgery	ns	0.0011 (**)	0.0012 (**)	0.0098 (**)	0.0042 (**)	ns	ns
HES 500 ml	ns	<0.0001 (****)	0.0001 (***)	0.0005 (***)	ns	ns	ns
HES 1000 ml	0.0156 (*)	0.0020 (**)	0.0039 (**)	ns	0.0020 (**)	ns	ns
HES end of surgery	ns	0.0027 (**)	0.0015 (**)	ns	0.0043 (**)	ns	ns

Significance level was set at $p < 0.017$, **$p < 0.01$, ***$p < 0.001$ and ****$p < 0.0001$

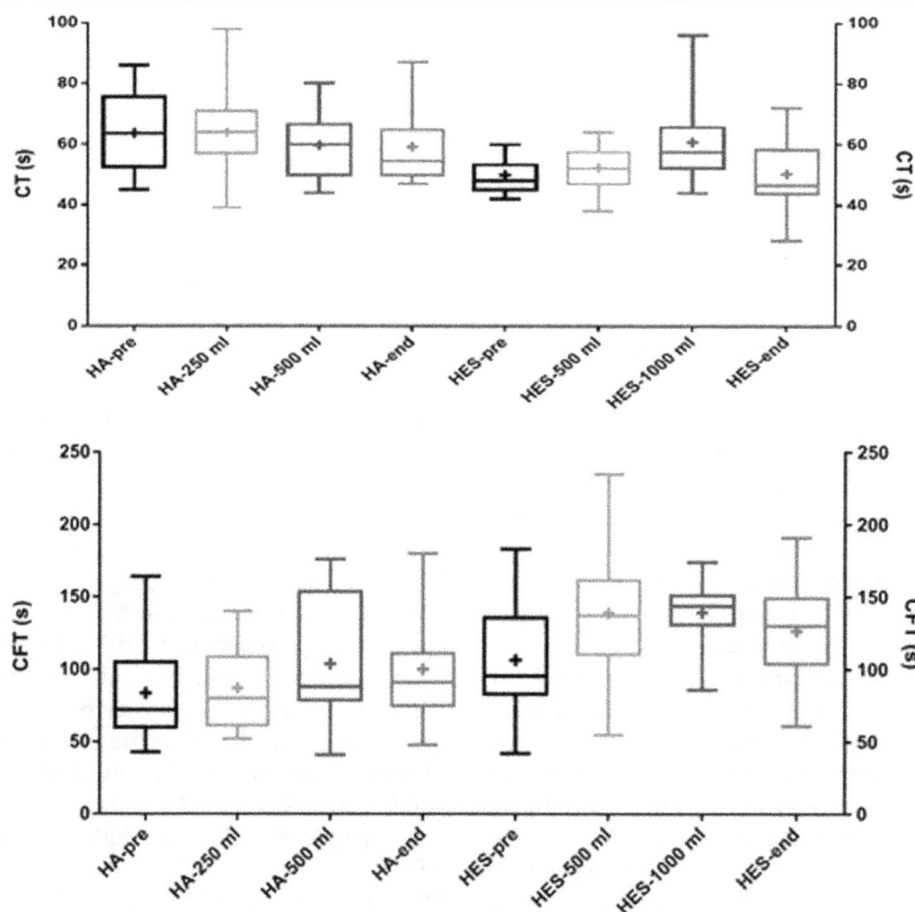

Fig. 1 ROTEM CT and CFT values of patients undergoing elective brain tumour neurosurgery. Blood samples were taken before the start of surgery, after receiving colloid infusions (human albumin (HA) or hydroxyethyl starch (HES)) 130/0.4 and at the end of surgery. *Boxplots* showing median and interquartile range with min-max whiskers and + signs identifying mean values

HES test group but almost none in the HA group. As seen in Fig. 1 and Table 2, CFT increased, and AA decreased with successive colloid infusions, which probably reflects a dilution effect on coagulation factors.

The difference in CFT and AA between test groups could be due to the different volumes of colloids given. Patients receiving HA were given an infusion of 500 ml in total, while those receiving HES had >double the volume, thus probably leading to a greater extent of initial dilution. Haemodilution could also explain why the CT parameter only changed after 1000 ml HES. The efficacy of volume replacement therapy depends on the initial plasma volume-expanding effect of the colloid and the duration of its effect. At the start of the present study, when HES data were collected, all patients received consecutive doses of 500 ml HES intra-operatively. However, with the new 5 % HA fluid regimen at our centre, very few patients received more than 500 ml for haemodynamic stabilisation and initial blood-loss replacement, probably due to a greater and enduring volume-expanding effect of HA as compared to HES

(Dubniks et al. 2009). However, the fluid therapy used in this study is only empiric-based. Future studies should involve blood/plasma volume measurements or cardiac output measurements to better evaluate the colloid insult on haemostasis.

MCF measures the amplification and propagation of the clot, dependent on fibrin polymerisation and platelet function. EXTEM- and FIBTEM-MCF are the most widely used parameters in clinical settings for assessing coagulation since they correlate strongly with traditional tests, most notably plasma fibrinogen (Theusinger et al. 2013; Haas et al. 2012). In our study, EXTEM-MCF decreased after the second volume infusion of HA, but already after the first volume of HES.

With FIBTEM-MCF, we observe a similar decrease, although it was now present after the first volume of HA. This is in accordance with previous studies, since colloids are known to affect coagulation through dilution as well as interaction with coagulation factors and fibrin polymerisation. HES has been especially well-documented to exert its effects on coagulation

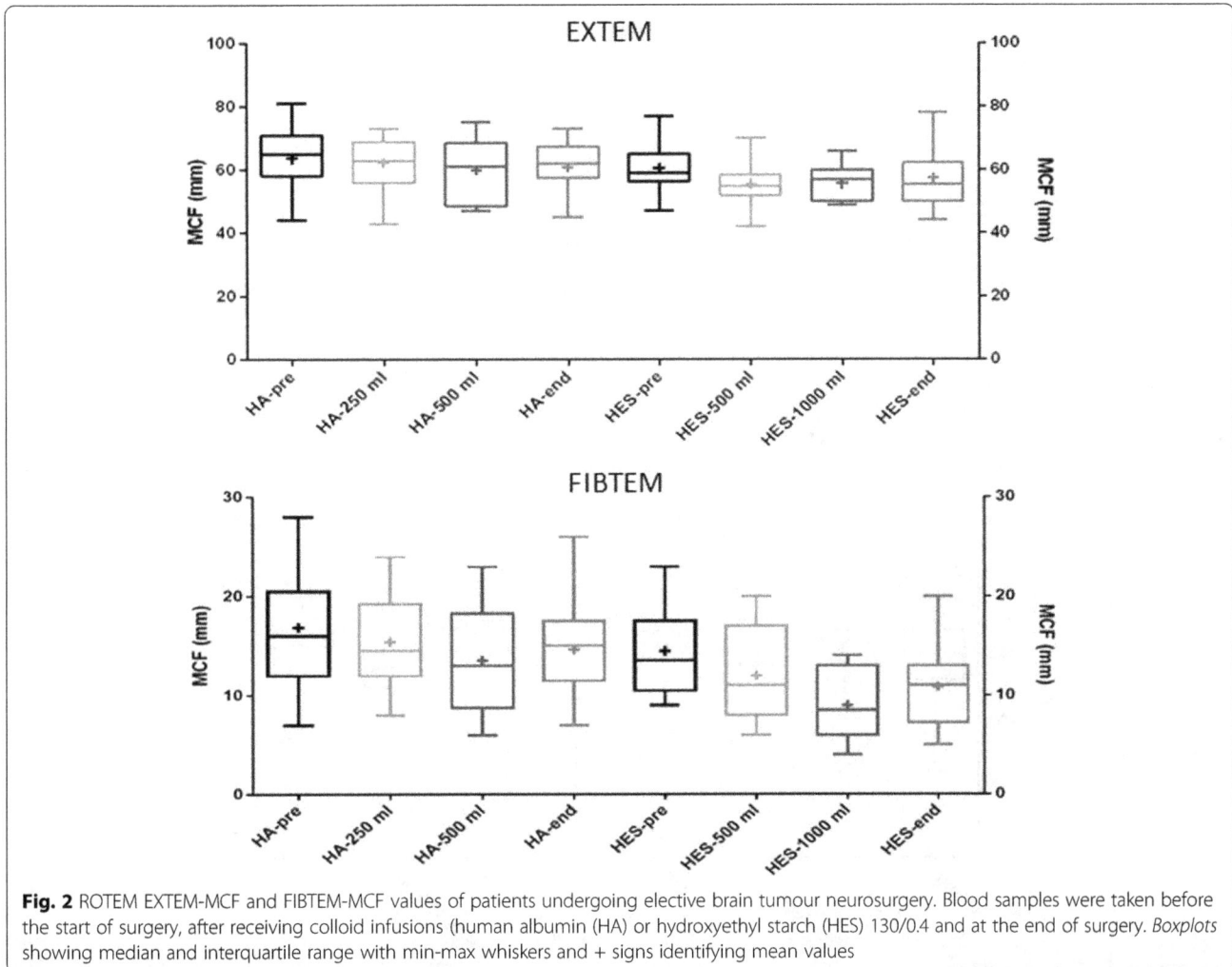

Fig. 2 ROTEM EXTEM-MCF and FIBTEM-MCF values of patients undergoing elective brain tumour neurosurgery. Blood samples were taken before the start of surgery, after receiving colloid infusions (human albumin (HA) or hydroxyethyl starch (HES) 130/0.4 and at the end of surgery. *Boxplots showing median and interquartile range with min-max whiskers and + signs identifying mean values*

by interacting with FXIII and fibrin polymerisation (Nielsen 2005). Fenger-Eriksen et al. showed that HES decreases coagulation factors (e.g. fibrinogen, FII, FX, FXIII) more than can be expected from haemodilution alone, suggesting that the resulting coagulopathy could be due to an acquired fibrinogen deficiency (Fenger-Eriksen et al. 2009).

The specific effects of HA on coagulation in vivo are not as well documented. Some studies imply that HA affects coagulation by decreasing platelet aggregation (Jorgensen & Stoffersen 1980; Kim et al. 1999). Another study showed that HA infusions are linked to decreased fibrinogen levels (Johnson et al. 1979); although, it is unclear whether this is merely an effect of haemodilution. Niemi et al. observed a hypercoagulative effect of HA haemodilution (Niemi & Kuitunen 1998), but this effect could not be reproduced in clinical settings (Niemi et al. 2005). In our study, the difference in volume required for MCF to be affected by each colloid might be accounted for by the different biochemical properties of

HES and HA. In clinical bleeding situations, FIBTEM-MCF of <10 mm can indicate plasma fibrinogen deficiency and prompts the use of fibrinogen concentrate or fresh-frozen plasma (Bolliger et al. 2012). The minimum values were especially low in the HES group where it registered as low as 4 mm.

However, we found no correlation between lower FIBTEM-MCF values and increased perioperative bleeding in our data, as blood losses were similar in both test groups.

For inter-group comparisons, several parameters differed between the test groups after the first colloid infusion. However, after the second infusion, no further changes could be seen. Furthermore, CT and FIBTEM-MCF both differed between groups at the end of surgery. The difference in CT was already present preoperatively, but the change in FIBTEM-MCF is possibly due to the more prominent effects of HES on clot stability; as discussed earlier, HES is known to weaken clot structure (Mittermayr et al. 2007). Previous studies

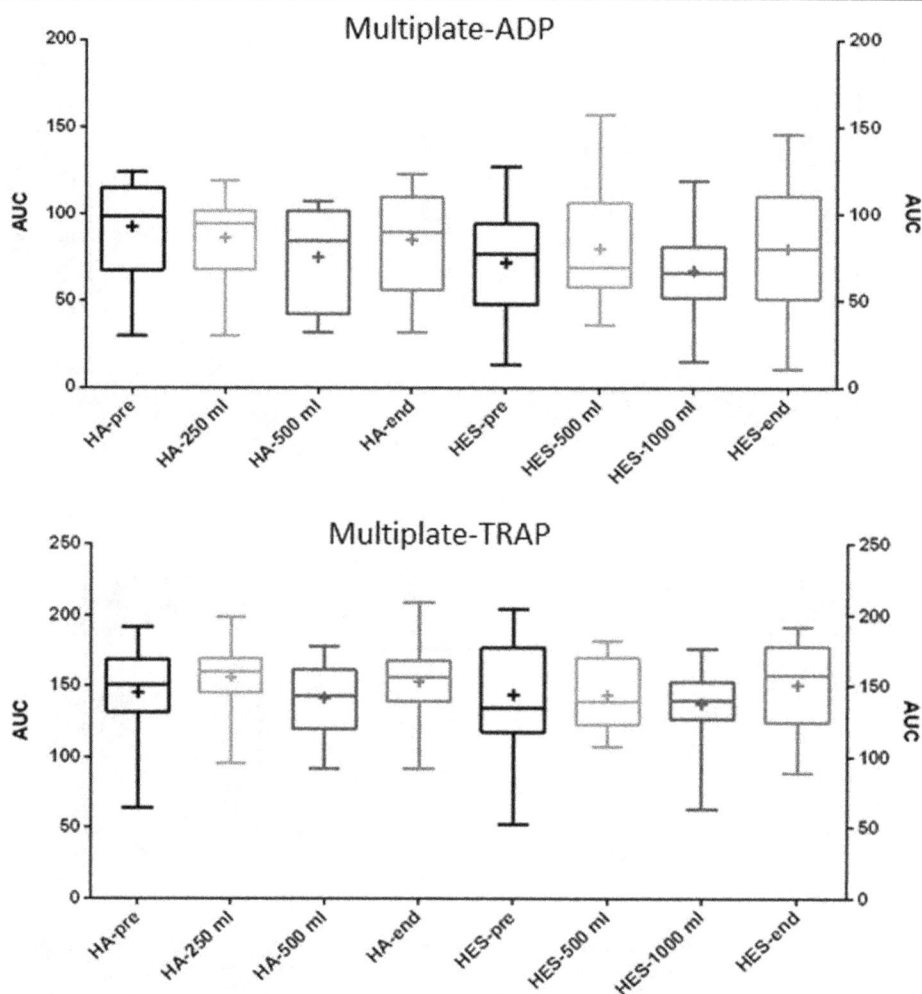

Fig. 3 Multiplate ADP and TRAP AUC values of patients undergoing elective brain tumour neurosurgery. Blood samples were taken before the start of surgery, after receiving colloid infusions (human albumin (HA) or hydroxyethyl starch (HES) 130/0.4 and at the end of surgery. *Boxplots* showing median and interquartile range with min-max whiskers and + signs identifying mean values

have found hypercoagulative ROTEM tracings at lower haemoglobin levels (Nagler et al. 2013; Solomon et al. 2013), but no such effect could be observed with certainty in our study.

At Lund University Hospital, 5 % HA is the preferred colloid for neurosurgery right now due to its ability to maintain plasma oncotic pressure. With a 20 % HA alleviation of cerebral oedema is possible (Jungner et al. 2010). However, it is hard to foresee changes in blood brain barrier that might contribute to oedema during elective brain tumour resection, so control of oncotic pressure with albumin for these types of patients is controversial.

In neurosurgery, haemostatic control poses a significant problem, as the balance between coagulation and bleeding must be maintained. If HA is to be preferred over HES, there might be a limitation to the appropriate volume of HA infusion. Either from haemodilution or another mechanism, HA seems to have an impact on coagulation. At Lund University Hospital, the upper limit of HA infusions is usually 500 ml for neurosurgical patients, with only a few receiving 750 ml. With regard to our data, infusions of these volumes might require monitoring with ROTEM or laboratory-based methods in order to detect coagulopathy and the need for fibrinogen or other transfusions. HA might be preferable in this regard since HA-induced coagulopathy is more easily reversed with fibrinogen concentrate than coagulopathy induced by HES, at least in vitro (Winstedt et al. 2013; Schlimp et al. 2013).

There are several limitations to this study. This study is not double-blinded or randomised. Initially, the aim was to study the safety of HES, as HES was our routine for haemodynamic stabilisation and initial blood-loss replacement in elective neurosurgery. This routine was later replaced by HA. It is underpowered to detect a correlation between our findings and clinical bleeding/postoperative complications. In ROTEM/Multiplate systems, results might not always correlate with clinical bleeding as there is no blood flow or endothelial interactions that affect coagulation in vivo.

We did not use the same amount of HA and HES. The patients received a mean of 375 ml HA but a mean of 861 ml HES, which is 230 % more fluid. From our very basic haemodynamic monitoring, there was an impression that the need for HA volume was much less than that of the HES volume. However, to measure this in an optimal way, we should have used blood-volume measurements or at least cardiac output monitoring. The volumes of HA and HES were not controlled by us, but by the anaesthetist in charge, trying to optimise MAP, systolic blood pressure, systolic blood pressure and PPV on top of replacing initial blood loss with 1–2 ml of the respective colloid for every millilitre of blood loss.

Dubnics M et al. have published two works on HES versus Albumin [Dubnics et al. 2007; Dubnics et al. 2009]. In short, one can say that they showed that 3 h after rescucitation with HES and HA (20 ml/kg) after bleeding in guinea pigs, plasma volume (PV) increased by 27 ml/kg in the HA group and 18 ml/kg in the HES group, equal to 1.5 times more HES needed to get the same PV-expanding effect. Corresponding PV expansion in a rat with increased permeability was 17 mL/kg for HA and 7 ml/kg of HES equal to 2.4 times as much HES albumin that needs to be given for the same PV expansion. Since the surgery, and bleeding is not likely to give the same greater permeability increase, it is more probable that the ratio for the conditions prevailing at neurosurgery are closer to 1.5 than 2.4, maybe 2.

The Saline protocol used by department may not be optimal, although we did not find any signs of hyperchloremic acidosis, hypernatremia or renal failure in our patients. Balanced crystalloids may be better [van Haren et al. 2014] from these aspects. Also, balanced crystalloids may be better than saline (and albumin) to maintain coagulation (Smith et al. 2015; Pathirana et al. 2015).

Finally, as this is a pilot study carried out during a limited period of time, the sample sizes are small, and conclusions must therefore be drawn with care regarding the preference of HA over HES as a neurosurgical fluid therapy. Nevertheless, as this study investigates clinically used fluid-therapy routines as opposed to fluid regimes designed a priori, the results are easier to apply to real-life clinical settings.

Conclusions

There were no clinically relevant differences concerning kidney function, bleeding or coagulation; although, ROTEM and Multiplate measurements indicated both inter- and intra-group statistical differences. Albumin had a certain impact on coagulation; especially after 500 ml infusion, the ROTEM changes are close to those induced by 1000 ml hydroxyethyl starch. Clot structure measured by ROTEM FIBTEM-MCF was significantly lower with HES at the end of surgery, but HES had been infused at higher volumes to maintain intra-operative haemodynamics. Unlike previous studies that focused on thromboelastography, we also used Multiplate to assess coagulation, but no significant changes could be detected other than after 500 ml HA infusion, and those changes were normalised by the end of surgery. HA seems to be a more favourable fluid for volume replacement in neurosurgical patients at restricted volumes of infusion; however, larger studies need to be carried out for more conclusive results and preferably with plasma volume measurements. Irrespective of the type of fluid regimen, intra-operative monitoring of coagulation during neurosurgery is recommended.

Abbreviations
AA: alpha angle; ADP: adenosine diphosphate; aPTT: activated thromboplastin time; AUS: area under curve; CFT: clot formation time; CT: clotting time; F: factor; HA: human albumin; HES: hydroxyethyl starch; MCF: maximal clot formation; PT: prothrombin time; ROTEM: rotational thromboelastometry; TRAP: thrombin receptor-activating peptide.

Competing interests
The authors declare that they have no competing interests.

Authors' contributions
NL performed the ROTEM and Multiplate analyses, compiled the statistics and prepared the tables and figures and took part in drafting the manuscript. SS collected clinical and other laboratory data from ROTEM/Multiplate and took part in drafting the final manuscript. BA is the director of neurosurgical anaesthesia, collected signed consent and took part in drafting the final manuscript. US planned, financed, prepared ethical committee application, informed patients and collected signed consents and took part in drafting the final manuscript. All authors have read and approved the final version of the manuscript.

Acknowledgements
The study was funded by Lund University ISEX/ALF funds for Ulf Schött.

Author details
[1]Department of Medicine, Växjö County Hospital, Växjö, Sweden.
[2]Department of Anaesthesia and Intensive Care, Lund University and Skane University Hospital, Lund S-22185, Sweden.

References
Agency EM. PRAC recommends suspending marketing authorisations for infusion solutions containing hydroxyethyl starch: European Medicines Agency; [cited 2013 Jun 14]. Available from: http://www.ema.europa.eu/ema/index.jsp?curl=pages/news_and_events/news/2013/06/news_detail_001814.jsp&mid=WC0b01ac058004d5c1.

Bolliger D, Seeberger MD, Tanaka KA. Principles and practice of thromboelastography in clinical coagulation management and transfusion practice. Transfus Med Rev. 2012;26:1–13.

Brenner T, Schmidt K, Delang M, Mehrabi A, Bruckner T, Lichtenstern C, et al. Viscoelastic and aggregometric point-of-care testing in patients with septic shock - cross-links between inflammation and haemostasis. Acta Anaesthesiol Scand. 2012;56:1277–90.

de Jonge E, Levi M, Büller HR, Berends F, Kesecioglu J. Decreased circulating levels of von Willebrand factor after intravenous administration of a rapidly degradable hydroxyethyl starch (HES 200/0.5/6) in healthy human subjects. Intensive Care Med. 2001;27:1825–9.

Dubniks M, Persson J, Grände PO. Plasma volume expansion of 5 % albumin, 4 % gelatin, 6 % HES 130/0.4, and normal saline under increased microvascular permeability in the rat. Intensive Care Med. 2007;33:293–9.

Dubniks M, Persson J, Grande PO. Comparison of the plasma volume-expanding effects of 6 % dextran 70, 5 % albumin, and 6 % HES 130/0.4 after hemorrhage in the guinea pig. J Trauma. 2009;67:1200–4.

Fenger-Eriksen C, Tønnesen E, Ingerslev J, Sørensen B. Mechanisms of hydroxyethyl starch-induced dilutional coagulopathy. J Thromb Haemost. 2009;7:1099–105.

Grande PO. The Lund concept for the treatment of patients with severe traumatic brain injury. J Neurosurg Anesthesiol. 2011;23:358–62.

Haas T, Spielmann N, Mauch J, Madjdpour C, Speer O, Schmugge M, et al. Comparison of thromboelastometry (ROTEM(R)) with standard plasmatic coagulation testing in paediatric surgery. Br J Anaesth. 2012;108:36–41.

Hahnenkamp K, Theilmeier G, Van Aken HK, Hoenemann CW. The effects of local anesthetics on perioperative coagulation, inflammation, and microcirculation. Anesth Analg. 2002;94:1441–7.

Hanke AA, Roberg K, Monaca E, Sellmann T, Weber CF, Rahe-Meyer N, et al. Impact of platelet count on results obtained from multiple electrode platelet aggregometry (Multiplate). Eur J Med Res. 2010;15:214–9.

Hartog CS, Reuter D, Loesche W, Hofmann M, Reinhart K. Influence of hydroxyethyl starch (HES) 130/0.4 on hemostasis as measured by viscoelastic device analysis: a systematic review. Intensive Care Med. 2011;37:1725–37.

Johnson SD, Lucas CE, Gerrick SJ, Ledgerwood AM, Higgins RF. Altered coagulation after albumin supplements for treatment of oligemic shock. Arch Surg. 1979;114:379–83.

Jorgensen KA, Stoffersen E. On the inhibitory effect of albumin on platelet aggregation. Thromb Res. 1980;17:13–8.

Jungner M, Grände PO, Mattiasson G, Bentzer P. Effects on brain edema of crystalloid and albumin fluid resuscitation after brain trauma and hemorrhage in the rat. Anesthesiology. 2010;112:1194–203.

Goh KY, Tsoi WC, Feng CS, Wickham N, Poon WS. Haemostatic changes during surgery for primary brain tumours. J Neurol Neurosurg Psychiatry. 1997;63:334–8.

Kim SB, Chi HS, Park JS, Hong CD, Yang WS. Effect of increasing serum albumin on plasma D-dimer, von Willebrand factor, and platelet aggregation in CAPD patients. Am J Kidney Dis. 1999;33:312–7.

Kind SL, Spahn-Nett GH, Emmert MY, Eismon J, Seifert B, Spahn DR, et al. Is dilutional coagulopathy induced by different colloids reversible by replacement of fibrinogen and factor XIII concentrates? Anesth Analg. 2013;117:1063–71.

Lang T, Bauters A, Braun SL, Pötzsch B, von Pape KW, Kolde HJ, et al. Multi-centre investigation on reference ranges for ROTEM thromboelastometry. Blood Coagul Fibrinolysis. 2005;16:301–10.

Levi M, Jonge E. Clinical relevance of the effects of plasma expanders on coagulation. Semin Thromb Hemost. 2007;33:810–5.

Mittermayr M, Streif W, Haas T, Fries D, Velik-Salchner C, Klingler A, et al. Hemostatic changes after crystalloid or colloid fluid administration during major orthopedic surgery: the role of fibrinogen administration. Anesth Analg. 2007;105:905–17.

Moral V, Aldecoa C, Asuero MS. Tetrastarch solutions: are they definitely dead? Br J Anaesth. 2013;111:324–7.

Nagler M, Kathriner S, Bachmann LM, Wuillemin WA. Impact of changes in haematocrit level and platelet count on thromboelastometry parameters. Thromb Res. 2013;131:249–53.

Nielsen VG. Colloids decrease clot propagation and strength: role of factor XIII-fibrin polymer and thrombin-fibrinogen interactions. Acta Anaesthesiol Scand. 2005;49:1163–71.

Niemi TT, Kuitunen AH. Hydroxyethyl starch impairs in vitro coagulation. Acta Anaesthesiol Scand. 1998;42:1104–9.

Niemi TT, Silvanto M, Rosenberg PH. Albumin induced hypercoagulability does not reduce blood loss in patients undergoing total hip arthroplasty. Scand J Surg. 2005;94:227–32.

Niemi TT, Suojaranta-Ylinen RT, Kukkonen SI, Kuitunen AH. Gelatin and hydroxyethyl starch, but not albumin, impair hemostasis after cardiac surgery. Anesth Analg. 2006;102:998–1006.

Pathirana S, Wong G, Williams P, Yang K, Kershaw G, Dunkley S, et al. The effects of haemodilution with albumin on coagulation in vitro as assessed by rotational thromboelastometry. Anaesth Intensive Care. 2015;43:187–92.

Perel P, Roberts I, Ker K. Colloids versus crystalloids for fluid resuscitation in critically ill patients. Cochrane Database Syst Rev. 2013;2:CD000567.

Roberts I, Blackhall K, Alderson P, Bunn F, Schierhout G. Human albumin solution for resuscitation and volume expansion in critically ill patients. Cochrane Database Syst Rev. 2011;11:CD001208.

Schlimp CJ, Cadamuro J, Solomon C, Redl H, Schöchl H. The effect of fibrinogen concentrate and factor XIII on thromboelastometry in 33 % diluted blood with albumin, gelatine, hydroxyethyl starch or saline in vitro. Blood Transfus. 2013;11:510–7.

Shore-Lesserson L, Manspeizer HE, DePerio M, Francis S, Vela-Cantos F, Ergin MA. Thromboelastography-guided transfusion algorithm reduces transfusions in complex cardiac surgery. Anesth Analg. 1999;88:312–9.

Smith CA, Gosselin RC, Utter GH, Galante JM, Young JB, Scherer LA, et al. Does saline resuscitation affect mechanisms of coagulopathy in critically ill trauma patients? An exploratory analysis. Blood Coagul Fibrinolysis. 2015;26:250–4.

Solomon C, Traintinger S, Ziegler B, Hanke A, Rahe-Meyer N, Voelckel W, et al. Platelet function following trauma. A multiple electrode aggregometry study. Thromb Haemost. 2011;106:322–30.

Solomon C, Rahe-Meyer N, Schöchl H, Ranucci M, Görlinger K. Effect of haematocrit on fibrin-based clot firmness in the FIBTEM test. Blood Transfus. 2013;11:412–8.

Theusinger OM, Schröder CM, Eismon J, Emmert MY, Seifert B, Spahn DR, et al. The influence of laboratory coagulation tests and clotting factor levels on Rotation Thromboelastometry (ROTEM(R)) during major surgery with hemorrhage. Anesth Analg. 2013;117:314–21.

Tynngård N, Berlin G, Samuelsson A, Berg S. Low dose of hydroxyethyl starch impairs clot formation as assessed by viscoelastic devices. Scand J Clin Lab Invest. 2014;74:344–50.

van Haren F, Zacharowski K. What's new in volume therapy in the intensive care unit? Best Pract Res Clin Anaesthesiol. 2014;28:275–83.

Winstedt D, Hanna J, Schott U. Albumin-induced coagulopathy is less severe and more effectively reversed with fibrinogen concentrate than is synthetic colloid-induced coagulopathy. Scand J Clin Lab Invest. 2013;73:161–9.

Zarychanski R, Abou-Setta AM, Turgeon AF, Houston BL, McIntyre L, Marshall JC, et al. Association of hydroxyethyl starch administration with mortality and acute kidney injury in critically ill patients requiring volume resuscitation: a systematic review and meta-analysis. JAMA. 2013;309:678–88.

18

Functional recovery is considered the most important target: a survey of dedicated professionals

Eirik K Aahlin[1,8]*, Maarten von Meyenfeldt[2], Cornelius HC Dejong[2], Olle Ljungqvist[3,4], Kenneth C Fearon[5], Dileep N Lobo[6], Nicolas Demartines[7], Arthur Revhaug[1,8], Stephen J Wigmore[5], Kristoffer Lassen[1,8] and on behalf of the Enhanced Recovery After Surgery (ERAS) Group

Abstract

Background: The aim of this study was to survey the relative importance of postoperative recovery targets and perioperative care items, as perceived by a large group of international dedicated professionals.

Methods: A questionnaire with eight postoperative recovery targets and 13 perioperative care items was mailed to participants of the first international Enhanced Recovery After Surgery (ERAS) congress and to authors of papers with a clear relevance to ERAS in abdominal surgery. The responders were divided into categories according to profession and region.

Results: The recovery targets 'To be completely free of nausea', 'To be independently mobile' and 'To be able to eat and drink as soon as possible' received the highest score irrespective of the responder's profession or region of origin. Equally, the care items 'Optimizing fluid balance', 'Preoperative counselling' and 'Promoting early and scheduled mobilisation' received the highest score across all groups.

Conclusions: Functional recovery, as in tolerance of food without nausea and regained mobility, was considered the most important target of recovery. There was a consistent uniformity in the way international dedicated professionals scored the relative importance of recovery targets and care items. The relative rating of the perioperative care items was not dependent on the strength of evidence supporting the items.

Keywords: Recovery, Perioperative care, ERAS, Fast track

Background

The Enhanced Recovery After Surgery (ERAS) Critical Pathway concept is based upon a protocol of care items applied perioperatively to achieve optimal stress reduction following surgery with subsequent reductions in overall morbidity and accelerated recovery [1]. The traditional concept dictates that all protocol items are of importance and synergistic effects on recovery are optimal when all items are implemented [1-3]. Recovery, however, is a compound term demanding the fulfilment of several indicators of well-being and is not clearly defined. At the same time,

implementing complex interventions like unabridged ERAS protocols is challenging and dependent on smooth cooperation of all groups of health professionals involved in patient care. If health workers from different regions and professions express significantly different views on what recovery implies and on the relative importance of the various ERAS protocol items in achieving this recovery, this may severely undermine successful implementation at ward and institution levels.

Francis D Moore defined surgical convalescence in 1958 in the following way: 'Convalescence includes all the interlocking physical, chemical, metabolic, and psychological factors commencing with the injury, or even slightly before the injury, and terminating only when the individual has returned to normal physical well-being, social and economic usefulness, and psychological habitus.' [4]. Whilst

* Correspondence: eirik.kjus.aahlin@unn.no
[1]Department of GI and HPB Surgery, University Hospital Northern Norway, Breivika, Tromsø, Norway
[8]Institute of Clinical Medicine, University of Tromsø, Tromsø, Norway
Full list of author information is available at the end of the article

FD Moore focused on the importance of functional recovery, length of hospital stay (LOS) has been the dominant outcome in convalescence research in later years [5].

We wanted to investigate how international experts and dedicated professionals view surgical convalescence today. We aimed to investigate differences and similarities on the views on central recovery targets and care items amongst the different professions and backgrounds.

Methods
Questionnaire
A questionnaire was developed by the authors specifically for this survey and consisted of two sets of questions:

- Set 1: The responders were asked to score eight different recovery targets on a scale from 1 to 11, where 1 was *not important* and 11 was *very important*.
- Set 2: The responders were also asked to score 13 care items on a similar scale according to the items' perceived importance in achieving recovery.

The targets and items are presented in Tables 1 and 2. The questionnaire was prepared for digital, web-based distribution by email (QuestBack®) and mailed to recipients between October and December 2012.

Participants
To reach potential opinion leaders in the respective surgical communities, we targeted two select groups of professionals:

- Group 1: Delegates to the first international ERAS congress in Cannes, France, in October 2012 were identified from the delegate list and subsequently contacted by email with the attached web-based questionnaire.

Table 1 Target for recovery

Target for recovery	Mean (SD)
To be completely free of nausea (not feeling or being sick)	9.88 (1.42)
To be independently mobile in hospital as soon as possible	9.72 (1.53)
To be able to eat and drink as soon as possible	9.59 (1.75)
To be able to return to all daily activities as soon as possible	9.28 (2.10)
To be completely free of pain at rest	9.27 (2.02)
To be completely free of pain upon movement	8.56 (2.8)
To be discharged from hospital as soon as possible	8.30 (2.28)
To be able to move the bowels as soon as possible	8.28 (2.61)

Mean rating of the recovery targets amongst all responders, listed in descending order of importance (scale 1 = not important, 11 = most important).

Table 2 Perioperative care item

Care item	Mean (SD)
Optimizing fluid balance	10.28 (1.22)
Preoperative counselling by nurse, anaesthetist and surgeon	10.26 (1.10)
Promoting early and scheduled mobilisation	10.24 (1.19)
Avoiding nasogastric tube after the operation	9.71 (1.86)
Allowing normal diet at will after the operation	9.70 (1.49)
Antimicrobial prophylaxis and skin preparation	9.62 (1.97)
Preoperative fasting kept at absolute minimum	9.41 (2.08)
Oral carbohydrate loading preoperatively	8.75 (2.40)
Stimulation of gut mobility	8.65 (2.35)
Avoiding a wound drain	8.56 (2.49)
Avoiding oral bowel preparation preoperatively	8.53 (2.45)
Using epidural analgesia for approximately 48 h postop	8.44 (2.78)
Avoiding preanaesthetic sedative medication	8.14 (2.57)

Mean rating of the care items amongst all responders, listed in descending order of importance (scale 1 = not important, 11 = most important).

- Group 2: A PubMed search was conducted on 13 October 2012 with the following search terms: ('enhanced recovery' OR 'critical pathway' OR 'fast track') AND ('surgery' OR 'operation' OR 'resection' OR '*ectomy'), for the latest 5 years in English. The resulting list of papers was hand searched to yield only papers with a clear relevance to ERAS in abdominal surgery. The first and last authors of the papers identified received a mail with the questionnaire, provided they were not already included in group 1.

Selection of recovery targets and care items
The eight recovery targets and 13 care items have been central in Enhanced Recovery guidelines [6-8] and consensus documents [9] and were chosen after consensus amongst the two senior authors.

Statistical analysis was performed with the SPSS (version 20) statistical package using purely descriptive statistics with calculation of mean score and standard deviation. Non-responders received two reminders per email. The recipients were asked their nationality and divided into regions according to UN definitions (http://unstats.un.org/unsd/methods/m49/m49regin.htm) and profession (physicians and nurses).

Ethical approval
This survey of attitudes of medical professionals did not affect patients or other individuals under treatment. The Regional Committee for Medical and Health Research Ethics did not consider formal ethical approval to be required.

Results

Emails with questionnaires were sent to a total of 311 individuals. In total, we received 165 responses, 121 congress participants and 44 authors. The response rate was 50% from both congress participants and authors. The responders were 103 men and 62 women. There were 87 surgeons, 30 anaesthetists, 28 nurses and 20 respondents with various backgrounds (administrators, dietitians, etc.). The responders' nationalities are presented in Table 3. Of the responders, 68% work primarily with colorectal surgery. The mean score of the recovery targets are presented in Table 1 and the mean score of the care items in Table 2. In both tables, the alternatives are presented in descending order of importance as scored by the responders.

Targets for recovery

Two targets had the highest mean score in all responder categories. These were 'To be completely free of nausea' and 'To be independently mobile'. Together with a third target, 'To be able to eat and drink as soon as possible', these three targets for recovery were consistently amongst the four targets with the highest mean score irrespective of professional or geographical responder categories. 'To be able to return to all daily activities as soon as possible' received the third highest score amongst the nurses (Table 4).

Relative importance of care item to achieve recovery

The following three care items were amongst the four care items with the highest mean score in all responder categories: 'Optimizing fluid balance', 'Preoperative counselling' and 'Promoting early and scheduled mobilisation'. The first two care items had the highest mean score in all categories. 'Avoiding nasogastric tube after the operation' received the third highest score amongst the responders from the world outside Europe (Table 5).

Discussion

The recovery targets which received the highest score according to importance in all groups of responders in our survey were 'To be completely free of nausea', 'To be independently mobile' and 'To be able to eat and drink

as soon as possible'. Amongst the 13 protocol care items listed, 'Optimizing fluid balance', 'Preoperative counselling' and 'Promoting early and scheduled mobilisation' were rated as those most important to achieve this recovery.

The present survey shows how targets for recovery and the relative importance of protocol items are perceived by a large international group of enhanced recovery protocol experts and dedicated professionals. Recruited from delegates to the first international ERAS conference and from principal authors of ERAS-related research literature, many of the responders were likely to be opinion leaders in their local and national perioperative pathway environment. As such, they constitute a body of experience and knowledge that probably reflects the current views held by health workers in a wider context. This is especially interesting when dealing with items where robust evidence is wanting. Our response rate is barely within acceptable limits in surveys of this kind [10], although a higher response rate would have been preferable.

The central finding is the similarities between different professions and regions in terms of scoring the most important recovery targets and care items. This could result from a *de facto* agreement or from bias in a sample of respondents drawn from similar backgrounds. This similarity is not statistically tested. Nevertheless, as stated above, this still indicates uniformity in how the relative importance of recovery targets and protocol care items are perceived and hence the attention this will receive in everyday practice across nations. Several international studies have documented incomplete implementation of various evidence-based Enhanced Recovery protocol items, such as avoidance of oral bowel preparation and nasogastric tube [11-13]. Whilst being long-standing core elements of Enhanced Recovery protocols, they are not consistently top rated in our survey.

'To be completely free of nausea', 'To be independently mobile' and 'To be able to eat and drink as soon as possible' are the recovery targets considered most important by the responders. Another survey amongst international experts concluded that a patient is ready for discharge when 'there is tolerance of oral intake, recovery of lower gastrointestinal function, adequate pain control with oral analgesia, ability to mobilize and self-care, and no evidence of complications or untreated medical problems' [14]. This is also consistent with the definition of a recovered patient, ready for discharge, used in both the earliest Enhanced Recovery studies and more recent ones [15,16]. Functional recovery, as in tolerance of food without nausea and regained mobility, is consistently considered the most important target for recovery and might be used when defining the recovered patient in future research and audits.

Table 3 Nationality

Region	Responders, n (%)
Northern Europe	91 (55.2)
Western Europe	22 (13.3)
Eastern and Southern Europe	18 (10.9)
America	19 (11.5)
Asia, Africa and Oceania	15 (9.1)
Total	165

The responders' nationality, divided into regions according to UN definitions.

Table 4 The highest ranked recovery targets

Physicians (n = 117)	Nurses (n = 28)	Europe (n = 131)	The world outside Europe (n = 34)
To be completely free of nausea (not feeling or being sick)	To be completely free of nausea (not feeling or being sick)	To be completely free of nausea (not feeling or being sick)	To be independently mobile in hospital as soon as possible
To be independently mobile in hospital as soon as possible	To be independently mobile in hospital as soon as possible	To be independently mobile in hospital as soon as possible	To be completely free of nausea (not feeling or being sick)
To be able to eat and drink as soon as possible	To be able to return to all daily activities as soon as possible	To be able to eat and drink as soon as possible	To be able to eat and drink as soon as possible

The three highest ranked recovery targets, according to profession and geographical region.

In a recent publication, recovery was divided into three distinct phases: the early (from the postoperative care unit to the ward), intermediate (from the ward to discharge) and late (from discharge to return to normal function) phases [17]. To be free of nausea, independently mobile and being able to eat and drink might serve as a common target for recovery in the intermediate phase. This is also consistent with the thinking of one of the pioneers in surgical recovery research, FD Moore, who divided recovery into four phases: the injury, the turning point, spontaneous nitrogen anabolism and fat redeposition [4]. 'The turning point' corresponds to the intermediate phase of surgical recovery, and the way FD Moore describes this phase has striking similarities to the most important targets for recovery in our survey: '...There is an increase in gastrointestinal function, with a return of peristalsis, the passage of flatus by the rectum, a desire for food....' [4]. The late phase of recovery, when the patient is discharged and struggle to regain normal function has received little attention in research and publications [5]. This phase might be especially important to patients and society, and it deserves to be investigated in studies with adequate follow-up length.

Interestingly, and somewhat surprising, was the finding that three of the targets and items which consistently received the highest score: 'Prevention of nausea', 'Preoperative counselling' and 'Early mobilisation', were the only items (together with *audit*) that were not supported by a Grade A recommendation in the 2009 ERAS consensus guidelines for colorectal surgery [9]. The level of evidence supporting these three targets and items was also considered low or very low in the latest guidelines

for perioperative care in elective pancreaticoduodenectomy, rectal/pelvic surgery and colonic surgery [6-8]. They were, however, strongly recommended [6-8].

This indicates that experts and dedicated professionals' views on target and/or care item importance are not necessarily linked to the level of evidence supporting it, as was also repeatedly the case in the recent guidelines [6-8]. Other surveys have shown that surgeons tend to have higher confidence in their own judgement than all other resources [18,19]. Surveys have also shown that there are frequent misconceptions about central terms in evidence-based medicine within the surgical community, like misconceptions concerning important aspects of evidence hierarchy and common terminology in study design [20]. In the era of evidence-based medicine, this serves as a reminder of the fact that there is no absolute relationship between perceived importance and established evidence.

Most targets and items were rated as important, indicating that our questionnaire lacks discriminatory power. However, any responder would be likely to think that one cannot have too much of a good thing and hence be unlikely to rate any target or item as 'not important'. Our data should be complemented with patients' ratings on the same targets and items. This would add to our understanding of the causes that impede successful implementation of protocols.

Our survey was intended to be a short mapping of the relative importance of central recovery targets and care items today as perceived by the international expertise. This could serve as a basis for more formal research aimed at creating common definitions of the different

Table 5 The highest ranked perioperative care items

Physicians (n = 117)	Nurses (n = 28)	Europe (n = 131)	The world outside Europe (n = 34)
Optimizing fluid balance	Preoperative counselling by nurse, anaesthetist and surgeon	Optimizing fluid balance	Preoperative counselling by nurse, anaesthetist and surgeon
Preoperative counselling by nurse, anaesthetist and surgeon	Promoting early and scheduled mobilisation	Promoting early and scheduled mobilisation	Optimizing fluid balance
Promoting early and scheduled mobilisation	Optimizing fluid balance	Preoperative counselling by nurse, anaesthetist and surgeon	Avoiding nasogastric tube after the operation

The three highest ranked perioperative care items, according to profession and geographical region.

phases of recovery. Such research might include the Delphi methodology, both in the selection of targets and items and in the further research process [21].

Conclusions

There was a striking uniformity in the way international expertise scored the relative importance of recovery targets and protocol items, and this rating was not dependent on the strength of supporting evidence. Functional recovery, as in tolerance of food without nausea and regained mobility, was considered the most important target for recovery and might be used as a definition of intermediate recovery in future research and audits. One definition of recovery that covers all phases and aspects might not be possible or even desirable.

Competing interests

All authors are members of the ERAS society. The authors declare that they have no other competing interests. No grant support was received.

Authors' contributions

EKA contributed to the study concepts, study design, data acquisition, data analysis and interpretation, quality control of data and algorithms, manuscript preparation, manuscript editing and manuscript review. MvM, CHCD, OL, KCF, DNL, ND and SJW contributed to the study concepts, study design, quality control of data and algorithms, manuscript editing and manuscript review. AR contributed to the study concepts, study design, quality control of data and algorithms, manuscript editing, manuscript preparation and manuscript review. KL contributed to the study concepts, study design, data acquisition, quality control of data and algorithms, manuscript preparation, manuscript editing and manuscript review. All authors read and approved the final manuscript.

Author details

[1]Department of GI and HPB Surgery, University Hospital Northern Norway, Breivika, Tromsø, Norway. [2]Department of Surgery, University Hospital Maastricht and NUTRIM School for Nutrition, Toxicology and Metabolism,, Maastricht, The Netherlands. [3]Department of Surgery, Örebro University Hospital, Örebro, Sweden. [4]Department of Molecular Medicine and Surgery, Karolinska Institutet, Stockholm, Sweden. [5]Clinical Surgery, University of Edinburgh, Royal Infirmary of Edinburgh, Edinburgh, UK. [6]Division of Gastrointestinal Surgery, Nottingham Digestive Diseases Centre National Institute for Health Research, Biomedical Research Unit, Nottingham University Hospitals, Queen's Medical Centre, Nottingham, UK. [7]Department of Visceral Surgery, University Hospital of Lausanne (CHUV), Lausanne, Switzerland. [8]Institute of Clinical Medicine, University of Tromsø, Tromsø, Norway.

References

1. Kehlet H, Wilmore DW: Evidence-based surgical care and the evolution of fast-track surgery. *Ann Surg* 2008, **248**:189–198.
2. Kehlet H: Multimodal approach to control postoperative pathophysiology and rehabilitation. *Br J Anaesth* 1997, **78**:606–617.
3. Wilmore DW, Kehlet H: Management of patients in fast track surgery. *BMJ* 2001, **322**:473–476.
4. MOORE FD: Getting well: the biology of surgical convalescence. *Ann N Y Acad Sci* 1958, **73**:387–400.
5. Neville A, Lee L, Antonescu I, Mayo NE, Vassiliou MC, Fried GM, Feldman LS: Systematic review of outcomes used to evaluate enhanced recovery after surgery. *Br J Surg* 2014, **101**:159–171.
6. Lassen K, Coolsen MM, Slim K, Carli F, de Aguilar-Nascimento JE, Schafer M, Parks RW, Fearon KC, Lobo DN, Demartines N, Braga M, Ljungqvist O, Dejong CH: Guidelines for perioperative care for

7. pancreaticoduodenectomy: Enhanced Recovery After Surgery (ERAS®) Society recommendations. *World J Surg* 2013, **37**:240–258.
7. Nygren J, Thacker J, Carli F, Fearon KC, Norderval S, Lobo DN, Ljungqvist O, Soop M, Ramirez J: Guidelines for perioperative care in elective rectal/pelvic surgery: Enhanced Recovery After Surgery (ERAS®) Society recommendations. *World J Surg* 2013, **37**:285–305.
8. Gustafsson UO, Scott MJ, Schwenk W, Demartines N, Roulin D, Francis N, McNaught CE, MacFie J, Liberman AS, Soop M, Hill A, Kennedy RH, Lobo DN, Fearon K, Ljungqvist O: Guidelines for perioperative care in elective colonic surgery: Enhanced Recovery After Surgery (ERAS®) Society recommendations. *World J Surg* 2013, **37**:259–284.
9. Lassen K, Soop M, Nygren J, Cox PB, Hendry PO, Spies C, von Meyenfeldt MF, Fearon KC, Revhaug A, Norderval S, Ljungqvist O, Lobo DN, Dejong CH: Consensus review of optimal perioperative care in colorectal surgery: Enhanced Recovery After Surgery (ERAS) Group recommendations. *Arch Surg* 2009, **144**:961–969.
10. Asch DA, Jedrziewski MK, Christakis NA: Response rates to mail surveys published in medical journals. *J Clin Epidemiol* 1997, **50**:1129–1136.
11. Hasenberg T, Keese M, Langle F, Reibenwein B, Schindler K, Herold A, Beck G, Post S, Jauch KW, Spies C, Schwenk W, Shang E: 'Fast-track' colonic surgery in Austria and Germany—results from the survey on patterns in current perioperative practice. *Colorectal Dis* 2009, **11**:162–167.
12. Kehlet H, Buchler MW, Beart RW Jr, Billingham RP, Williamson R: Care after colonic operation—is it evidence-based? Results from a multinational survey in Europe and the United States. *J Am Coll Surg* 2006, **202**:45–54.
13. Lassen K, Hannemann P, Ljungqvist O, Fearon K, Dejong CH, von Meyenfeldt MF, Hausel J, Nygren J, Andersen J, Revhaug A: Patterns in current perioperative practice: survey of colorectal surgeons in five northern European countries. *BMJ* 2005, **330**:1420–1421.
14. Fiore JF Jr, Bialocerkowski A, Browning L, Faragher IG, Denehy L: Criteria to determine readiness for hospital discharge following colorectal surgery: an international consensus using the Delphi technique. *Dis Colon Rectum* 2012, **55**:416–423.
15. Basse L, Hjort JD, Billesbolle P, Werner M, Kehlet H: A clinical pathway to accelerate recovery after colonic resection. *Ann Surg* 2000, **232**:51–57.
16. Vlug MS, Bartels SA, Wind J, Ubbink DT, Hollmann MW, Bemelman WA: Which fast track elements predict early recovery after colon cancer surgery? *Colorectal Dis* 2012, **14**:1001–1008.
17. Lee L, Tran T, Mayo NE, Carli F, Feldman LS: What does it really mean to "recover" from an operation? *Surgery* 2014, **155**:211–216.
18. Kitto S, Villanueva EV, Chesters J, Petrovic A, Waxman BP, Smith JA: Surgeons' attitudes towards and usage of evidence-based medicine in surgical practice: a pilot study. *ANZ J Surg* 2007, **77**:231–236.
19. Kitto SC, Peller JC, Villanueva EV, Gruen RL, Smith JA: Rural surgeons' attitudes towards and usage of evidence-based medicine in rural surgical practice. *J Eval Clin Pract* 2011, **17**:678–683.
20. Poolman RW, Sierevelt IN, Farrokhyar F, Mazel JA, Blankevoort L, Bhandari M: Perceptions and competence in evidence-based medicine: are surgeons getting better? A questionnaire survey of members of the Dutch Orthopaedic Association. *J Bone Joint Surg Am* 2007, **89**:206–215.
21. Keeney S, Hasson F, McKenna HP: A critical review of the Delphi technique as a research methodology for nursing. *Int J Nurs Stud* 2001, **38**:195–200.

Incidence, outcome, and attributable resource use associated with pulmonary and cardiac complications after major small and large bowel procedures

Lee A Fleisher[1*] and Walter T Linde-Zwirble[2]

Abstract

Background: Complications increase the costs of care of surgical patients. We studied the Premier database to determine the incidence and direct medical costs related to pulmonary complications and compared it to cardiac complications in the same cohort.

Methods: We identified 45,969 discharges in patients undergoing major bowel procedures. Postoperative pulmonary and cardiac complications were identified through the use of International Classification of Diseases, Ninth Edition, Clinical Modification (ICD-9-CM) codes and through the use of daily resource use data. Pulmonary complications included pneumonia, tracheobronchitis, pleural effusion, pulmonary failure, and mechanical ventilation more than 48 h after surgery. Cardiac complications included ventricular fibrillation, acute myocardial infarction, cardiogenic shock, cardiopulmonary arrest, transient ischemia, premature ventricular contraction, and acute congestive heart failure.

Results: Postoperative pulmonary complications (PPC) or postoperative cardiac complications (PCC) were present in 22% of cases; PPC alone was most common (19.0%), followed by PPC and PCC (1.8%) and PCC alone (1.2%). The incremental cost of PPC is large ($25,498). In comparison, PCC alone only added $7,307 to the total cost.

Conclusions: The current study demonstrates that postoperative pulmonary complications represent a significant source of morbidity and incremental cost after major small intestinal and colon surgery and have greater incidence and costs than cardiac complications alone. Therefore, strategies to reduce the incidence of these complications should be targeted as means of improving health and bending the cost curve in health care.

Keywords: Colectomy, Surgery, Postoperative, Pulmonary complications, Myocardial infarction, Cardiac arrest, Pneumonia, Cost

Background

During the past decade, there has been a marked decrease in surgical mortality [1]. This decrease appears to be related in part to better treatment of complications in some hospitals since perioperative complications remain high and continue to be a significant source of both decreased health and increased costs after surgery [2].

Beginning in the 1970s, there was a concerted effort to identify patients at increased risk of perioperative cardiovascular morbidity and mortality and to identify strategies to reduce these complications. This has led to the development and publication of formal Guidelines on Perioperative Cardiovascular Evaluation and Management for Noncardiac Surgery and incorporation of specific therapies into public performance measurement [3]. In contrast to cardiovascular disease, the evaluation and management of perioperative pulmonary complications has not had the same degree of concerted effort to either identify those at risk or implement additional risk reduction strategies.

* Correspondence: lee.fleisher@uphs.upenn.edu
[1]Department of Anesthesiology and Critical Care, Perelman School of Medicine, Leonard Davis Institute of Health Economics, University of Pennsylvania, 3400 Spruce Street, Dulles 680, Philadelphia, PA 19104, USA
Full list of author information is available at the end of the article

The absence of a concerted focus on perioperative pulmonary complications may in part be due to the lack of recognition of their incidence and their economic burden [4]. An additional issue is related to the definition of pulmonary complications since there is wide variability in manifestations of complications: from minor aspiration to pneumonia to overt sepsis. Assessing the impact of pulmonary complications is also difficult since a pulmonary complication may lead to cardiovascular collapse with resultant cardiac morbidity or mortality. Pulmonary complications may also be the final common pathway for major morbidity or mortality in patients with other complications such as non-pulmonary infectious complications. Given the lack of concerted attention in this important area of health-care outcomes, we analyzed an enriched administrative dataset to determine the incidence and direct medical costs related to pulmonary complications in order to provide more focused attention on the problem and provide an impetus to identify cost-effective risk-reducing strategies and compared it to cardiac complications in the same cohort.

Methods

Case selection

We constructed the study cohort using the 2008 Premier Hospital Discharge database. The Premier database (Premier, Inc., Charlotte, NC, USA) includes information on all inpatients and hospital-based outpatients treated in more than 600 US hospitals. The database includes patient demographic data and diagnosis codes; the date-stamped log of all invoiced items, including procedures, medications, laboratory orders, diagnostic, and therapeutic services; as well as devices used by individual patients. The cohort of interest consisted of all discharges, age 18 years and older, in the Medicare Severity DRGs 329–331, major small and large bowel procedures. For each case, we extracted the following: demographic characteristics; principal diagnosis group (neoplasm, colitis/diverticulitis, other); Charlson-Deyo co-morbidities; postoperative pulmonary and cardiac complications; postoperative length of stay (LOS); postoperative intensive care unit (ICU) use; postoperative ICU LOS; total hospital costs; and national projection weights.

Identification of postoperative complications

Postoperative pulmonary and cardiac complications were identified through the use of International Classification of Diseases, Ninth Edition, Clinical Modification (ICD-9-CM) codes in any secondary coding space and through the use of daily resource use data. Pulmonary complications included pneumonia (481, 482, 485, 486); tracheobronchitis (494.1, 466, 464.1); pleural effusion (511.1, 511.8, 511.9); pulmonary failure (518.81, 518.84); and mechanical ventilation more than 48 h after surgery

(from daily resource use). Cardiac complications included ventricular fibrillation (427.4); acute myocardial infarction (410.X1); cardiogenic shock (785.51); cardiopulmonary arrest (427.5); transient ischemia (411.1, 411.89); premature ventricular contraction (PVC) (427.6); and acute congestive heart failure (428.21, 428.31, 428.41).

Case-mix adjustment

We constructed a case-mix adjustment model to characterize the impact of preoperative characteristics on the incidence of postoperative complications and estimate the attributable effects of PPC and PCC on resource use and outcome. We constructed an analysis of variance model using patients with no PPC and no PCC to predict total cost as a function of age group; principal diagnosis group (neoplasm—150–59, 183, 188, 195, 197, 209, 211, 214, 228, 230–35, 239; colitis/diverticulitis—555–569; and other); and Charlson-Deyo co-morbidity. We chose cost and not mortality risk as a severity measure because hospital mortality is very low in those without postoperative complications. The predicted cost equation was applied to all cases, both those with and without postoperative complications, and subjects were characterized by quintiles of preoperative severity.

Resource use and outcome presentation

Overall mortality and resource use was presented directly and also parsed into a base value, what was expected had there been no postoperative complications, and an incremental effect, the difference between the total and base values.

Statistical analysis

We compared continuous data using the Mann–Whitney U test and categorical data by chi-squared or Fisher's exact test as appropriate. We organized patient data by the presence of postoperative complications (PPC only, PCC only, neither PPC nor PCC, and both PPC and PCC) and by quintiles (Q) of preoperative severity. We generated national estimates using Premier-supplied weights. We constructed the databases in FoxPro (Microsoft Corp, Redmond, WA, USA) and conducted analyses in Data Desk (Data Description, Ithaca, NY, USA).

Results

We identified 45,969 discharges with major small and large bowel procedures. The average age was 62.9 years and 45.1% were male. Descriptive characteristics are provided in Table 1. Colitis/diverticulitis was the most common principal diagnosis (43.7%), followed by neoplasm (39.3%) and other (17.0%). More than a third of the cohort (37.2%) had at least one Charlson-Deyo co-morbidity, with diabetes being the most common (15.8%) followed

Table 1 Major small and large bowel procedure cohort characteristic, overall and by postoperative complication group

Variables	All (n = 45,969)	No PPC/PCC (n = 35,875)	PPC alone (n = 8,744)	PCC alone (n = 547)	PPC and PCC (n = 803)
Rate (%)		78.0	19.0	1.2	1.8
Hospital mortality (%)	3.6	0.7	11.9	12.6	36.1
Age (mean, years)	62.9	61.3	67.8	73.7	74.5
Age group (%)					
18–34	5.4	6.2	3.2	0.9	0.6
35–54	23.8	26.5	15.6	6.2	5.7
55–64	21.3	22.3	18.5	14.3	10.8
65–74	22.2	21.7	23.7	23.9	25.7
75–84	19.7	17.6	26.0	35.8	37.0
85+	7.5	5.8	12.9	18.8	20.2
Sex, male (%)	45.1	45.0	45.3	49.2	46.8
Race (%)					
White	70.2	70.2	69.7	72.4	71.5
Black	10.4	10.0	12.0	11.2	12.0
Other	19.4	19.8	18.3	16.5	16.6
Charlson-Deyo co-morbidity (%)					
Diabetes	15.8	14.6	19.9	22.7	24.7
Complicated diabetes	1.4	1.1	2.3	2.2	3.1
Chronic pulmonary disease	8.0	5.9	16.0	12.6	16.6
Chronic renal disease	6.4	4.4	12.9	14.1	21.2
Neoplasm	5.7	5.0	8.5	5.3	7.2
Metastatic neoplasm	13.1	12.6	14.6	14.6	14.1
Cerebrovascular disease	1.1	0.9	1.9	1.5	2.7
Dementia	0.3	0.2	0.6	1.1	0.6
Prior myocardial infarction	4.0	3.5	5.0	11.5	10.5
Para- and quadriplegia	0.4	0.3	0.9	0.9	1.4
Peripheral vascular disease	3.1	2.3	5.5	9.9	9.2
Chronic rheumatic disease	2.2	1.9	3.2	2.5	3.2
Mild liver disease	0.9	0.7	1.7	1.1	1.7
Severe liver disease	0.4	0.2	1.1	0.4	1.2
HIV	0.1	0.1	0.1	0.0	0.0
Any co-morbidity	37.2	34.1	47.2	53.2	55.8
Mean number	0.6	0.5	0.9	1.0	1.2

by metastatic neoplasm (13.1%) and chronic pulmonary conditions (8.0%).

Incidence and survival

Pulmonary or cardiac complications were present in 22% of cases; PPC alone was most common (19.0%), followed by PPC and PCC (1.8%) and PCC alone (1.2%). Those with postoperative complications were older and had a greater co-morbid burden than those that did not.

Those with PPC alone had 11.9% mortality and accounted for nearly two thirds (63.6%) of hospital deaths (Figure 1).

PCC alone cases had a similar mortality (12.6%) but accounted for only 4.2% of deaths. Those with PPC and PCC had the highest mortality (36.1%), though only 1.3% of the cohort accounted for 17.7% of deaths.

Individual complications

Respiratory failure was the most common postoperative complication, being present in one in eight patients with 21.8% mortality (Table 2). Other pulmonary complications ranged from 0.4% incidence (pneumothorax) to 6.1% (MV48). Overall, 20.8% of patients had at least one

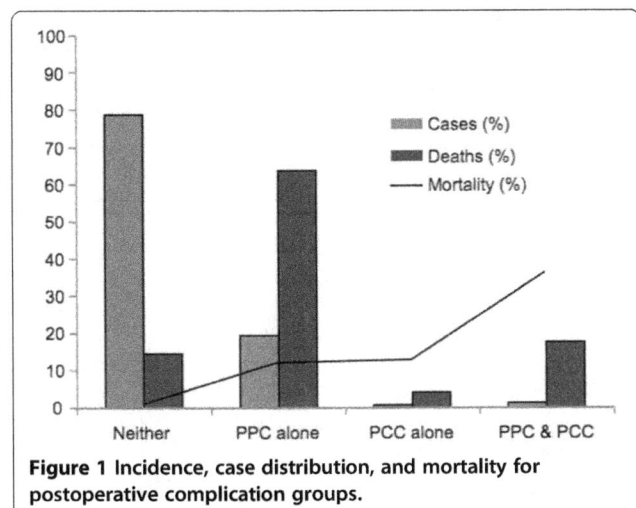

Figure 1 Incidence, case distribution, and mortality for postoperative complication groups.

PPC with a combined hospital mortality of 13.9%. Cardiac complications (2.9% incidence) were seven times less frequent than pulmonary complications, but with higher hospital mortality (26.6%). Acute myocardial infarction (AMI) was the most common PCC but occurred in only 1.2% of patients.

Severity model

The average cost of those without PPC and PCC increased with age ($2,732 more for those over 85 compared to

Table 2 Incidence and hospital mortality for postoperative complications

Complications	Cases (% of group)	Rate (%)	Mortality (%)
Pulmonary			
Pneumonia	2,249 (23.6)	4.9	14.4
Tracheobronchitis	434 (4.5)	0.9	6.2
Pleural effusion	1,584 (16.6)	3.4	13.7
Pulmonary collapse	3,499 (36.7)	7.6	6.2
Pneumothorax	189 (2.0)	2.0	24.9
Respiratory failure	5,686 (59.6)	12.4	21.8
MV48[a]	2,807 (29.4)	6.1	28.5
Any pulmonary	9,547	20.8	13.9
Cardiac			
Ventricular fibrillation	63 (4.7)	0.1	61.9
AMI	570 (42.2)	1.2	26.7
Cardiogenic shock	64 (4.7)	0.1	57.8
Cardiopulmonary arrest	220 (16.3)	0.5	70.9
Transient ischemia	47 (3.5)	0.1	2.1
PVC	367 (27.2)	0.8	6.0
Acute CHF	175 (13.0)	0.4	14.9
Any cardiac	1,350	2.9	26.6

[a]Mechanical ventilation more than 48 h after surgery.

those under 35), principal diagnosis of colitis/diverticulitis ($2,487 more than neoplasm), and co-morbidity (diabetes $1,091; peripheral vascular disease $1,493; cerebrovascular disease $4,792; chronic pulmonary disease $1,044; rheumatic disease $1,544; complex diabetes $2,700; para- and quadriplegia $3,422; chronic renal disease $6,046; and severe liver disease $8,706). The rate of postoperative complications increased greatly across the quintiles of severity (Table 3), increasing from 11.0% in the first quintile to 41.7% in the fifth quintile. While PPC alone tripled from 10.5% in Q1 to 34.7% in Q5, the rate of PCC alone and PPC and PCC increased by more than a factor of ten from Q1 to Q5.

Hospital mortality and resource use by severity quintiles

The base mortality increased from 0.1% in Q1 to 2.2% in Q5 for an overall value of 0.7% (Table 3). This is dwarfed by the incremental mortality associated with PPC alone (11.2% absolute), PCC alone (12.0%), and PPC and PCC (35.5%) (Figure 2). While the base cost increased by $5,909 between Q1 and Q5, the incremental cost of PPC is large ($25,498) but increased only modestly from $22,199 in Q1 to $26,508 in Q5 (Figure 3). In comparison, PCC alone only added $7,307 to the total cost. Overall, the incremental cost of PPC is 153% of the mean base cost.

In contrast to mortality and cost, the base ICU use rate increased greatly from 6.0% in Q1 to 23.3% in Q5. Those with postoperative complications had much greater ICU use. Postoperative ICU use for those with PPC rose from 48% in Q1 to 76% in Q5. This is much greater than PCC alone and less than PPC and PCC, which in Q5 had an ICU use rate of 83.2%. Base postoperative floor LOS ranged from 5.9 days in Q1 to 7.6 days in Q5 with a mean of 6.4 days. PPC alone added 3.5 days, greater than PCC alone (1.3 days) and PPC and PCC (2.8 days). Base postoperative ICU LOS was modest varying only from 0.2 days in Q1 to 0.7 in Q5. The incremental postoperative ICU LOS varied little by preoperative severity but could be large: adding 1.1 ICU days for PCC, 4.5 ICU days for PPC, and 7.1 ICU days for those with PPC and PCC.

National projections

Projecting to US national levels, there were 308,798 major small and large bowel procedure discharges in 2008, with 59,980 with PPC alone, 3,739 with PCC alone, and 5,295 with PPC and PCC. The expected number of hospital deaths in the absence of PPC and PCC was 2,370, only 21% of the observed 11,157 deaths. The expected cost in the absence of postoperative complications was $5.25B, 75% of the observed $6.99B. Similarly, in the absence of PPC and PCC, we would have expected 51.5% of the observed ICU use, 90% of postoperative floor days, and 25% of ICU days to have been used. In summary, PCC alone was associated with 3.8% of

Table 3 Association between preoperative severity, postoperative complications, and outcomes

Severity quintiles	Q1	Q2	Q3	Q4	Q5	Total
	(n = 8,403)	(n = 9,976)	(n = 8,846)	(n = 9,174)	(n = 9,574)	(n = 45,969)
Complication rate (%)						
PPC alone	10.5	14.5	13.9	20.3	34.7	19.0
PCC alone	0.2	1.3	0.8	1.3	2.2	1.2
PPC and PCC	0.3	1.1	1.0	1.4	4.7	1.7
Any complication	11.0	16.9	15.7	23.0	41.7	21.9
Base mortality (%)	0.1	0.4	0.3	0.7	2.2	0.7
Incremental mortality (%)						
PPC alone	5.2	7.9	8.3	8.5	15.8	11.2
PCC alone	3.1	7.5	6.4	8.7	15.6	12.0
PPC and PCC	13.5	35.0	33.8	32.9	36.3	35.5
Base cost ($)	14,875	15,438	16,017	17,462	20,784	16,672
Incremental cost ($)						
PPC alone	22,199	24,199	24,658	26,817	26,508	25,498
PCC alone	5,524	5,528	9,070	4,057	9,765	7,307
PPC and PCC	45,308	48,950	38,096	30,884	31,394	34,872
Base ICU use (%)	6.0	9.0	8.2	11.8	23.3	11.0
Incremental ICU use (%)						
PPC alone	42.0	45.7	50.2	54.0	52.7	54.0
PCC alone	9.8	24.9	33.1	20.4	25.2	28.5
PPC and PCC	71.2	67.1	75.3	68.3	59.9	70.6
Base post-op ICU LOS (days)	0.2	0.2	0.2	0.3	0.7	0.3
Incremental post-op ICU LOS (days)						
PPC alone	3.0	4.0	3.7	4.6	5.0	4.5
PCC alone	0.4	0.7	1.0	0.6	1.4	1.1
PPC and PCC	7.5	8.0	7.5	6.7	6.5	7.1
Base post-op floor LOS (days)	5.9	6.3	6.4	6.6	7.6	6.5
Incremental post-op floor LOS (days)						
PPC alone	3.0	4.0	3.7	4.6	5.0	4.5
PCC alone	0.4	0.7	1.0	0.6	1.4	1.1
PPC and PCC	7.5	8.0	7.5	6.7	6.5	7.1

deaths, PPC and PCC with 16.4% of deaths, and PPC alone with 58.5% of all deaths.

Discussion

The current study demonstrates that postoperative pulmonary complications represent a significant source of morbidity and incremental cost after major small intestinal and colon surgery and have greater incidence and costs than cardiac complications alone. Although PPC alone was associated with a high incidence of mortality (11.9%), the combination of PPC and PCC together was associated with the greatest risk. The incidence increased with increasing age until 85 years of age, with over 20% of all patients experiencing some form of pulmonary complication.

The high incidence of pulmonary complications is consistent with studies utilizing the American College of Surgeons National Surgical Quality Improvement Program (ACS NSQIP), although the actual rate is higher than that in their selected population of hospitals [5]. This may reflect differences in the definition of PPC we used, which included a larger group of diagnoses, or it may reflect differences between hospitals enrolled in a quality improvement program compared to a more random sample. Importantly, we observed a 4.9% incidence of postoperative pneumonia and 6.1% incidence of mechanic ventilation greater than 24 h, which is consistent with other studies. For example, Kennedy and colleagues reported a 25.4% incidence of complications for surgery for

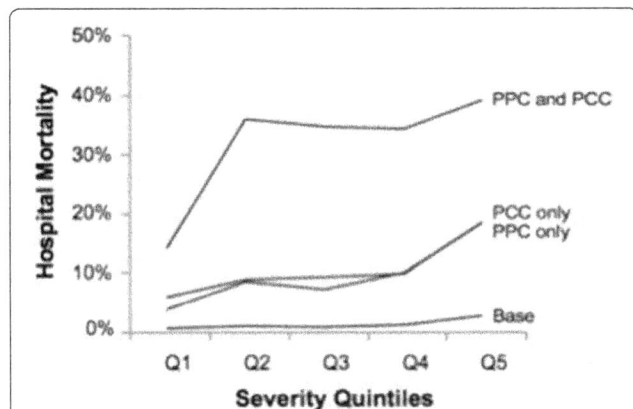

Figure 2 Base and incremental mortalities for postoperative complication groups by preoperative severity groups.

colon cancer, with respiratory complications being the second most common complication after superficial site infection [6]. In contrast, Arozullah and colleagues observed a 1.5% incidence of postoperative pneumonia in a mixed group of major noncardiac surgery at 100 Veterans Administration Medical Centers [7]. The lower incidence of pneumonia in this population may reflect the type of surgery compared to a cohort of major abdominal surgery in our study.

We observed a high mortality associated with PPC, particularly those with concomitant PCC. Arozullah and colleagues observed a 21% incidence of 30-day mortality in those patients with pneumonia compared to our 14.4% incidence of in-hospital mortality. Jencks and colleagues demonstrated that patients with postoperative pneumonia have a high incidence of readmission, and therefore, our in-hospital mortality rate may not reflect the true 30-day incident [8]. Additionally, we observed a more contemporary cohort of non-Veterans Administration Medical

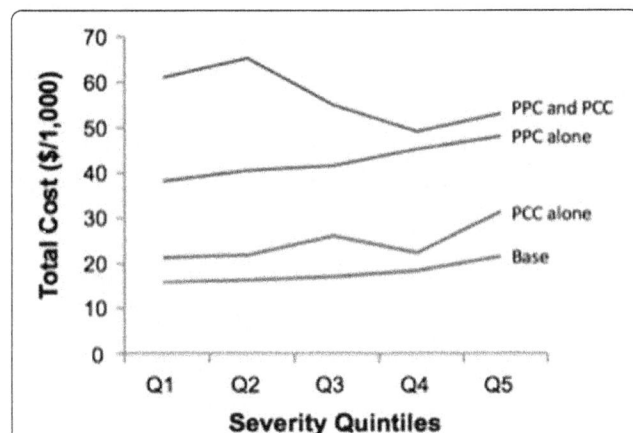

Figure 3 Base and incremental costs for postoperative complication groups by preoperative severity groups.

Centers, and they may actually have a better failure-to-rescue rate.

We observed that postoperative cardiac complications continue to occur at low rates (2.9% overall incidence with 1.2% incidence of AMI) but are associated with a high mortality rate. This is consistent with other studies. For example, Dimick and colleagues at the University of Michigan found the incidence of 30-day cardiovascular complications to be 1% overall in a cohort of general and vascular surgery patients [9]. A 26.6% in-hospital mortality is consistent with most contemporary studies and suggests that while decreasing in frequency, cardiac complications still carry a significant mortality. When evaluating the mortality rate for either complication, it is important to isolate solitary complications from those that are combined.

PPC was associated with a significant increased length of stay and overall costs. Dimick and colleagues demonstrated a $62,704 average increment in costs in those patients with PPC in a mixed cohort of patients [9]. Khan and colleagues reported an increased hospital length of stay of 89% and increased costs by 55%, which is more consistent with our findings [10]. Thompson and colleagues studied abdominal surgical patients and demonstrated an increased hospital length of stay of 11 days and charges of $31,000 associated with PPC [11]. Short and colleagues utilized Medicare claims for the years 2005 through 2009 in six cancer resections and assessed the rate of complications using the Agency for Healthcare Research and Quality Patient Safety Indicators (PSI) [12]. They found that the rate of postoperative respiratory failure was 2.58% and increased costs by >50% for all cancer resections. Vaughan-Sarrazin and colleagues looked at cost of complications in general surgery patients in the Veterans Administration NSQIP as a means of building a business case for improving surgical quality [13]. The average cost for patients with no complication was $22,000, while the total costs for patients with a pulmonary embolism was $62,726 and increased to more than $115,000 for patients with failure to wean from the ventilator within 48 h of operation.

The significant medical and economic burden of postoperative pulmonary or cardiopulmonary complications clearly suggest that increased attention should be directed at reducing this complication. We included an analysis of cardiac complications in order to assess the importance of pulmonary complications in perspective. The past decade has seen numerous studies published which have evaluated interventions to reduce cardiac complications of noncardiac surgery [3]. Similar studies are lacking in the area of reducing the incidence and burden of pulmonary complications. Shander and colleagues have recently reported on a patient safety summit dedicated to risk-reducing and preventive strategies [4]. They have emphasized the paucity of data regarding such strategies as well as discussed potential technologies and strategies to reduce the incidence of ventilator-associated pneumonia.

Our study has several limitations related to the use of administrative claims to assess burden and costs of disease. By using the Premier database, we have the distinct advantage of daily resource utilization and an enriched set of diagnostic codes. However, we still have the inherent limitation of any such dataset with regard to the accuracy of the codes and inclusions of all potentially relevant variables. For example, we did not analyze smoking status given the inaccuracy of this variable in discharge data. With respect to outcome measures, hospitals may have different definitions of the individual outcomes and surveillance for such outcomes. We also made some assumptions regarding the sequence of cardiac versus respiratory complications that could influence our findings.

Conclusions

We have demonstrated that postoperative pulmonary complications, either in isolation or in tandem with postoperative cardiac complications, occur at a high incidence after intestinal surgery and are associated with significant mortality and costs. Therefore, strategies to reduce the incidence of these complications should be targeted as means of improving health and bending the cost curve in health care.

Competing interests

Dr. Linde-Zwirble received funding to purchase the Premier database and consulting fees to demonstrate the value of the database from Covidien, which manufactures products which could be used to reduce perioperative pulmonary complications. The Department of Anesthesiology and Critical Care at the University of Pennsylvania has received grants and equipment from Covidien, but Dr. Fleisher has not received any direct research funds or honorarium.

Authors' contributions

LAF conceived of the study, participated in its design and analysis, and drafted the manuscript. WTLZ participated in the design of the study, performed the statistical analysis, and helped to draft the manuscript. Both authors read and approved the final manuscript.

Acknowledgements

The authors wish to acknowledge the assistance of Jonathan Bloom, M.D., and Doug Hansell, M.D., in the original concept of the study. Dr. Linde-Zwirble received funding from Covidien.

Author details

[1]Department of Anesthesiology and Critical Care, Perelman School of Medicine, Leonard Davis Institute of Health Economics, University of Pennsylvania, 3400 Spruce Street, Dulles 680, Philadelphia, PA 19104, USA. [2]ZD Associates, Perkasie, PA, USA.

References

1. Finks JF, Osborne NH, Birkmeyer JD: **Trends in hospital volume and operative mortality for high-risk surgery.** N Engl J Med 2011, **364:**2128–2137.
2. Ghaferi AA, Birkmeyer JD, Dimick JB: **Variation in hospital mortality associated with inpatient surgery.** N Engl J Med 2009, **361:**1368–1375.
3. Fleisher LA, Fleischmann KE, Auerbach AD, Barnason SA, Beckman JA, Bozkurt B, Davila-Roman VG, Gerhard-Herman MD, Holly TA, Kane GC, Marine JE, Nelson TM, Spencer CC, Thompson A, Ting HH, Uretsky BF, Wijeysundera DN: **ACC/AHA guideline on perioperative cardiovascular evaluation and management of patients undergoing noncardiac surgery: a report of the American College of Cardiology/American Heart Association task force on practice guidelines.** J Am Coll Cardiol 2014.
4. Shander A, Fleisher LA, Barie PS, Bigatello LM, Sladen RN, Watson CB: **Clinical and economic burden of postoperative pulmonary complications: patient safety summit on definition, risk-reducing interventions, and preventive strategies.** Crit Care Med 2011, **39:**2163–2172.
5. Gupta H, Gupta PK, Fang X, Miller WJ, Cemaj S, Forse RA, Morrow LE: **Development and validation of a risk calculator predicting postoperative respiratory failure.** Chest 2011, **140:**1207–1215.
6. Kennedy GD, Rajamanickam V, O'Connor ES, Loconte NK, Foley EF, Leverson G, Heise CP: **Optimizing surgical care of colon cancer in the older adult population.** Ann Surg 2011, **253:**508–514.
7. Arozullah AM, Khuri SF, Henderson WG, Daley J: **Development and validation of a multifactorial risk index for predicting postoperative pneumonia after major noncardiac surgery.** Ann Intern Med 2001, **135:**847–857.
8. Jencks SF, Williams MV, Coleman EA: **Rehospitalizations among patients in the Medicare fee-for-service program.** N Engl J Med 2009, **360:**1418–1428.
9. Dimick JB, Chen SL, Taheri PA, Henderson WG, Khuri SF, Campbell DA Jr: **Hospital costs associated with surgical complications: a report from the private-sector National Surgical Quality Improvement Program.** J Am Coll Surg 2004, **199:**531–537.
10. Khan NA, Quan H, Bugar JM, Lemaire JB, Brant R, Ghali WA: **Association of postoperative complications with hospital costs and length of stay in a tertiary care center.** J Gen Intern Med 2006, **21:**177–180.
11. Thompson DA, Makary MA, Dorman T, Pronovost PJ: **Clinical and economic outcomes of hospital acquired pneumonia in intra-abdominal surgery patients.** Ann Surg 2006, **243:**547–552.
12. Short MN, Aloia TA, Ho V: **The influence of complications on the costs of complex cancer surgery.** Cancer 2014, **120:**1035–1041.
13. Vaughan-Sarrazin M, Bayman L, Rosenthal G, Henderson W, Hendricks A, Cullen JJ: **The business case for the reduction of surgical complications in VA hospitals.** Surgery 2011, **149:**474–483.

How fast can glucose be infused in the perioperative setting?

Robert G. Hahn

Abstract

Background: How the initial infusion rate of glucose solution should be set to avoid hyperglycemia in the perioperative setting is unclear.

Methods: Computer simulations were performed based on data from seven studies where the kinetics of glucose was calculated using a one-compartment model. Glucose had been infused intravenously on 44 occasions to volunteers and on 256 occasions to surgical patients at various stages of the perioperative process. The rates that yield plasma glucose concentrations of 7, 9, and 12 mmol/l were calculated and standardized to a 5 % glucose solution infused in a subject weighing 70 kg.

Results: The lowest infusion rates were found during surgery and the first hours after surgery. No more than 0.5 ml/min of glucose 5 % could be infused if plasma glucose above 7 mmol/l was not allowed, while 2 ml/min maintained a steady state concentration of 9 mmol/l. Intermediate infusion rates could be used in the preoperative period and 1–2 days after moderate-sized surgery (e.g., hysterectomy or hip replacement). Here, the half-lives averaged 30 min, which means that plasma glucose would rise by another 25 % if a control sample is taken 1 h after a continuous infusion is initiated. The highest infusion rates were found in non-surgical volunteers, where 8 ml/min could be infused before 9 mmol/l was reached.

Conclusions: Computer simulations suggested that rates of infusion of glucose should be reduced by 50 % in the perioperative period and a further 50 % on the day of surgery in order to avoid hyperglycemia.

Keywords: Blood glucose, Metabolism glucose, Pharmacokinetics, Hyperglycemia

---

Background

Intravenous glucose is the hallmark of maintenance fluid therapy to prevent starvation and provide free water for intracellular hydration. However, practices differ regarding its use in the perioperative period. Oral intake is the recommended type of carbohydrate administration in routine patients, but various reasons may call for the use of intravenous glucose both before and after surgery. Providing intravenous glucose carries the risk of inducing hyperglycemia, which promotes postoperative infection (Hahn and Hahn 2011; Sieber et al. 1987; Kwon et al. 2013; Frisch et al. 2010; Hanazaki et al. 2009; Lipshutz and Gropper 2009) and osmotic diuresis (Doze and White 1987). Very high glucose concentrations lead to more pronounced cerebral damage in the event of cardiac arrest (Myers and Yamaguchi 1977; Siemkowicz 1985).

Infusion rates that provide effective fluid and nutritional support therapy while avoiding hyperglycemia might be difficult to determine in the perioperative setting, as glucose turnover becomes impaired as part of the trauma response (Ljunggren et al. 2014a). Plasma glucose should be measured to guide adjustments of the infusion rate, but the point at which the check best reflects the risk of hyperglycemia is unclear to most clinicians.

The aim of the present work was to predict how fast glucose can be infused to reach specific concentrations of plasma glucose at defined points in time during the perioperative period in non-diabetic patients. These rates may serve as approximations of how initial infusion rates should be set, depending on the level to which the plasma glucose can be allowed to rise.

The hypothesis was that infusion rates should be reduced by at least 50 % as compared to healthy humans during and after surgery. To indicate the degree by which

---

Correspondence: Robert.hahn@sodertaljesjukhus.se
Research Unit at Södertälje Hospital, 152 86 Södertälje, Sweden

the rates should be modified, computer simulations were performed based on kinetic data from seven previous studies of glucose administration performed at various stages of the perioperative period (Sjöstrand and Hahn 2003; Hahn et al. 2011; Hahn et al. 2013; Ljunggren and Hahn 2012; Sjöstrand and Hahn 2004; Sicardi Salomón et al. 2006; Strandberg and Hahn 2005).

Methods

This study is based on 321 infusion experiments, performed between 2002 and 2012, in which glucose was administered by intravenous infusion. The subjects were 26 volunteers and 161 patients in various stages of the perioperative process. All subjects gave their consent for participation after being informed about the purpose of the study. The results have been published in seven previous reports (Sjöstrand and Hahn 2003; Hahn et al. 2011; Hahn et al. 2013; Ljunggren and Hahn 2012; Sjöstrand and Hahn 2004; Sicardi Salomón et al. 2006; Strandberg and Hahn 2005). Four of them excluded patients with any disease (Sjöstrand and Hahn 2003; Hahn et al. 2011; Sjöstrand and Hahn 2004; Strandberg and Hahn 2005), and three excluded patients with disease of importance to glucose and fluid turnover (Hahn et al. 2013; Ljunggren and Hahn 2012; Sicardi Salomón et al. 2006).

Ethics

The appropriate Ethics Committee approved the protocol for each of the studies. These were the Ethics Committee of Huddinge Hospital (Sjöstrand and Hahn 2003; Sjöstrand and Hahn 2004; Strandberg and Hahn 2005) and, later, the Regional Ethics Committee of Stockholm (Hahn et al. 2011; Hahn et al. 2013; Ljunggren and Hahn 2012; Sicardi Salomón et al. 2006). The approval numbers and the dates of decision were 258/00 (June 5, 2000) (Sjöstrand and Hahn 2003), 2007/1670-31 (January 30, 2008) (Hahn et al. 2011), 2011/1141-31/3 (September 28, 2011) (Hahn et al. 2013), 2008/1691-31/4 (September 28, 2011) (Ljunggren and Hahn 2012), 429/97 (January 12, 1998) (Sjöstrand and Hahn 2004), 19/03 (February 11, 2003) (Sicardi Salomón et al. 2006) and 34/99 (March 29, 1999) (Strandberg and Hahn 2005). The chairpersons were Lennart Kaijser (Sjöstrand and Hahn 2003; Sjöstrand and Hahn 2004; Strandberg and Hahn 2005), Hans Glaumann (Sicardi Salomón et al. 2006), Olof Forssberg (Hahn et al. 2011), Håkan Julius (Hahn et al. 2013), and Annika Marcus (Ljunggren and Hahn 2012).

Procedures and measurements

All subjects were in the fasting state, which means that no food or sugar-containing beverages had been ingested for at least 4 h. Experiments started in the morning, and the only fluid given was a solution containing glucose 2.5 % (Sjöstrand and Hahn 2003; Sjöstrand and Hahn 2004; Sicardi Salomón et al. 2006; Strandberg and Hahn 2005) or 30 % (Hahn et al. 2011; Hahn et al. 2013; Ljunggren and Hahn 2012). The fluid with the low glucose concentration was buffered and half-isotonic with regard to electrolytes (sodium 70, chloride 45, and acetate 25 mmol/l), while the other solution contained only glucose. Infusion times varied between 1 and 80 min, and the total amount of glucose was usually between 200 and 300 mg/kg (Table 1). General anesthesia was used in the patients where the glucose kinetics was studied during ongoing surgery. Pain relief was enhanced by thoracic epidural anesthesia in nine of these patients who underwent major abdominal surgery.

Plasma glucose concentrations in venous blood were measured on 7–20 occasions, using the glucose oxidase method. Duplicate samples were usually drawn at baseline and ensured a coefficient of variation of 1.2–1.5 %.

Calculations

Kinetic analyses and simulations were made according to a one-compartment model implemented in MATLAB 4.2 (MathWorks Inc., Natick, MA). Simulations employed mean and individual data from the seven studies to predict the infusion rates required to reach and to maintain each one of three predetermined concentrations of plasma glucose (7, 9, and 12 mmol/l). The infusion rates required to reach these targets within 30 min were also calculated. The equations used are specified in the Appendix.

Insulin resistance was estimated by the Homeostatic Model Assessment of Insulin Resistance (HOMA-IR), which was the product of the plasma concentrations of glucose (mmol/l) and insulin (pmol/) just before the infusion started (Ljunggren and Hahn 2012). These data were available in all studied except one (Sicardi Salomón et al. 2006). No correction for units was made, but HOMA-IR was ^{10}log-transformed to obtain a linear correlation with the hyperinsulinemic glucose clamp (Borai et al. 2007; Ljunggren et al. 2014b).

Data are presented as the means (standard deviation).

Results

The characteristics of the studied cohorts are presented in Table 1. Twenty-one experiments were excluded because of incomplete data, leaving 300 experiments to be included in the final analysis.

Plasma glucose from representative series of experiments is shown in Fig. 1.

The volume of distribution (V_d), clearance (CL), and HOMA-IR for each study group is shown in Table 1.

The infusion rates of glucose 5 % predicted to reach and maintain steady state levels of 7, 9, and 12 mmol/l in a subject weighing 70 kg based on each experiment separately are illustrated graphically in Fig. 2 and also given in Table 2, left.

Table 1 Data on the groups used for the simulations. The results are given as the mean (SD)

Study group	Experiments (N)	Age (years)	Body weight (kg)	Female/ males	Glucose load (g/kg)	Plasma glucose baseline (mmol/l)	Plasma insulin baseline (pmol/l)	^{10}log HOMA-IR[a]	V_d/BW (ml/kg)	CL/BW (ml/ (kg min))	Half-life[b] (min)	Reference
Healthy volunteers	44	29 (7)	73 (14)	8/18[c]	0.25–0.62	5.0 (0.4)	35 (23)	2.15 (0.33)	164 (74)	8.7 (3.4)	15 (8)	Sjöstrand and Hahn (2003); Hahn et al. (2011)
1 day before hip replacement surgery	82	68 (9)	82 (15)	54/28	0.20–0.30	5.2 (0.7)	62 (50)	2.38 (0.35)	164 (29)	4.7 (1.8)	28 (11)	Hahn et al. (2013); Ljunggren and Hahn (2012)
During hernia surgery	9	37 (16)	80 (11)	0/9	≈0.20	5.7 (0.4)	–	–	152 (24)	1.6 (0.3)	66 (13)	Sicardi Salomón et al. (2006)[d]
During laparoscopic cholecystectomy	20	40 (8)	75 (10)	14/6	0.25–0.47	5.0 (0.6)	45 (26)	2.29 (0.25)	121 (19)	2.8 (0.7)	33 (12)	Sjöstrand and Hahn (2004); Sicardi Salomón et al. (2006)[d]
During open abdominal surgery	9	69 (6)	63 (11)	4/5	≈0.20	5.7 (1.1)	–	–	190 (34)	1.5 (0.7)	110 (67)	Sicardi Salomón et al. (2006)[d]
2–3 h after hip replacement surgery	60	68 (9)	83 (15)	41/9	0.20	5.9 (1.1)	47 (28)	2.35 (0.34)	174 (34)	3.3 (0.9)	38 (11)	Ljunggren and Hahn (2012)
1 day after hip replacement surgery	82	68 (9)	82 (15)	41/19	0.20–0.30	6.3 (0.8)	66 (44)	2.55 (0.27)	170 (31)	3.7 (1.3)	35 (13)	Hahn et al. (2013); Ljunggren and Hahn (2012)
2 days after hysterectomy	15	50 (5)	70 (9)	15/0	0.31	6.2 (0.7)	35 (16)	2.28 (0.25)	147 (41)	6.1 (12)	17 (5)	Strandberg and Hahn (2005)

[a]The ^{10}log of (P-glucose × P-insulin). For crude HOMA-IR, the product should be divided by 156 to correct for units (22.5 if insulin is reported in mU l^{-1}) where 1 = normal

[b]The half-life was obtained as 0.693 V_d/CL

[c]Six males underwent four experiments each

[d]The study divided the kinetics into infusion and postinfusion phase. The kinetics from the infusion was used here

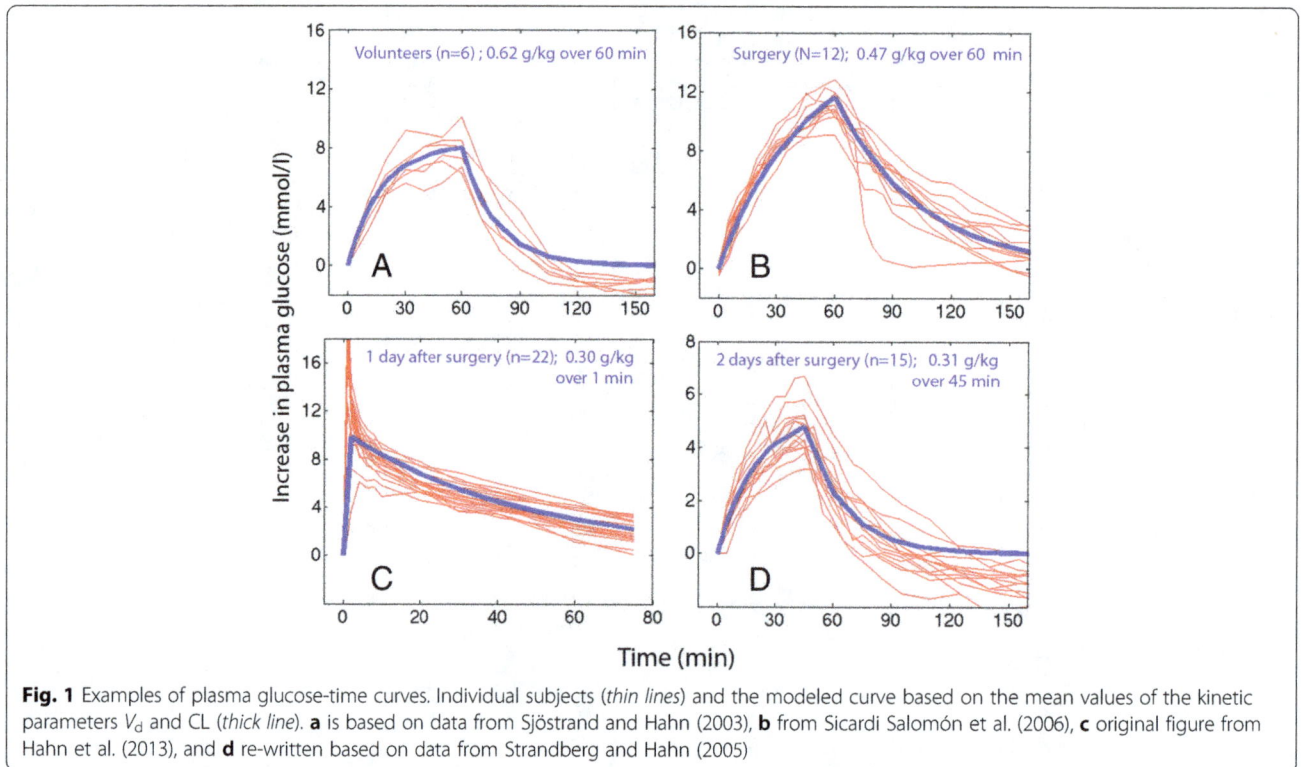

Fig. 1 Examples of plasma glucose-time curves. Individual subjects (*thin lines*) and the modeled curve based on the mean values of the kinetic parameters V_d and CL (*thick line*). **a** is based on data from Sjöstrand and Hahn (2003), **b** from Sicardi Salomón et al. (2006), **c** original figure from Hahn et al. (2013), and **d** re-written based on data from Strandberg and Hahn (2005)

The infusion rates required to reach 7, 9, and 12 mmol/l within 30 min are shown in Table 2, right. After 30 min, each concentration can be maintained by reducing the rate of infusion to the one shown in Table 2, left. In all groups, the appropriate reduction is to 50–70 % of the rates needed to obtain the concentration (Fig. 3a).

HOMA-IR correlated poorly with the kinetic parameters obtained during the infusion experiments and also with the simulated maximum infusion rates (Fig. 3b–e).

Discussion

Limits for the infusion rate of intravenous glucose are warranted, as studies demonstrate that, otherwise, patients are at risk of becoming markedly hyperglycemic (Sieber et al. 1987; Doze and White 1987). The consequences are dependent on the duration of the hyperglycemia and become worse in diabetics. Plasma glucose >10 mmol/l clearly increases the risk of postoperative infection, but there is also a higher likelihood of acute renal failure and death (Kwon et al. 2013; Frisch et al. 2010; Hanazaki et al. 2009; Lipshutz and Gropper 2009). Osmotic diuresis develops when plasma glucose is 12–15 mmol/l, which implies that the kidneys lose control of the fluid and electrolyte excretion.

The infusion rates suggested here are intended to be a guide for how to begin intravenous glucose therapy if hyperglycemia is to be avoided. They are calculated for glucose 5 %. Anesthetists who use glucose 2.5 % simply double the rates.

Main results

The results show that the anesthetist has to consider at least a fourfold modification in infusion rate of glucose solution to account for the fact that hyperglycemia develops more easily in conjunction with surgery.

The infusion rates were clustered in three groups. The lowest were found during surgery and during the first hours after surgery (Table 2). Here, the calculated rates required to avoid plasma glucose >7 mmol/l were so low (0.5–1.5 ml/min) that providing glucose in this setting is hardly meaningful. A 1-l bag of glucose 5 % would need to be administered over 11–33 h to avoid hyperglycemia. In contrast, a rate of infusion of 2 ml/min would be possible if plasma glucose of 9 mmol/l was acceptable. That corresponds to an infusion time of 8 h for a 1-l bag.

The intermediate rates are found in the preoperative period and 2 days after surgery. Here, plasma glucose of 7 mmol/l could still easily be exceeded, if 9 mmol/l would be acceptable, glucose could be infused twice as fast as during surgery (1 l over 4 h). Finally, glucose can apparently be given to healthy individuals at an even higher rate without causing hyperglycemia.

Another way to administer glucose is by using a two-step strategy consisting of a more rapid initial infusion after which the rate is reduced to maintain a predetermined steady-state concentration. In the present series of simulations, we used 30 min as a reasonable time

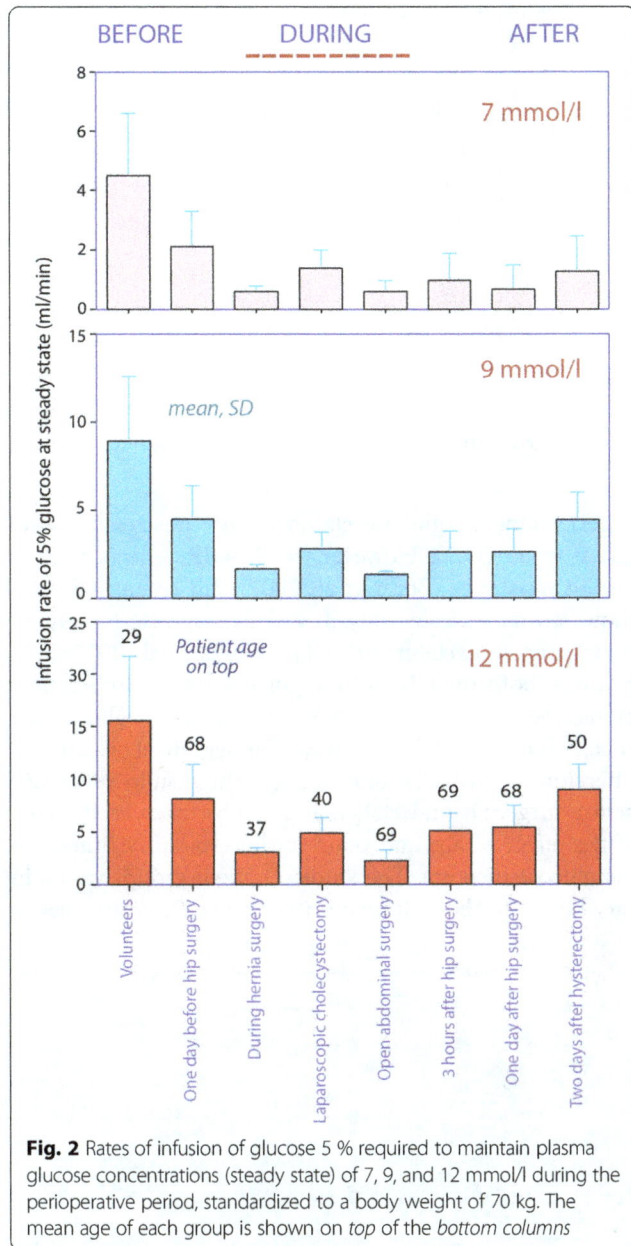

Fig. 2 Rates of infusion of glucose 5 % required to maintain plasma glucose concentrations (steady state) of 7, 9, and 12 mmol/l during the perioperative period, standardized to a body weight of 70 kg. The mean age of each group is shown on *top* of the *bottom columns*

glucose takes place after *one* half-life, which is roughly 30 min in less stressful surgery such as laparoscopic cholecystectomy. As the final steady state takes about four half-lives to reach, the clinician would have to wait as long as 2–2.5 h until the maximum plasma glucose concentration is obtained. Therefore, a useful approach would be to take a control sample after 1 h, which roughly corresponds to two half-lives in the perioperative setting, and to consider that then the plasma glucose will increase by another 25 % if no adjustment to the infusion rate is made. This simple rule does not seem to be useful during open abdominal surgery as the half-life is much longer and also associated with greater variability.

Limitations due to the studied cohorts

The patients included in this report are representative for a large proportion of the surgical population, while the suitable infusion rates may possibly be different in younger subjects and in special conditions. The studied patients were all in good health, which is an ethical requirement since the protocols involved volume loading that expanded the plasma volume by 10–15 %. No previous study has been performed which suggests suitable initial infusion rates for glucose in these groups of patients. The lack is probably explained by a well-spread belief that each patient must be evaluated individually because the plasma glucose responses to glucose infusions vary too much. Therefore, the existing literature offers surprisingly little guidance on this topic. However, the cohorts shown in Fig. 1 illustrate that the between-patient variation in plasma glucose is quite small in the perioperative period and that very good predictions can be made by taking the modeled average parameter values in a one-compartment model (thick blue lines) represent the individual plasma concentrations (thin red lines).

Open abdominal surgery was the only exception to this rule. The marked variability in the plasma glucose responses to exogenous glucose in this group could possibly be explained by variable efficiency of the thoracic epidural anesthesia to block the trauma response. In any event, repeated measurements of plasma glucose are warranted to guide glucose therapy if needed during this type of surgery.

Patients with diabetes, sepsis, and steroid treatment also need more individualized glucose administration and monitoring. Naturally, non-diabetic patients who receive intravenous insulin require much larger amounts of glucose than indicated here (Berndtson et al. 2008). The glucose metabolism shows that circadian rhythm responses may be greater to feeding during the dark period of the day (Kalsbeek et al. 2014).

Insulin resistance and HOMA-IR

Insulin resistance is the key mechanism for the slowing of glucose turnover during and after surgery (Ljunggren

period for glucose loading. Most of the study groups would require quite similar amounts of glucose to raise the plasma glucose level—approximately 2–3 ml/min to increase the concentration to 7 mmol/l within 30 min in a subject weighing 70 kg. Most of the variability in infusion rates depicted in Table 2, right, is due to differences in baseline glucose, while between-patient differences in glucose kinetics become more apparent when attempting to maintain steady state.

A practical question is at which point in time a control blood sample should be taken when a check for hyperglycemia is desired in an individual patient. Such information is possible to derive from the half-lives given in Table 1. For a continuous infusion, half of the increase in plasma

Table 2 Rates of infusion of glucose 5 % required for reaching various predetermined target steady-state concentrations of plasma glucose (left) and rates of infusion required to reach the target within 30 min (right)

Study group	Infusion rate (ml/min) at steady state			Infusion rate (ml/min) to reach target after 30 min		
	7 mmol/l	9 mmol/l	12 mmol/l	7 mmol/l	9 mmol/l	12 mmol/l
Healthy volunteers	4.5 (2.1)	8.9 (3.7)	15.5 (6.2)	5.7 (2.6)	11.3 (4.3)	19.7 (7.1)
1 day before hip replacement surgery	2.1 (1.2)	4.5 (1,9)	8.1 (3.3)	3.7 (1.5)	7.8 (2.0)	14.0 (2.8)
During hernia surgery	0.6 (0.2)	1.6 (0.3)	3.0 (0.5)	2.3 (0.9)	5.7 (1.4)	10.9 (2.3)
During laparoscopic cholecystectomy	1.4 (0.6)	2.8 (0.9)	4.9 (1.4)	2.7 (1.3)	5.6 (1.5)	9.9 (2.1)
During open abdominal surgery	0.6 (0.4)	1.3 (0.2)	2.2 (1.1)	2.3 (1.6)	5.5 (1.8)	10.3 (2.5)
2–3 h after hip replacement surgery	1.0 (0.9)	2.6 (1.2)	5.1 (1.7)	2.1 (2.2)	6.0 (2.4)	11.7 (2.9)
1 day after hip replacement surgery	0.7 (0.8)	2.6 (1.3)	5.4 (2.1)	1.4 (1.6)	5.2 (1.9)	11.1 (2.6)
2 days after hysterectomy	1.3 (1.2)	4.4 (1.6)	9.0 (2.4)	1.8 (1.5)	6.1 (1.7)	12.6 (2.5)

All rates are adapted for subjects weighing 70 kg. Data are the mean (SD). Calculations begin with the actual baseline plasma glucose level of each subject

et al. 2014a). Inactivity-induced impairment of cardiorespiratory fitness can induce some degree of insulin resistance even before surgery (Larsen et al. 2012). Another mechanism that raises plasma glucose is increased gluconeogenesis caused by psychological stress and surgical trauma. In our kinetic model, the summary effect of all these factors consists in a reduction of CL and a slightly raised plasma glucose concentration at baseline (Table 1).

The HOMA-IR did not reveal great differences between the groups and was of little or no help as a guide to the choice of infusion rates that avoid hyperglycemia. The HOMA-IR indicates insulin resistance as measured by the hyperinsulinemic glucose clamp in the "unstressed" state (Borai et al. 2007). However, HOMA-IR reflects hepatic insulin resistance (Borai et al. 2007) and recent evidence shows an increase by only 3–4 % in response to surgery (Ljunggren and Hahn 2012; Ljunggren et al. 2014b). In contrast, both the CL and the glucose clamp are strongly influenced by peripheral (skeletal muscle) insulin resistance, which might be doubled (Ljunggren et al. 2014a). Therefore, HOMA-IR only reflects the insulin resistance before surgery is undertaken and can be taken as an index of the effect of age and poor cardiorespiratory fitness on the glucose disposal. The studied patient groups varied in age, but only the volunteers (mean age 29 years) had a

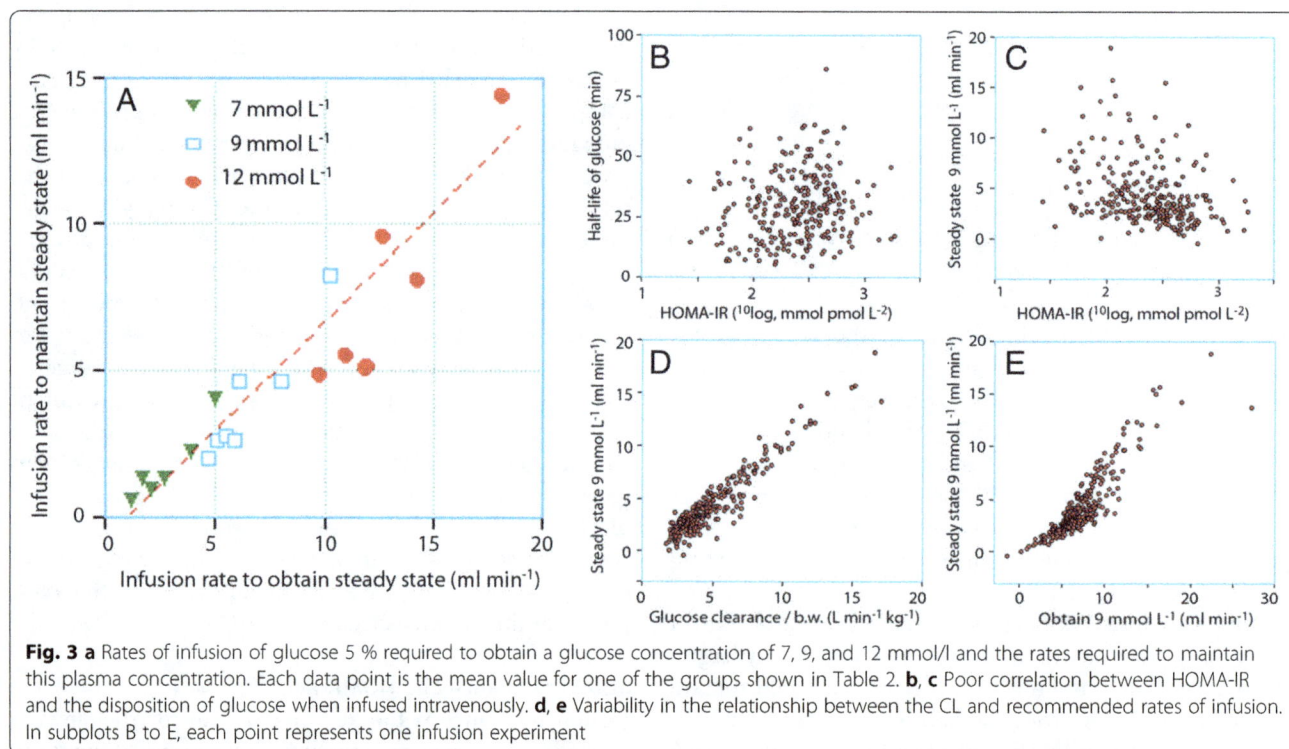

Fig. 3 a Rates of infusion of glucose 5 % required to obtain a glucose concentration of 7, 9, and 12 mmol/l and the rates required to maintain this plasma concentration. Each data point is the mean value for one of the groups shown in Table 2. **b, c** Poor correlation between HOMA-IR and the disposition of glucose when infused intravenously. **d, e** Variability in the relationship between the CL and recommended rates of infusion. In subplots B to E, each point represents one infusion experiment

markedly lower insulin resistance than the others (Table 1). The disappearance rate of glucose is 10–15 % higher after a test meal in young as compared to old men and women, a difference that can be related mostly to insulin resistance (Basu et al. 2006). The incidence of diabetes type 2 also increases with age, but no such patients were included in this compilation.

The kinetic model

The one-compartment kinetic model used here has been criticized for being simplistic and overlooking the endogenous glucose production, but it still offered excellent curve fits in individual subjects during the vast majority of the time period required for the glucose disposal. One of the downsides is that higher than modeled plasma glucose levels sometimes occur during the first minutes after a bolus infusion (Fig. 1c). This short "overshoot" can be studied by multi-compartment modeling (Ferranini et al. 1985) but is of limited relevance to the anesthetist who provides glucose as a continuous infusion at a low speed. Another issue is that slight hypoglycemia often develops 30–45 min after a glucose infusion given to a subject with high insulin sensitivity (Fig. 1a, d). This "undershoot" was not considered here and can be avoided clinically by gradual reduction of the infusion rate.

The one-compartment model is linear for glucose (Sjöstrand and Hahn 2003), which means that the predicted plasma glucose concentrations become similar regardless of whether the V_d and CL used for the simulation are derived from experiments providing small or large amounts of glucose, and regardless of whether the infusion time is long or short. In this report, V_d was larger for a 1-min injection compared to infusions, but the half-life of the glucose was still quite similar regardless of the infusion time (Table 1).

Conclusions

Computer simulations based on kinetic data from seven studies suggested infusion rates that should be avoided to limit the risk of hyperglycemia in the perioperative period. Healthy volunteers can take infusion rates at least four times higher than patients on the day of surgery, and preoperative patients can take infusion rates twice as high. On the day of surgery, the acceptable rates are so low that infusing a glucose solution is hardly meaningful. Only very small amounts of glucose and free water can be provided at this time without imposing a risk of hyperglycemia.

Appendix

A single-compartment kinetic model analyzed all plasma glucose data. Here, the relationship between the rate of infusion R_o, the volume of distribution V_d, and clearance

CL was calculated using the following differential equation (Sjöstrand and Hahn 2003):

$$\frac{d(C-C_b)}{dt} = \frac{R_o}{V_d} - \frac{CL}{V_d}(C(t)-C_b) \tag{1}$$

where C is the plasma glucose at time t and C_b is the baseline level. The solutions to this differential equation before Eq. 2 and after Eq. 3 infusion are as follows:

$$(C(t)-C_b) = \frac{R_o}{CL}\left(1-e^{-CL\times t/V_d}\right) \tag{2}$$

$$(C(t)-C_b) = \frac{R_o}{CL}\left(1-e^{-CL\times T/V_d}\right)e^{-CL\times(t-T)/V_d} \tag{3}$$

where T is the infusion time. The optimal values of V_d and CL were estimated for each experiment separately via a Gauss-Newton least-squares regression routine applied to Eqs. 2 and 3, which had been entered into the MATLAB computer program.

In the same MATLAB environment, calculations were used to simulate the expected plasma glucose concentration at any time t in experiments not performed. The infusion rate (R_o) needed to maintain a steady-state concentration (C_{ss}) was obtained as

$$R_o = CL \times BW \times (C_{ss}-C_b) \times 0.0036 \tag{4}$$

where BW is the body weight (as CL is expressed per kilo body weight), C_b is the baseline glucose concentration for a group or individual, while 0.0036 converts mmol/min to ml/min of a glucose 5 % solution (the molar weight for glucose of 180 g is divided by 50 mg, which is the content of 1 ml of glucose 5 %).

The infusion rate required to reach a pre-determined plasma concentration $C(t)$ within a certain time t was obtained as follows (in this study, t was set to 30 min):

$$R_o = \frac{CL \times BW(C(t)-C_b) \times 0.0036}{(1-e^{-CL\times t/V_d})} \tag{5}$$

Equation 5 is a re-arrangement of Eq. 2 where t is set to 30 min. Equation 4, in turn, is a special case of Eq. 5 where the expression in the denominator approaches 1.0.

Abbreviations
CL: clearance; HOMA-IR: homeostatic model assessment of insulin resistance; V_d: volume of distribution.

Competing interests
The authors declare that they have no competing interests.

Author's contributions
RH was responsible for the study idea, data analysis, and manuscript writing.

Acknowledgements
The author is indebted to the co-authors of the seven manuscripts that contain the kinetic data used for the present report. The work was supported by Mats Kleberg Foundation (dnr 2015-00132).

References

Basu R, Dalla Man C, Campioni M, Basu A, Klee G, Toffolo G, et al. Effects of age and sex on postprandial glucose metabolism. Differences in glucose turnover, insulin secretion, insulin action, and hepatic insulin extraction. Diabetes. 2006;55:2001–14.

Berndtson D, Olsson J, Hahn RG. Hypovolaemia after glucose-insulin infusions in volunteers. Clin Sci. 2008;115:371–8.

Borai A, Livingstone C, Ferns GAA. The biochemical assessment of insulin resistance. Ann Clin Biochem. 2007;44:324–42.

Doze VA, White PF. Effects of fluid therapy on serum glucose levels in fasted outpatients. Anesthesiology. 1987;66:223–6.

Ferranini E, Dougles JD, Cobelli C, Toffolo G, Pilo A, DeFronzo RA. Effect of insulin on the distribution and disposition of glucose in man. J Clin Invest. 1985;76:357–64.

Frisch A, Hudson M, Chandra P, et al. Prevalence and clinical outcome of hyperglycemia in the perioperative period in noncardiac surgery. Diabetes Care. 2010;33:1783–8.

Hahn RG, Hahn RG. Crystalloid fluids. In: Hahn RG, editor. Clinical Fluid Therapy in the Perioperative Setting. Cambridge: Cambridge University; 2011. p. 1–10.

Hahn RG, Ljunggren S, Larsen F, Nyström T. A simple intravenous glucose tolerance test for assessment of insulin sensitivity. Theor Biol Med Model. 2011;8:12.

Hahn RG, Nyström T, Ljunggren S. Plasma volume expansion from the intravenous glucose tolerance test before and after hip replacement surgery. Theor Biol Med Model. 2013;10:48.

Hanazaki K, Maeda H, Okabayashi T. Relationship between perioperative glycemic control and postoperative infections. World J Gastroenterol. 2009;15:4122–5.

Kalsbeek A, la Fleur S, Fliers E. Circadian control of glucose metabolism. Mol Metab. 2014;3:372–83.

Kwon S, Thompson R, Dellinger P, Yanez D, Farrohki E, Flum D. Importance of perioperative glycemic control in general surgery: a report from the surgical care and outcomes assessment program. Ann Surg. 2013;257:8–14.

Larsen FJ, Anderson M, Ekblom B, Nyström T. Cardiorespiratory fitness predicts insulin action and secretion in healthy individuals. Metabolism. 2012;61:12–6.

Lipshutz AK, Gropper MA. Perioperative glycemic control. An evidence-based review. Anesthesiology. 2009;110:408–21.

Ljunggren S, Hahn RG. Oral nutrition or water loading before hip replacement surgery; a randomized clinical trial. Trials. 2012;13:97.

Ljunggren S, Hahn RG, Nyström T. Insulin sensitivity and beta-cell function after carbohydrate oral loading in hip replacement surgery: a double-blind, randomised controlled clinical trial. Clin Nutr. 2014a;33:392–8.

Ljunggren S, Nyström T, Hahn RG. Accuracy and precision of commonly used methods for quantifying surgery-induced insulin resistance. Prospective observational study. Eur J Anaesth. 2014b;31:110–6.

Myers RE, Yamaguchi S. Nervous system effects of cardiac arrest in monkeys. Preservation of vision. Arch Neurol. 1977;34:65–74.

Sicardi Salomón Z, Rodhe P, Hahn RG. Progressive reduction of glucose clearance during surgery. Acta Anaesthesiol Scand. 2006;50:848–54.

Sieber FE, Smith DS, Traystman RJ, Wollman H. Glucose: a reevaluation of its intraoperative use. Anesthesiology. 1987;67:72–81.

Siemkowicz E. The effect of glucose upon restitution after transient cerebral ischemia: a summary. Acta Neurol Scand. 1985;71:417–27.

Sjöstrand F, Hahn RG. Validation of volume kinetic analysis of glucose 2.5 % solution given by intravenous infusion. Br J Anaesth. 2003;90:600–7.

Sjöstrand F, Hahn RG. Volume kinetics of glucose 2.5 % solution during laparoscopic cholecystectomy. Br J Anaesth. 2004;92:485–92.

Strandberg P, Hahn RG. Volume kinetics of glucose 2.5 % solution and insulin resistance after abdominal hysterectomy. Br J Anaesth. 2005;94:30–8.

21

Observational study of the effects of age, diabetes mellitus, cirrhosis and chronic kidney disease on sublingual microvascular flow

Toby Reynolds[1], Amanda Vivian-Smith[1], Shaman Jhanji[2] and Rupert M Pearse[3*]

Abstract

Background: Sidestream dark field (SDF) imaging has been used to demonstrate microcirculatory abnormalities in a variety of critical illnesses. The microcirculation is also affected by advancing age and chronic comorbidities. However, the effect of these conditions on SDF microcirculatory parameters has not been well described.

Methods: SDF images were obtained from five groups of 20 participants: healthy volunteers under the age of 25, healthy volunteers over the age of 55, and clinic patients over the age of 55 with one of diabetes mellitus, cirrhosis and stage 5 chronic kidney disease. Microcirculatory parameters between the groups were then compared for significance using analysis of variance for parametric and the Kruskal-Wallis test for non-parametric data.

Results: Median microvascular flow index was 2.85 (interquartile range 2.75 to 3.0) for participants aged <25, 2.81 (2.66 to 2.97) for those aged >55, 2.88 (2.75 to 3.0) for those with diabetes mellitus, 3.0 (2.83 to 3.0) for those with cirrhosis and 3.0 (2.78 to 3.0) for those with chronic kidney disease (P for difference between groups = 0.14). Similarly, there were no significant differences in the proportion of perfused vessels and perfused vessel density between the groups.

Conclusions: Older age, diabetes, and chronic kidney and liver disease need not be considered confounding factors for comparison of SDF microcirculatory parameters in the critically ill.

Keywords: Microvascular flow, Sidestream dark field imaging, Age, Diabetes mellitus, Cirrhosis, Chronic kidney disease

Background

Critical illness is often accompanied by abnormalities of the microcirculation [1]. Persistent alterations such as heterogeneity of flow and microvascular shunting can lead to tissue hypoxia and are associated with organ failure and death [2-4], while impaired microvascular flow in the perioperative period is associated with the development of complications [5]. Improving systemic measures of perfusion can be accompanied by improved microcirculatory parameters [6] but the relationship between the two is not always straightforward [7,8], including during vasopressor treatment [9,10]. Monitoring the microcirculation may thus help evaluate an individual patient's tissue perfusion [7,11].

The novel techniques of orthogonal polarisation spectral (OPS) imaging [12], and more recently sidestream dark field (SDF) imaging [13] allow imaging of the microcirculation *in vivo* in a way that was previously technically difficult. Research using these techniques has helped characterise the sublingual microcirculation in various acute diseases, and describe the changes in microcirculatory parameters following acute physiological changes or administration of pharmacological therapies. However, the influence of existing chronic conditions on microcirculatory assessments made using SDF and OPS imaging has not been well studied. Advancing age, diabetes mellitus, cirrhosis, and end-stage renal failure are commonly found in critically ill perioperative patients [14,15]. All have well recognised associations with an abnormal microvasculature, and altered microvascular flow has been demonstrated using other techniques [16-19]. In order to interpret

* Correspondence: r.pearse@qmul.ac.uk
[3]Barts and The London School of Medicine and Dentistry, Queen Mary's University of London, Turner Street, London E1 2AD, UK
Full list of author information is available at the end of the article

current and future clinical studies of the microcirculation using SDF and OPS imaging, it is essential to determine whether stable patients with advanced age and these chronic diseases exhibit changes in sublingual microvasculature when assessed using these techniques. The objective of this study was to help provide this understanding by evaluating sublingual microvascular flow using SDF imaging in healthy older volunteers and in patients with diabetes, cirrhosis and chronic kidney disease (CKD).

Methods

Study design

This was a single centre, observational study based at a university hospital, and was approved by East London and the City Research Ethics Committee (ref. 09/H0704/3). Patients aged over 55 years with one of either diabetes (diagnosed >2 years), cirrhosis (confirmed by liver biopsy or expert hepatology opinion) or CKD (stage 5 by estimated glomerular filtration rate, but not on dialysis) were identified from amongst those attending diabetology, hepatology or nephrology outpatient clinics. Healthy volunteers aged either under 25 or over 55 years without medical disease were identified from among hospital staff and their relatives. All participants gave written informed consent. Exclusion criteria were pregnancy, age 18 years and refusal of consent.

Data collection

Sublingual microvascular flow was evaluated using sidestream dark field imaging with a x5 objective lens (Microscan, Microvision Medical, Amsterdam, Netherlands) [20]. Image acquisition and subsequent blinded analysis was performed according to published consensus criteria [21]. SDF images were obtained from at least three sublingual areas. Microvascular flow index (MFI) was calculated after dividing each image into four equal quadrants. Quantification of flow was determined using an ordinal scale (0: no flow, 1: intermittent flow, 2: sluggish flow, 3: normal flow) for small (<20 μm) and large (>20 μm) vessels. MFI is the average score of all quadrants for a given category of vessel size. Vessel density was calculated by inserting a grid of three equidistant horizontal and three equidistant vertical lines over the image. Vessel density is equal to the number

of vessels crossing these lines divided by their total length. Flow was then categorised as present, intermittent or absent to calculate the proportion of perfused vessels (PPV) and thus the perfused vessel density (PVD), an estimate of functional capillary density (FCD). Analysis of the videos was performed by a single, blinded observer (TR). Additional data collected for all participants included age, weight, gender, past medical history, current medications, pulse rate, sublingual temperature, heart rate and blood pressure. In diabetic patients the most recent HbA1c percentage result was recorded. In patients with cirrhosis the current Child-Turcotte-Pugh score was recorded. In patients with renal disease, the creatinine clearance was estimated from plasma creatinine using the four-variable modified diet in renal disease method [22].

Statistical analysis

Data from a previous study, performed locally, demonstrated a difference in MFI of 0.3 prior to major abdominal surgery in those patients who went on to develop complications after surgery compared to those who did not [5]. Assuming a type I error rate of 5% (two-tailed) and a type II error rate of 10% using this previous data, 20 patients would be required in each group to detect a difference in MFI of 0.26 (SD ± 0.25). We therefore aimed to recruit 20 participants in each group. Parametric data are presented as mean (standard deviation, SD) and non-parametric data are presented as median (interquartile range, IQR). Variable distributions were assessed for normality using the Kolmogorov-Smirnov test. The primary outcome measure of this study was a difference in small vessel MFI between the groups. Secondary outcome measures were differences in PPV and PVD for small vessels. Differences between groups were tested using analysis of variance (ANOVA) for parametric data and the Kruskal-Wallis test for non-parametric data. Significance was set at $P < 0.05$. Statistical calculations were performed in SPSS (SPSS Inc, Chicago, IL, USA).

Results

One hundred participants were recruited between September 2010 and July 2011. Adequate video footage was obtained in 98 participants (20 aged <25 years, 20

Table 1 Baseline participant data

	Age <25 years	Age >55 years	Diabetes mellitus	Cirrhosis	Chronic kidney disease
Male	10 (50%)	9 (45%)	10 (50%)	12 (67%)	14 (70)
Age (years)	24 (23–25)	61 (60–65)	64 (62–72)	60 (57–66)	71 (64–74)
Body mass index (kg/m2)	21.9 (20.9–24.9)	24.7 (23.0–29.0)	29.4 (24.8–32.9)	24.8 (23.7–26.9)	28.0 (24.6–33.3)
Sublingual temperature (°C)	36.5 (36.3–37.0)	36.4 (36.0–36.7)	36.2 (36.0–36.5)	36.6 (36.2–37.2)	36.5 (36.5–36.8)
Mean arterial pressure (mmHg)	93 (91–96)	100 (93–109)	92 (88–102)	98 (89–106)	98 (89–106)
Heart rate (bpm)	72 (63–82)	75 (65–83)	72 (62–86)	74 (64–92)	70 (65–80)

Data presented as n (%) or median (IQR). n = 20 for all groups except cirrhosis where n = 18.

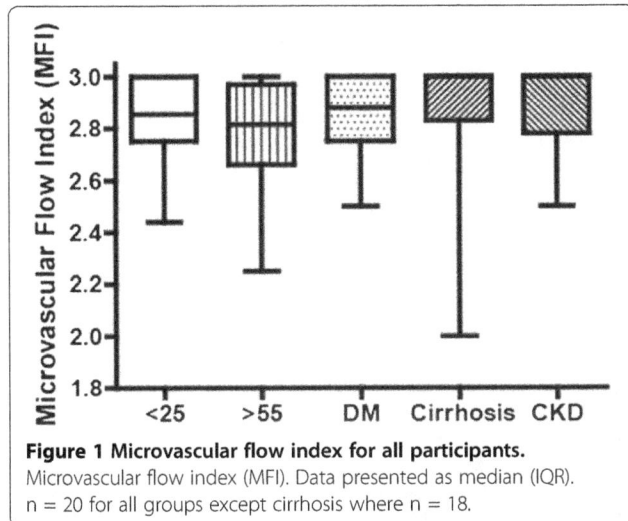

Figure 1 Microvascular flow index for all participants.
Microvascular flow index (MFI). Data presented as median (IQR). n = 20 for all groups except cirrhosis where n = 18.

aged >55 years, 20 with diabetes, 18 with cirrhosis, and 20 with stage 5 CKD). Participant characteristics and baseline clinical data are displayed in Table 1. All the healthy young participants had no medical problems, were non-smokers and declared no regular medication use. Two healthy older participants took medication for hypothyroidism (normal thyroid function tests), two were smokers, two took statins and two took antihypertensive medication, all for primary prevention of cardiovascular disease. All diabetic patients suffered from type 2 diabetes, nine took insulin and 15 took antihypertensive medication. The mean glycated haemoglobin (HbA1c) for patients with diabetes was 8.8% (SD 1.7%). For participants with cirrhosis, three took propranolol for variceal bleeding prophylaxis, and eight took other antihypertensive medication. The cause of cirrhosis was viral in 11 cases, alcohol-related in five cases, medication-related in one case and cryptogenic in one case. Seventeen patients were Child-Pugh-Turcotte score A and one was score B. For patients with stage 5 CKD, this was due to intrinsic renal disease in seven cases, polycystic kidney disease in one case, reflux nephropathy in one case, drug toxicity in one case, and hypertension in ten cases. All were taking antihypertensive medication. The mean estimated glomerular filtration rate was 11.5 ml/min (SD 2.9).

A median of 3 (IQR 2 to 4) clips were analysed for each patient. For small vessels (<20 μm), there were no

statistically significant differences in MFI, PPV and PVD between the groups (Figure 1 and Table 2). This finding was repeated in a secondary analysis that excluded the two hypertensive participants from the healthy >55 group. Baseline sublingual large vessel (>20 μm) MFI was median 3.0 (IQR 2.9 to 3.0) and PPV was median 1.0 (IQR 0.97 to 1.0), suggesting good quality image capture unaffected by pressure artefact.

Discussion

The principal finding of this study was that sublingual SDF imaging does not demonstrate statistically significant differences in MFI, PPV and PVD between healthy young volunteers, healthy older volunteers, and patients with diabetes, cirrhosis and end-stage renal failure. MFI was lower in older volunteers and higher in those with cirrhosis and renal failure, and PVD was higher in patients with diabetes, cirrhosis and renal failure. However, none of these trends reached significance.

There is little doubt that age, diabetes, cirrhosis and renal disease do cause alterations to the microvasculature. Diabetes, particularly type 2 diabetes, is associated with increased capillary density. This has been recently demonstrated using SDF imaging of the labial microcirculation [23]. Our results showed a trend towards an increased PVD that was not statistically significant. Similarly, our results indicated a non-significant trend towards higher PVD and MFI values in cirrhotic and CKD patients. In cirrhosis, vasodilatory mediators promote arteriovenous shunting, eventually leading to the development of a hyperdynamic circulation. Cirrhotic patients show an exaggerated post-ischaemic hyperaemia response, which has been interpreted as evidence that the peripheral microvasculature is predisposed to vasodilatation [24]. Sheikh and colleagues recorded seemingly low MFI values in their comparison of SDF analysis of compensated, decompensated and septic cirrhotic patients [25], but as their study did not include any healthy patients, comparison with our own results is not possible. Using nailfold microscopy, Thang and colleagues found a trend towards reduced capillary density in CKD stage 5 patients compared to controls, although this did not reach significance [26]. Bemelmans and colleagues compared MFI in dialysis patients before and after dialysis [27]. The baseline MFI values they

Table 2 SDF microvascular flow parameters for all participants

	Age <25 years	Age >55 years	Diabetes mellitus	Cirrhosis	Chronic kidney disease	P value
MFI	2.85 (2.75–3.0)	2.81 (2.66–2.97)	2.88 (2.75–3.0)	3.0 (2.83–3.0)	3.0 (2.78–3.0)	0.14
PPV	0.92 (0.06)	0.88 (0.09)	0.92 (0.07)	0.89 (0.08)	0.91 (0.05)	0.46
PVD	8.04 (1.49)	8.02 (0.96)	9.17 (1.70)	8.51 (1.43)	8.38 (1.36)	0.08

PPV in %, PVD in mm^{-1}. Data presented as mean (SD) or median (IQR). n = 20 for all groups except cirrhosis where n = 18. MFI, microvascular flow index; PPV, proportion of perfused vessels; PVD, perfused vessel density.

found are similar to those we report, but without a control group in their study, comparison is not possible.

We found that microvascular flow as measured by SDF parameters was not significantly different when subjects were older or had comorbid diabetes, chronic kidney disease or cirrhosis. It is possible that a much larger study than ours may have identified differences between these groups and young, healthy subjects using SDF parameters. It is also possible that alternative techniques may have detected differences that were not apparent using SDF imaging. However, our aim was to identify important confounding effects in the use of SDF parameters to assess for acute changes in the microcirculation of critically ill patients. Assessment of the microcirculation specifically using SDF imaging has generated significant research interest in perioperative medicine and critical care, in part because this technique can be used *in vivo* with minimal disruption to the subject and could potentially form an important part of bedside clinical evaluation. In calculating our sample size, we specified an effect size equal to a 0.26 difference in MFI, on the basis that effect sizes of this magnitude have been seen in previous studies of critically ill patients. Thus we believe our results show that no such confounding effects need be taken into account.

We cannot rule out the possibility that pre-existing microvascular dysfunction not apparent on SDF imaging may predispose patients with chronic diseases to SDF-detectable microvascular flow alterations when they become acutely unwell. Further research would be needed to investigate the importance of any such effect.

Conclusions

Advancing age, diabetes mellitus, chronic kidney disease and cirrhosis do not appear to cause changes in sublingual microvascular flow assessed by sidestream dark field imaging in stable patients.

Abbreviations

CKD: chronic kidney disease; FCD: functional capillary density; IQR: interquartile range; MFI: microvascular flow index; OPS: orthogonal polarisation spectral; PPV: proportion of perfused vessels; PVD: perfused vessel density; SD: standard deviation; SDF: sidestream dark field.

Competing interests

The authors declare they have no competing interests.

Authors' contributions

TR, AVS, SJ and RP contributed to the study conception and design. TR and AVS recruited participants, recorded and analysed the data. TR and SJ performed the statistical analysis. TR, AVS, SJ and RP contributed to interpretation of the data and drafting the manuscript. All authors read and approved the final manuscript.

Authors' information

RP is a National Institute for Health Research (UK) Clinician Scientist.

Acknowledgements

This study was supported with a grant from the Isaac Schapera Trust for Medical Research. The funding body had no role in study design, collection, analysis, or interpretation of data, preparation of the manuscript or in the decision to submit the manuscript for publication.
We thank Professor Magdi Yaqoob, Professor Graham Foster and Dr Tahseen Chowdhury for their assistance in recruiting participants to this study.
SJ acknowledges UK National Health Service funding to the Royal Marsden/Institute of Cancer Research National Institute for Health Research (UK) Biomedical Research Centre.
Elements of this study were presented at the 33rd International Symposium on Intensive Care and Emergency Medicine in abstract form.

Author details

[1]Adult Critical Care Unit, Royal London Hospital, Barts Health NHS Trust, Whitechapel Rd, London E1 1BB, UK. [2]Intensive Care Unit, Royal Marsden Hospital, Fulham Road, London SW3 6JJ, UK. [3]Barts and The London School of Medicine and Dentistry, Queen Mary's University of London, Turner Street, London E1 2AD, UK.

References

1. Spronk PE, Zandstra DF, Ince C: **Bench-to-bedside review: sepsis is a disease of the microcirculation.** *Crit Care* 2004, **8:**462–468.
2. De Backer D, Creteur J, Preiser J-C, Dubois M-J, Vincent J-L: **Microvascular blood flow is altered in patients with sepsis.** *Am J Respir Crit Care Med* 2002, **166:**98–104.
3. Sakr Y, Dubois M-J, De Backer D, Creteur J, Vincent J-L: **Persistent microcirculatory alterations are associated with organ failure and death in patients with septic shock.** *Crit Care Med* 2004, **32:**1825–1831.
4. Spanos A, Jhanji S, Vivian-Smith A, Harris T, Pearse RM: **Early microvascular changes in sepsis and severe sepsis.** *Shock* 2010, **33:**387–391.
5. Jhanji S, Lee C, Watson D, Hinds C, Pearse RM: **Microvascular flow and tissue oxygenation after major abdominal surgery: association with post-operative complications.** *Intensive Care Med* 2009, **35:**671–677.
6. Jhanji S, Vivian-Smith A, Lucena-Amaro S, Watson D, Hinds CJ, Pearse RM: **Haemodynamic optimisation improves tissue microvascular flow and oxygenation after major surgery: a randomised controlled trial.** *Crit Care* 2010, **14:**R151.
7. Elbers PWG, Ince C: **Mechanisms of critical illness - classifying microcirculatory flow abnormalities in distributive shock.** *Crit Care* 2006, **10:**221.
8. Elbers PWG, Prins WB, Plokker HWM, van Dongen EPA, van Iterson M, Ince C: **Electrical cardioversion for atrial fibrillation improves microvascular flow Independent of blood pressure changes.** *J Cardiothorac Vasc Anesth* 2012, **26:**799–80.
9. Jhanji S, Stirling S, Patel N, Hinds CJ, Pearse RM: **The effect of increasing doses of norepinephrine on tissue oxygenation and microvascular flow in patients with septic shock.** *Crit Care Med* 2009, **37:**1961–1966.
10. Dubin A, Pozo MO, Casabella CA, Pálizas F Jr, Murias G, Moseinco MC, Kanoore Edul VS, Pálizas F, Estenssoro E, Ince C: **Increasing arterial blood pressure with norepinephrine does not improve microcirculatory blood flow: a prospective study.** *Crit Care* 2009, **13:**R92.
11. Bangash M, Pearse RM: **Microcirculation.** In *Encyclopedia of intensive care medicine.* Edited by Vincent JL, Hall JB. London: Springer; 2012:1395–1399.
12. Mathura KR, Vollebregt KC, Boer K, De Graaff JC, Ubbink DT, Ince C: **Comparison of OPS imaging and conventional capillary microscopy to study the human microcirculation.** *J Appl Physiol* 2001, **91:**74–78.
13. Goedhart PT, Khalilzada M, Bezemer R, Merza J, Ince C: **Sidestream Dark Field (SDF) imaging: a novel stroboscopic LED ring-based imaging modality for clinical assessment of the microcirculation.** *Opt Express* 2007, **15:**15101–15114.
14. Knaus WA, Wagner DP, Draper EA, Zimmerman JE, Bergner M, Bastos PG, Sirio CA, Murphy DJ, Lotring T, Damiano A: **The APACHE III prognostic system. Risk prediction of hospital mortality for critically ill hospitalized adults.** *Chest* 1991, **100:**1619–1636.
15. Esper AM, Martin GS: **The impact of comorbid conditions on critical illness.** *Crit Care Med* 2011, **39:**2728–2735.

16. Poole D, Behnke B, Musch T: **Capillary hemodynamics and oxygen pressures in the aging microcirculation.** *Microcirculation* 2006, **13:**289–299.

17. Granger DN, Rodrigues SF, Yildirim A, Senchenkova EY: **Microvascular responses to cardiovascular risk factors.** *Microcirculation* 2010, **17:**192–205.

18. Sherman IA, Pappas SC, Fisher MM: **Hepatic microvascular changes associated with development of liver fibrosis and cirrhosis.** *Am J Physiol* 1990, **258:**H460–H465.

19. Stewart J, Kohen A, Brouder D, Rahim F, Adler S, Garrick R, Goligorsky MS: **Noninvasive interrogation of microvasculature for signs of endothelial dysfunction in patients with chronic renal failure.** *Am J Physiol Heart Circ Physiol* 2004, **287:**H2687–H2696.

20. Boerma EC, Mathura KR, van der Voort PHJ, Spronk PE, Ince C: **Quantifying bedside-derived imaging of microcirculatory abnormalities in septic patients: a prospective validation study.** *Crit Care* 2005, **9:**R601–R606.

21. De Backer D, Hollenberg S, Boerma C, Goedhart P, Büchele G, Ospina-Tascon G, Dobbe I, Ince C: **How to evaluate the microcirculation: report of a round table conference.** *Crit Care* 2007, **11:**R101.

22. Levey AS, Coresh J, Greene T, Stevens LA, Zhang YL, Hendriksen S, Kusek JW, Van Lente F, Chronic Kidney Disease Epidemiology Collaboration: **Using standardized serum creatinine values in the modification of diet in renal disease study equation for estimating glomerular filtration rate.** *Ann Intern Med* 2006, **145:**247–254.

23. Djaberi R, Schuijf JD, de Koning EJ, Wijewickrama DC, Pereira AM, Smit JW, Kroft LJ, de Roos A, Bax JJ, Rabelink TJ, Jukema JW: **Non-invasive assessment of microcirculation by sidestream dark field imaging as a marker of coronary artery disease in diabetes.** *Diab Vasc Dis Res* 2013, **10:**123–134. Epub 2012 May 23.

24. Thomson SJ, Cowan ML, Forton DM, Clark SJ, Musa S, Grounds M, Rahman TM: **A study of muscle tissue oxygenation and peripheral microcirculatory dysfunction in cirrhosis using near infrared spectroscopy.** *Liver Int* 2010, **30:**463–471. Epub 2009 Nov 16.

25. Sheikh MY, Javed U, Singh J, Choudhury J, Deen O, Dhah K, Peterson MW: **Bedside sublingual video imaging of microcirculation in assessing bacterial infection in cirrhosis.** *Dig Dis Sci* 2009, **54:**2706–2711.

26. Thang OH, Serné EH, Grooteman MP, Smulders YM, ter Wee PM, Tangelder GJ, Nubé MJ: **Capillary rarefaction in advanced chronic kidney disease is associated with high phosphorus and bicarbonate levels.** *Nephrol Dial Transplant* 2011, **26:**3529–3536. Epub 2011 Mar 17.

27. Bemelmans RH, Boerma EC, Barendregt J, Ince C, Rommes JH, Spronk PE: **Changes in the volume status of haemodialysis patients are reflected in sublingual microvascular perfusion.** *Nephrol Dial Transplant* 2009, **24:**3487–3492.

22

Perioperative acute kidney injury

Stacey Calvert[1] and Andrew Shaw[2*]

Abstract

Acute kidney injury (AKI) is a serious complication in the perioperative period, and is consistently associated with increased rates of mortality and morbidity. Two major consensus definitions have been developed in the last decade that allow for easier comparison of trial evidence. Risk factors have been identified in both cardiac and general surgery and there is an evolving role for novel biomarkers. Despite this, there has been no real change in outcomes and the mainstay of treatment remains preventive with no clear evidence supporting any therapeutic intervention as yet. This review focuses on definition, risk factors, the emerging role of biomarkers and subsequent management of AKI in the perioperative period, taking into account new and emerging strategies.

Keywords: Acute kidney injury, Biomarkers, Perioperative, Pharmacological interventions, Risk stratification

Review

Introduction

Acute kidney injury (AKI) occurs in 1% to 5% of all hospital admissions, and in the perioperative period has serious implications, being consistently associated with (unacceptably) high mortality, morbidity and a more complicated hospital course with associated cost implications. This is particularly the case when renal replacement therapy (RRT) is required [1-22]. It is widely recognized that AKI requiring dialysis is an independent risk factor for death [1-3]; more recently, however, even minimal increases in serum creatinine have been associated with an increase in both short and long-term mortality, regardless of whether partial or full recovery of renal function has occurred at the time of discharge [4-11]. This risk of death is independent from other postoperative complications and co-morbidities [7-9]. AKI is related to the subsequent development and progression of chronic kidney disease (CKD) and the need for future dialysis, most notably in those with a degree of pre-existing renal impairment [11-15], but also in those who have apparent recovery following an episode of AKI [7]. Despite an increase in our knowledge of AKI and advances in other relevant areas over the last two decades (including intensive care, delivery of dialysis and surgical techniques), there have been no significant changes in these outcomes [12,15-17]. As such, identification of risk factors, close monitoring of renal function and early adoption of both preventive

measures and treatments remain important considerations for those taking care of perioperative patients who are likely to develop AKI.

Incidence

Surgery remains a leading cause of AKI in hospitalized patients (the incidence ranges from 18% to 47% depending on the definition used) [17,18]. This has been best researched in the cardiac surgery setting where it has been shown that up to 15% of patients exposed to cardiopulmonary bypass (CPB) will develop AKI, with 2% requiring RRT [23]. Depending on the criteria used to define AKI and the postoperative period studied, mortality ranges from 1% to 30% [5,24] although this is consistently higher, approaching 80%, if RRT is required [2,17,24]. AKI is not limited to cardiac surgery although its incidence outside of this setting is often underappreciated. Kheterpal *et al.* demonstrated that in patients without pre-existing renal disease, approximately 1% of major non-cardiac surgery was complicated by AKI, with an eight-fold increase in 30-day mortality [20,23]. This incidence is comparable to other notable postoperative complications including major adverse cardiac events (MACE) and venous thromboembolism [23].

In the intensive care setting, the Beginning and Ending Supportive Therapy for the Kidney (BEST Kidney) investigators confirmed major surgery as the second leading cause of AKI (in 34%) in this cohort of patients, with overall hospital mortality of 60.3% [1]. Analysis of data from the United Kingdom Intensive Care National Audit

* Correspondence: andrew.shaw@duke.edu
[2]Dept of Anesthesiology and Critical Care Medicine, Duke University Medical Center/Durham VAMC, Durham, USA
Full list of author information is available at the end of the article

and Research Centre Case Mix program supports this, showing surgical admissions accounted for 16.4% of admissions with severe AKI in the first 24 hours (with elective and emergency cases accounting for 5.6% and 10.8%, respectively). In that study, defining severe AKI as creatinine >300 μmol/l and/or urea >40 mmol/l has restricted the patient cohort and potentially, therefore, may limit its generalizability [25]. Elsewhere, it has been reported that one third of patients with AKI require a critical care admission at some point in their care [14].

Definition

Although AKI has been the focus of much research over the past decades, lack of a consensus definition has been a major factor hampering clinical research and comparison of trial data [1,12,13,22,26,27]. There are now two major classifications of AKI in use. The Acute Dialysis Quality Initiative (ADQI) Group introduced the RIFLE (Risk, Injury, Failure, Loss and End-stage) classification system in 2004, which defines three grades of severity and two outcomes, in an effort to standardize the definition [7,12,28,29]. This has subsequently been validated in a number of studies [7,29-35]. The Acute Kidney Injury Network (AKIN) group proposed refinements to this criteria, outlining AKI as abrupt (occurring within 48 hours) and using a smaller change in serum creatinine from baseline in patients who are optimally hydrated to define AKI [12,28,29], following recognition of emerging evidence demonstrating the clinical importance of small increases

in serum creatinine [5-9]. No clear advantages between these criteria have been demonstrated and despite these recommendations, definitions of AKI continue to vary [29]. The Kidney Disease: Improving Global Outcomes (KDIGO) workgroup has recently reviewed these criteria and published a single definition for use in both clinical practice and research. AKI is defined when any of the following three criteria are met; an increase in serum creatinine by 50% in seven days, an increase in serum creatinine > 0.3 mg/dL in 48 hours or oliguria. The severity is staged according the criteria outlined in Table 1 [36].

Recognition is often still delayed and more recently, the role of electronic reporting systems has been successfully tested in the UK with the aim of alerting clinicians early to the presence of AKI, appreciating the impact of small increases in creatinine from baseline that previously may have been considered as fluctuations remaining within the normal range. In turn, this should allow for timely intervention and improved overall patient care [37].

RIFLE, AKIN and KDIGO all diagnose AKI according to serum creatinine and urine output as outlined in Table 1. This, however, is not without its limitations, as serum creatinine is neither sensitive nor specific, tending to represent a functional change rather than being a true marker of kidney injury and is well known to be affected by multiple factors including age, ethnicity, gender, muscle mass, total body volume, medications and protein intake

Table 1 Classification of acute kidney injury by RIFLE, AKIN and KIDGO criteria [12,28,36]

Stage	Glomerular filtration rate (GFR) criteria	Urine output criteria
RIFLE classification		
Risk	Serum creatinine increased x 1.5 or GFR decrease >25%	<0.5 ml/kg/hr for ≥ 6 hours
Injury	Serum creatinine increased x 2 or GFR decrease >50%	<0.5 ml/kg/hr for ≥ 12 hours
Failure	Serum creatinine increased x 3 or GFR decrease ≥ 75% or an absolute serum creatinine ≥ 354 μmol/L with an acute rise ≥ 4 μmol/L	<0.3 ml/kg/hr for ≥ 24 hours or anuria for ≥12 hours
Loss	Persistent AKI, requiring RRT for > 4 weeks	
End-stage kidney disease	Requiring dialysis > 3 months	
AKIN classification		
Stage 1	Serum creatinine increased ≥26.2 μmol/L or x 0.5 to 2 baseline	<0.5 ml/kg/hr for ≥ 6hours
Stage 2	Serum creatinine increased x 2 to 3 baseline	<0.5 ml/kg/hr for ≥ 12 hours
Stage 3	Serum creatinine increased > x 3 baseline or serum creatinine ≥ 354 μmol/L with an acute rise ≥ 44 μmol/L or initiation of RRT	<0.3 ml/kg/hr for ≥ 24 hours or anuria for ≥12 hours
KDIGO classification		
Stage 1	Serum creatinine increased x 1.5 to 1.9 baseline or by ≥ 26.2 μmol/L	<0.5 ml/kg/hr for 6 to 12 hours
Stage 2	Serum creatinine increased x 2 to 2.9 baseline	<0.5 ml/kg/hr for ≥ 12 hours
Stage 3	Serum creatinine increased > x 3 baseline or serum creatinine ≥ 354 μmol/L with an acute rise ≥ 44 μmol/L or initiation of RRT	<0.3 ml/kg/hr for ≥ 24 hours or anuria for ≥12 hours

AKIN, Acute Kidney Injury Network; *KDIGO*, Kidney Disease: Improving Global Outcomes.

[16,38]. Given that a reduction in glomerular filtration rate (GFR) greater than 50% can occur before this is reflected in serum creatinine [16,39,40], the ability to detect AKI prior to a change in serum creatinine would represent a significant advance in the management of AKI. As such, the American Society of Nephrology set identification and characterization of biomarkers for AKI as a key research area in 2005 [41].

Risk factors

There have been a number of studies investigating the risk factors associated with the development of AKI, from which several factors, both patient and procedure related, have been consistently associated in both cardiac and non-cardiac surgery (Table 2) [3,20,23,24,42-45]. Patient related factors are often more strongly associated with postoperative mortality than surgical factors. These include age, hypertension, diabetes mellitus, cardiac failure, peripheral vascular disease, cerebrovascular disease and pre-existing chronic kidney disease [3,23,24,42-44]. Perhaps the most important of these is the latter, with rates of AKI requiring dialysis approaching 30% in patients with pre-existing kidney disease undergoing cardiac surgery [7,17,24,42-44]. That said, there remain risk factors specific to certain types of surgery which are associated with postoperative AKI, including prolonged CPB time, combined valve and coronary artery bypass graft (CABG) surgery, increased aortic cross-clamp time during vascular surgery and increased intra-abdominal pressure in major abdominal surgery [2,17,46]. Unsurprisingly, many of these risk factors are associated with either poor renal perfusion or decreased renal reserve and few are correctable prior to surgery.

Integral to improving outcomes, however, is the ability to identify high risk patients, not only allowing for earlier intervention and optimal subsequent management, but

Table 2 Factors associated with the development of AKI

Patient related factors	Surgical factors
Age	Duration of surgery
Hypertension	Intra-peritoneal surgery
Diabetes Mellitus	Length of CPB
Chronic Obstructive Pulmonary Disease	Cross clamp time
LVF, EF <40%	Hemolysis (cardiac surgery)
Chronic kidney disease	Hemodilution (cardiac surgery)
Emergency surgery	Use of IABP (cardiac surgery)
Sepsis	
Peripheral vascular disease	
Cerebrovascular disease	
Ascites	

EF, ejection fraction; *IABP*, Intra-aortic balloon pump; *LVF*, left ventricular function.

also identification of cohorts of patients in which new treatments can be studied. Several groups have, therefore, sought to develop risk stratification indexes in both cardiac and general surgery [23,24,42,45,47]. Kheterphal *et al.* developed a General Surgery AKI Risk Index after evaluating almost 76,000 general surgical patients, which also included a validation sample. A score is given for each patient, based on nine separate preoperative risk factors, following which patients are categorized into one of five classes. Class I (determined by having zero to two risk factors) has an incidence of AKI of 0.2%; in contrast to Class V (>6 risk factors) which confers an AKI risk of 9.5% [23]. Although useful in highlighting risk factors, further validation over multiple centers is crucial, with similar single center risk scoring systems post-cardiac surgery having been shown to underestimate the true incidence of AKI, despite taking into account demographic variation [47].

Novel biomarkers

An ideal biomarker would be highly sensitive and specific for AKI, responding consistently and rapidly to injury, with normal ranges for age, race and gender established and levels that correlate to severity as well as having biological stability and a reliable, quick and cost effective assay for detection [48,49]. It would also be useful to determine the extent of interpersonal variation attributable to genetic factors and the impact of confounding clinical factors [48]. The area under the receiver-operating characteristic curve (AUC_{ROC}) is used to assess the performance of a diagnostic biomarker, with a value greater than 0.75 demonstrating good discriminatory value and greater than 0.90 demonstrating excellent discrimination.

A current challenge is that novel biomarkers are being compared to serum creatinine as the 'gold standard' when it is the very weakness of serum creatinine as a sensitive and specific marker that prompted research into this area. Indeed, many authors have made this exact point in their opening statements [50]. More than 20 different biomarkers have been identified in recent years, predominantly in studies of post-cardiac surgery. However, most current focus is on neutrophil gelatinase-associated lipocalin (NGAL), kidney injury molecule – 1 (KIM-1), IL-18 and cystatin-C. At present these remain experimental and need validation in larger studies prior to transition into clinical practice [38]. It is highly likely that several other biomarkers will also be introduced into clinical practice over the next few years.

NGAL

NGAL has generated significant interest in recent years, particularly in AKI following cardiac surgery, although its use is not restricted to this cohort of patients [39,51-53]. In patients with normal renal function, NGAL is almost undetectable in either urine or plasma, yet animal studies clearly demonstrated that NGAL is markedly upregulated early following ischemic injury [54]. In subsequent clinical studies, urinary NGAL has been shown to be both sensitive and specific in predicting postoperative AKI in pediatric patients undergoing cardiac surgery [43,51,52]. Similarly, plasma NGAL measured at two hours post-CPB correlated strongly with severity and duration of AKI, with an AUC_{ROC} of 0.96, sensitivity of 0.84 and specificity of 0.94 [39]. In an adult population, this result has been less consistent [51,52] with Wagener *et al.* demonstrating an AUC_{ROC} of 0.61 and sensitivity of 0.39 in urinary NGAL measured 18 hours post-surgery [52]. Likewise, raised plasma NGAL levels have been clearly demonstrated in AKI following CPB surgery, however again with a low sensitivity thereby limiting its use as a single biomarker in the prediction of AKI [55]. It has been proposed that this poor sensitivity may be in part due to the current limitations of defining AKI using serum creatinine [52], although it should also be noted that patients who develop AKI also tend to have a longer CPB time. Although this has been clearly demonstrated to be a risk factor, it also raises the possibility that NGAL (particularly plasma NGAL) could actually reflect length of CPB/degree of inflammation versus degree of kidney injury [39]. Many of these studies have, however, excluded patients with pre-existing renal dysfunction. A *post-hoc* subgroup analysis has attempted to address this and although these results must be interpreted with a degree of caution, they do show that the use of urinary NGAL is significantly influenced by pre-existing renal function, with no clear relationship between postoperative urinary NGAL and the development of AKI in patients with a GFR < 60 ml/minute [56]. This suggests that the relationship between NGAL and AKI is complex and is likely to be different in the setting of CKD [57].

KIM-1

KIM-1 is a type 1 transmembrane glycoprotein, undetectable in normal kidney tissue, which has been shown to be markedly upregulated following injury secondary to ischemia and nephrotoxins in a variety of both animal and human studies, with a soluble form readily detectable in the urine [58]. Early human studies demonstrated a clear increase in KIM-1 protein expression at biopsy that correlated with high urinary levels, detectable prior to cast formation, following ischemic injury [58]. Since then, KIM-1 has been shown to be a highly sensitive marker for AKI in patients undergoing cardiac surgery [59] and, alongside another urinary biomarker, N-acetyl-β-(D)-glucosaminidase, high levels have been associated with adverse outcomes including the need for renal replacement therapy and death [60].

IL-18

The cytokine IL-18 has also been shown to be an early biomarker for AKI in a variety of clinical situations, including in patients with CKD [61-65]. Post-CPB surgery, urinary IL-18 was detectable four to six hours post-surgery, peaking at 12 hours with an AUC_{ROC} of 0.75 and remaining elevated over the next 24 to 28 hours (AUC_{ROC} at 24 hours 0.75) [61]. In addition, there is a correlation between peak levels and increased severity of AKI and mortality [63,64]. Unsurprisingly, given the role of IL-18 as a pro-inflammatory cytokine, levels are higher in cohorts of patients with sepsis than in those without [64].

Cystatin C

Cystatin C is a cysteine protease inhibitor produced by all nucleated cells. Given that it is freely filtered by the glomerulus, undergoes almost complete tubular reabsorption and is not secreted by renal tubules, it is desirable as a marker of GFR [40,66-68]. However, serum cystatin C levels have been shown to be affected by the use of steroids, thyroid dysfunction, age, gender and CRP independent of GFR [40,66,67]. A prospective study looking at 72 patients undergoing cardiac surgery demonstrated no clear association between AKI and plasma cystatin C although an early and persistent increase in urinary cystatin C was associated with AKI, and the level excreted correlated with the severity of AKI. This suggests that in this cohort of patients, urinary cystatin C may be more useful [67].

Importantly, many studies to date have excluded patients with CKD, who have been consistently demonstrated to be at high risk for AKI in the perioperative period [20] and these biomarkers must therefore first be characterized over a range of baseline values, with more information required to identify and explain clinical factors that may confound their performance in the perioperative period [38-40,51-57,67]. It is unlikely that any single biomarker would be sufficient for accurate diagnosis and risk stratification of AKI but rather that the way forward would be to develop a panel of biomarkers which, used in conjunction, would allow for assessment of disease severity and risk alongside earlier diagnosis [40,49,59,61]. This faces its own challenges and as yet there is insufficient information as to which combinations to recommend for use. More work is clearly needed in this area, with the ultimate aim being earlier recognition of AKI, thereby allowing for progress to be made in its subsequent treatment.

Pathophysiology of AKI

Etiologically, AKI is divided into pre-renal, intrinsic or renal, and post-renal causes, in surgery representing 30%

to 60%, 20% to 40% and 1% to 10% of cases, respectively [17] (Table 3). Renal hypoperfusion is often the initial insult in perioperative AKI, which importantly can lead to a reduction in medullary blood flow [17,46,69]. The outer medulla with its high metabolic demands (medullary oxygen extraction approaches 90%) is particularly vulnerable to both hypoperfusion and hypoxia, both in patients with known CKD whose underlying reserve is reduced but also in patients with normal preoperative renal function [69-71]. Interestingly, in acute respiratory distress syndrome (ARDS) it is increasingly recognized that the disease process, for example, pulmonary versus extra-pulmonary causes, impacts the course of the disease and whether the same could be said for AKI remains to be seen [72].

Animal models have been developed, predominantly based on ischemia-reperfusion injury or drug-induced injury, which have significantly improved our understanding of AKI, especially with regard to the role of inflammation. This is thought to be especially important in AKI associated with CPB surgery [73]. In clinical practice, ischemia-reperfusion injury can occur secondary to either general hypoperfusion or specific actions, for example, cross-clamping of the aorta in vascular surgery. Interventions that are beneficial in animal models, however, have not yet been shown to be effective in clinical practice [74,75].

Histologically, there is still a paucity of information available, in part due to the invasive nature of renal biopsies that are often not undertaken in patients in whom AKI is presumed secondary to pre-renal factors [74]. In biopsies that have been obtained, and from post-mortem findings, there is a clear disparity seen between the clinical scenario and the pathological findings [74]. This, in turn, supports the concept of cytopathic hypoxia leading to cellular shutdown versus cell necrosis or apoptosis [75].

Management of AKI
The goals in management of AKI include preservation of existing renal function as well as prevention of acute complications (hyperkalemia, acidosis, volume overload) and the need for long-term renal replacement therapy. Avoidance of AKI remains the cornerstone of management while research continues into effective treatment options.

Preventive measures
Fluids and goal directed therapy
Maintenance of normal renal perfusion is perhaps the most important prophylactic measure, with 80% of patients experiencing postoperative AKI having an episode of hemodynamic instability in the perioperative period [17,46]. The use of fluids in this period is therefore vital although this should be approached with caution as there are equally important recognized postoperative complications associated with excess fluid including poor wound healing and increased duration of mechanical ventilation [76,77]. There is increasing evidence that a positive fluid balance in both surgical and critical care patients is associated with an increase in intra-abdominal hypertension which, in turn, has a detrimental effect on renal function [77-79]. Furthermore, hyperchloremia is often associated with over-zealous fluid resuscitation with 0.9% saline and has been associated with a decrease in renal blood flow [77]. Importantly, studies comparing conservative versus liberal fluid strategies have not seen an increase in the incidence in AKI or an increased need for RRT in the conservative arms [77].

There has, however, been no randomized controlled trial (RCT) directed at addressing the role of fluid hydration in the prevention of AKI in surgical patients [80] and this task often falls to junior members of the team. A targeted approach with titration to specified end-points may in fact be more appropriate [77,81].

Goal directed therapy (GDT) is a strategy that involves the use of fluids, packed red cells and inotropes to reach target hemodynamic parameters including cardiac output and oxygen delivery to prevent organ dysfunction [46,82,83]. Many high risk surgical patients (both elective and emergency) are admitted to the ICU in the

Table 3 Summary of causes of AKI defined etiologically

Pre-renal	Intrinsic renal disease	Post-renal
Hypovolemia, for example, hemorrhage, diarrhea, vomiting	Ischemia from prolonged hypoperfusion	Obstructive causes, for example, prostatic hypertrophy, renal stones, urethral strictures, pelvic masses
Hypotension, for example, sepsis	Glomerular disease, for example, glomerulonephritis, TTP, DIC	
Low cardiac output state, for example, CCF, cardiac tamponade	Nephrotoxins, for example, aminoglycosides, NSAIDs, radiological contrast	
Impaired renal autoregulation, for example, renal artery stenosis, ACEi/ARB/NSAIDs	Metabolic abnormalities, for example, hypercalcemia	
	Rhabdomyolysis, for example, crush injuries, burns	

ACEi, angiotensin converting enzyme inhibitor; ARB, angiotensin recreptor blocker; CCF, congestive cardiac failure; DIC, disseminated intravascular coagulation; TTP, thrombotic thrombocytopenic purpura.

perioperative period, often with many comorbidities and GDT in this time period has been associated with fewer complications (including AKI) and improved mortality [84]. In 2009, a meta-analysis demonstrated that AKI is significantly reduced by perioperative hemodynamic optimization, whether done in the pre-, intra- or post-operative period [46]. This is particularly relevant when resources for pre-operative optimization are limited. Of note, meeting physiological values was as 'reno-protective' as meeting supra-normal values, which itself may be associated with other complications although this remains a point of debate [46].

The use of sodium bicarbonate has been addressed in cardiac surgery. Following on from work supporting the use of urinary alkanization in contrast nephropathy, a pilot RCT in 100 post-CPB surgical patients showed a reduction in the incidence of AKI in patients receiving sodium bicarbonate versus a placebo saline infusion although no changes were demonstrated in either the need for RRT or mortality [85]. Further trials in this area are ongoing/promising.

Avoidance of nephrotoxic agents

A number of different medications commonly used in the perioperative period have potentially harmful effects on renal function. Angiotensin-converting enzyme inhibitors (ACEi) and angiotensin receptor blockers (ARB) and NSAIDs are among drugs known to affect renal autoregulation. Whether or not to continue ACEi/ARB in the perioperative period remains under debate although a meta-analysis has shown ACEi confer no protective benefits in this time period [86].

NSAIDs can also cause interstitial nephritis and their association with the development of AKI led to recommendations from the Medicines and Healthcare Products Regulatory Agency suggesting that they should be avoided in all patients with hypovolemia and sepsis regardless of renal function [87]. Antibiotics can lead to AKI by either direct injury, for example aminoglycosides in high concentrations, thereby necessitating monitoring of drug levels, or secondary to an acute interstitial nephritis, for example penicillins, quinolones and cephalosporins.

The role of intravenous contrast in AKI is well recognized and where its use is unavoidable, the minimum possible dose should be given as well as using the newer iso-osmolar and low-osmolar non-ionic contrast, now recognized to be less toxic [88,89]. Surgery should be postponed in stable patients with contrast-induced AKI. Whether oral N-acetylcysteine confers any protective benefit in this situation remains controversial [90].

Hemodilution and transfusion in cardiac surgery

Specific to cardiac surgery, the roles of hemodilution and transfusion have also been studied. There is a known association between AKI and erythrocyte transfusion in cardiac surgery [91-94]. More recently, a single center study has both confirmed this and suggested that the level of pre-operative anemia also has an impact, being associated with a more pronounced increase in the incidence of AKI [95]. There is, however, ongoing work into the role of erythropoietin (EPO) in this setting, with a small pilot trial confirming its effectiveness although a larger trial is required before this could be recommended [96]. Hemodilution is induced in the setting of cardio-pulmonary bypass surgery, in theory decreasing blood viscosity and improving microcirculatory flow in the presence of both hypoperfusion and hypothermia. However, this has been associated with a significant increase in the incidence of AKI and, as such, current guidelines underline the importance of limiting hemodilution, with the Society of Thoracic Surgeons and the Society of Cardiovascular Anaesthesiologists recommending maintenance of hematocrit >21% and hemoglobin >7 g/dl [91,97-100].

Pharmacological interventions

There have been many attempts to find pharmacological interventions in the management of AKI, with the ongoing challenge regarding the use of standard definitions and end-points making it difficult to directly compare trial evidence. Until recently there have been no drugs that have consistently been demonstrated to confer benefit, although there is now some emerging evidence in the setting of cardiac surgery [80,86].

Dopamine

Dopamine has been extensively used and its place debated over the years, with much of the early enthusiasm driven by the assumption that increased renal blood flow seen with low-dose dopamine is beneficial in the management of AKI [101-103]. A meta-analysis published in 2001, however, demonstrated no benefit using dopamine for either the prevention or treatment of AKI. This recommendation followed identification and analysis of 58 studies, 24 of which reported the outcomes reviewed (including 17 RCTs) [102]. This was further supported in a systematic literature review, last updated in 2008 [86].

Fenoldopam

Fenoldopam is a selective DA-1 agonist which to date has had mixed results when used in the management of AKI [80,104,105]. In cardiac surgery, however, fenoldopam was shown to consistently reduce the need for RRT and mortality, although its use is potentially complicated by systemic hypotension [80,106]. This undesirable side effect may be improved with the use of intra-renal infusions, an innovative/emerging strategy which to date has proven successful in case reports although further trial information with a larger number of patients is required [105].

Diuretics (furosemide/mannitol)

While use of diuretics may improve urine output in the setting of acute kidney injury, again there is no evidence to support that they confer any improvement in outcomes measured (including need for RRT and mortality) [80,101,107]. Furthermore, use of furosemide has been shown to be not only ineffective but also detrimental, associated with higher postoperative serum creatinine levels in cardiac patients [80,102,108]. Of note, mannitol is often added to the priming solution used in CPB surgery. Although initially shown to confer some preventive benefits in children undergoing CPB surgery, these results have not been reproduced in repeat studies, with a suggestion that mannitol is actually associated with increased tubular injury when given in combination with dopamine [81,106,108,109].

Atrial natriuretic peptide (ANP)

ANP is produced by cardiac atria in response to atrial dilatation and its properties as an endogenous diuretic and natriuretic substance led to further evaluation of ANP as another potential therapy. Early RCTs showed a benefit in only a sub-group of oliguric patients which was not reproduced in follow up studies and systemic hypotension was noted to be a complicating factor [110-113]. A significant reduction in the need for RRT was, however, seen in postcardiac surgical patients with decompensated congestive cardiac failure (CCF) who received low-dose infusions of recombinant human ANP. Of note, the lower dose infusion was associated with a decrease in the incidence of systemic hypotension, which in itself may contribute to the change in results seen [113,114]. Outside of cardiac surgery, there is at present no perceived benefit with ANP [80,114].

Nesiritide (recombinant human β natriuretic peptide)

Nesiritide is another cardiac natriuretic peptide that is currently under evaluation. Initial results in both cardiac and abdominal aneurysm repair surgery have shown potential protective benefits with an overall reduction in mortality, however, there is a possible association with increased mortality in acutely decompensated heart failure [114-116]. Overall, nesiritide warrants further investigation before recommendations/conclusions can be confidently made [114-116].

Theophylline

Theophylline, an adenosine antagonist, in theory is proposed to preserve renal blood flow by attenuating vasoconstriction of renal vessels [117,118]. Several small studies have been conducted using theophylline in contrast-induced nephropathy; however, a meta-analysis in 2005 was inconclusive and recommended that a RCT in this area with a defined hydration protocol would be of benefit [117]. In the setting of CPB surgery, an infusion of theophylline conferred no benefit in reducing the incidence of AKI [118].

N-acetylcysteine

The role of N-acetlycysteine, an antioxidant most commonly used to enhance formation of glutathione after paracetamol overdose, has not been shown to confer any protective benefits in the perioperative period [119,120]. As mentioned above, there may be some role for this agent in contrast-induced nephropathy [90].

Glycemic control

A landmark study in 2001 demonstrated tight glycemic control and showed improved outcomes in an Intensive Therapy Unit setting, with a 41% reduction in AKI requiring RRT [121]. This has, therefore, sparked renewed focus in this area; however, subsequent studies have not reproduced these benefits [122]. More recently, in cardiac surgery, while severe intraoperative and early postoperative hyperglycemia was associated with poorer outcomes (including an increased incidence of AKI), incremental decreases in mean glucose concentrations did not show consistent improvements in outcomes [123]. Given the inconsistent results seen, the concept of tight glycemic control needs further reassessment, with development of strategies that focus on avoiding large variations in blood glucose and hypoglycemia [122,123].

Prophylactic RRT

There is currently insufficient evidence to support the use of prophylactic RRT in high-risk patients undergoing major surgery. Indeed it seems somewhat counterproductive to dialyze someone in order to prevent dialysis. A single center study in which 44 patients were randomized either to receive prophylactic dialysis or postoperative dialysis if indicated did,,however, show both a decrease in mortality (4.8% versus 30.4%) and in AKI requiring RRT [124]. An effect size this large is statistically very unlikely in practice. Similarly, in the setting of contrast nephropathy, a small single center RCT showed that prophylactic hemofiltration was associated with a decrease in both mortality and morbidity although these findings are limited by the lack of standardized hydration protocols and use of N-Acetyl Cysteine in this trial [125]. However, more evidence is required before this invasive strategy can be recommended.

RRT in established AKI

Many of the goals of modern treatment are to prevent AKI; when established, however, RRT then plays an important role in the subsequent management, with approximately 15% of patients in intensive care with AKI receiving dialysis [126]. Despite decades of research and debate, this remains an area where there is no clear consensus as to the optimal timing, modality or dose of RRT, yet it is recognized as a significant factor affecting outcome in critically ill patients [1,11,127,128]. Earlier studies suggested a benefit to higher dose hemodialysis or hemofiltration [127] although this was not confirmed in follow up studies and the debate rages on [128-131].

Conclusions

AKI is a serious and often under-appreciated complication in the perioperative period, with even small rises in serum creatinine associated with both increased morbidity and mortality. The use of risk stratification indices should help in the identification of high risk patients, useful both for clinical practice and on-going research. Recent advances have been made in the field of biomarkers although this work has yet to be translated into clinical practice and the mainstay of treatment remains preventive, aiming to keep patients optimally hydrated while avoiding nephrotoxic agents. There are no pharmacological agents yet with proven benefits in the management of AKI although there is some emerging evidence favoring the use of fenoldopam and ANP in the setting of cardiac surgery, with novel techniques in the delivery of agents helping to overcome systemic side effects.

Abbreviations

ACEi: Angiotensin converting enzyme inhibitor; AKI: Acute kidney injury; AKIN: Acute Kidney Injury Network; ANP: Atrial natriuretic peptide; ARB: Angiotensin receptor blocker; ARDS: Acute respiratory distress syndrome; AUC_ROC: Area under the receiver operating characteristic curve; CABG: Coronary artery bypass graft; CCF: Congestive cardiac failure; CKD: Chronic kidney disease; CPB: Cardiopulmonary bypass; DIC: Disseminated intravascular coagulation; EF: Ejection fraction; EPO: Erythropoietin; GDT: Goal directed therapy; GFR: Glomerular filtration rate; IABP: Intra-aortic balloon pump; Il-18: Interleukin-18; KDIGO: Kidney Disease Improving Global Outcomes; KIM-1: Kidney injury molecule-1; LVF: Left ventricular function; MACE: Major adverse cardiac events; NGAL: Neutrophil gelatinase-associated lipocalin; NSAIDs: Non-steroidal anti-inflammatory drugs; RIFLE: Risk Injury, Failure, Loss and End-stage; RCT: Randomized controlled trial; RRT: Renal replacement therapy; TTP: Thrombotic thrombocytopenic purpura.

Competing interests

The authors declare that they have no competing interests.

Author details

¹St George's Hospital, London, SW17 0QT, UK. ²Dept of Anesthesiology and Critical Care Medicine, Duke University Medical Center/Durham VAMC, Durham, USA.

Authors' contributions

SC wrote the first draft. SC and AS edited and finalized the review. Both authors read and approved the final manuscript.

References

1. Uchino S, Kellum JA, Bellomo R, Doig GS, Morimatsu H, Morgera S, Schetz M, Tan I, Bouman C, Macedo E, Gibney N, Tolwani A, Ronco C: **Acute renal failure in critically ill paitents: a multinational, multicenter study.** *JAMA* 2005, **294**:813–818.
2. Chertow GM, Levy EM, Hammermeister KE, Grover F, Daley J: **Independent association between acute renal failure and mortality following cardiac surgery.** *Am J Med* 1998, **104**:343–348.
3. Thaker CV, Kharat V, Blanck S, Leaonard AC: **Acute kidney injury after gastric bypass surgery.** *Clin J Am Soc Nephrol* 2007, **2**:426–430.
4. Loef BG, Epema AH, Smilde TD, Henning RH, Ebels T, Navis G, Stegeman CA: **Immediate postoperative renal function deterioration in cardiac surgical patients predicts in-hospital mortality and long-term survival.** *J Am Soc Nephrol* 2005, **16**:195–200.
5. Lassnigg A, Schmidlin D, Mouhieddine M, Bachmann LM, Druml W, Bauer P, Hiesmayr M: **Minimal changes of serum creatinine predict poor prognosis in patients after cardiothoracic surgery: a prospective cohort study.** *J Am Soc Nephrol* 2004, **15**:1597–1605.
6. Ishani A, Nelson D, Clothier B, Schult T, Nugent S, Greer N, Slinin Y, Ensrud KE: **The magnitude of acute serum creatinine increase after cardiac surgery and the risk of chronic kidney disease, progression of kidney disease, and death.** *Arch Intern Med* 2011, **171**:226–233.
7. Hobson CE, Yavas S, Segal MS, Schold JD, Tribble CG, Layon AJ, Bihorac A: **Acute kidney injury is associated with increased long-term mortality after cardiothoracic surgery.** *Circulation* 2009, **119**:2444–2453.
8. Bihorac A, Yavas S, Subbiah S, Hobson CE, Schold JD, Gabrielli A, Layon AJ, Segal MS: **Long term risk of mortality and acute kidney injury during hospitalization after major surgery.** *Ann Surg* 2009, **249**:851–858.
9. Lafrance JP, Miller DR: **Acute kidney injury associates with increased long-term mortality.** *J Am Soc Nephrol* 2010, **21**:345–352.
10. Palevskky PM: **Epidemiology of acute renal failure: the tip of the Iceberg.** *Clin J Am Soc Nephrol* 2006, **2006**:6–7.
11. Mehta RL, Pascual MT, Soroko S, Savage BR, Himmelfarb J, Ikizler TA, Paganini EP, Chertow GM: **Spectrum of acute renal failure in the intensive care unit: the PICARD experience.** *Kidney Int* 2004, **66**:1613–1621.
12. Mehta RL, Kellum JA, Shah AV, Molitoris BA, Ronco C, Warnock DG, Levin A, the Acute Kidney Injury Network: **Acute Kidney Injury Network: report of an initiative to improve outcome in acute kidney injury.** *Crit Care* 2007, **11**:R31.
13. Metnitz PG, Krenn CG, Steltzer H, Lang T, Ploder J, Lenz K, Le Gall JR, Druml W: **Effect of acute renal failure requiring renal replacement therapy on outcome in critically ill patients.** *Crit Care Med* 2002, **30**:2051–2058.
14. Liano F, Junco E, Pascual J, Madero R, Verde E: **The spectrum of acute renal failure in the intensive care unit compared with that seen in other settings. The Madrid Acute Renal Failure Study Group.** *Kidney Int* 1998, **66**:S16–S24.
15. Druml W: **Long term prognosis of patients with acute renal failure: is intensive care worth it?** *Intensive Care Med* 2005, **31**:1145–1147.
16. Mehta RL, Chertow GM: **Acute renal failure definitions and classification: time for change?** *J Am Soc Nephrol* 2003, **14**:2178–2187.
17. Carmichael P, Carmichael AR: **Acute renal failure in the surgical setting.** *ANZ J Surg* 2003, **73**:144–153.
18. Shusterman N, Strom BL, Murray TG, Morrison G, West SL, Maislin G: **Risk factors and outcome of hospital acquired acute renal failure. Clinical epidemiologic study.** *Am J Med* 1987, **83**:65–71.
19. Liangos O, Wald R, O'Bell JW, Price L, Pereira BJ, Jabor BL: **Epidemiology and outcomes of acute renal failure in hospitalized patients: a national survey.** *Clin J Am Soc Nephrol* 2006, **1**:43–51.
20. Kheterpal S, Tremper KK, Englesbe MJ, O'Reilly M, Shanks AM, Fetterman DM, Rosenberg AL, Swartz RD: **Predictors of postoperative acute renal failure after noncardiac surgery in patients with previously normal renal function.** *Anesthesiology* 2007, **107**:892–902.
21. Xue JL, Daniels F, Star RA, Kimmel PL, Eggers PW, Molitoris BA, Himmelfarb J, Collins AJ: **Incidence and mortality of acute renal failure in medicare beneficiaries, 1992–2001.** *J Am Soc Nephrol* 2006, **17**:1135–1142.
22. Chertow GM, Burdick E, Honour M, Bonventre JV, Bates DW: **Acute kidney injury, mortality, length of stay, and costs in hospitalized patients.** *J Am Soc Nephrol* 2005, **16**:3365–3370.

23. Kheterpal S, Tremper KK, Heung M, Rosenberg AL, Englesbe M, Shanks AM, Campbell DA: Development and validation of an acute kidney injury risk index for patients undergoing general surgery. *Anesthesiology* 2009, **110**:505–515.

24. Chertow GM, Lazarus M, Christiansen CL, Cook F, Hammermeister KE, Grover F, Daley J: Preoperative renal risk stratification. *Circulation* 1997, **95**:878–884.

25. Kolhe NV, Stevens PE, Crowe AV, Lipkin GW, Harrison DA: Case mix, outcome and activity for patients with severe acute kidney injury during the first 24 hours after admission to an adult general critical care unit: application of predictive models from a secondary analysis of the ICNARC Case Mix Programme database. *Crit Care* 2008, **12**(Suppl 1):S2.

26. Bellomo R, Kellum JA, Ronco C: Defining acute renal failure: physiological principles. *Intensive Care Med* 2006, **30**:33–37.

27. Bellomo R, Kellum JA, Ronco C: Defining and classifying acute renal failure: from advocacy to consensus and validation of the RIFLE criteria. *Intensive Care Med* 2009, **11**:409–413.

28. Bellomo R, Ronco C, Kellum JA, Mehta RL, Palevsky P: Acute renal failure: definition, outcome measures, animal models, fluid therapy and information technology needs: the Second International Consensus Conference of the Acute Dialysis Quality Initiative (ADQI) Group. *Crit Care* 2004, **8**:R204–R212.

29. Bagshaw SM, George C, Bellomo R: A comparison of the RIFLE and AKIN criteria for acute kidney injury in critically ill patients. *Nephrol Dial Transplant* 2008, **23**:1569–1574.

30. Abosaif NY, Tolba YA, Heap M, Russel J, El Nahas AM: The outcome of acute renal failure in the intensive care unit according to RIFLE: model application, sensitivity, and predictability. *Am J Kidney Dis* 2005, **46**:1038–1048.

31. Hoste EA, Clermont G, Kerston A, Ventataraman R, Angus DC, De Bacquer D, Kellum JA: RIFLE criteria for acute kidney injury are associated with hospital mortality in critically ill patients: a cohort analysis. *Crit Care* 2006, **10**:R73.

32. Kuitunen A, Vento A, Suojaranta-Ylinen R, Pettila V: Acute renal failure after cardiac surgery: evaluation of the RIFLE criteria. *Ann Thorac Surg* 2006, **81**:542–546.

33. Uchino S, Bellomo R, Goldsmith D, Bates S, Ronco C: An assessment of RIFLE criteria for acute renal failure in hospitalized patients. *Crit Care Med* 2006, **34**:1913–1917.

34. Ostermann M, Chang RW: Acute kidney injury in the intensive care unit according to RIFLE. *Crit Care Med* 2007, **35**:1837–1845.

35. O'Riordan A, Wong V, McQuillan R, McCormick PA, Hegarty JE, Watson AJ: Acute renal disease, as defined by the RIFLE criteria, post-liver transplantation. *Am J Transplant* 2007, **7**:168–176.

36. Disease K, Improving Global Outcomes (KDIGO) Acute Kidney Injury Work Group: KDIGO Clinical Practice Guidelines for Acute Kidney Injury. *Kidney Int Suppl* 2012, **2**:1–138.

37. Selby NM, Crowley L, Fluck RJ, McIntyre CW, Monaghan J, Lawson H, Kohle NV: Use of electronic results reporting to diagnose and monitor AKI in hospitalized patients. *Clin J Am Soc Nephrol* 2012, **7**:533–540.

38. Coca SG, Yalavarthy R, Concato J, Parikh CR: Biomarkers for the diagnosis and risk stratification of acute kidney injury: a systematic review. *Kidney Int* 2007, **73**:1008–1016.

39. Dent CL, Ma Q, Dastrala S, Bennett M, Mitsnefes MM, Barasch J, Devarajan P: Plasma neutrophil gelatinase-associated lipocalin predicts acute kidney injury, morbidity and mortality after pediatric cardiac surgery: a prospective uncontrolled cohort study. *Crit Care* 2007, **11**:R127.

40. Herget-Rosenthal S, Marggraf G, Husing J, Goring F, Petruck F, Janssen O, Philipp T, Kribben A: Early detection of acute renal failure by serum cystatin C. *Kidney Int* 2004, **66**:1115–1122.

41. American Society of Nephrology Renal Research Report. *J Am Soc Nephrol* 2005, **16**:1886–1890.

42. Thakar CV, Arrigain S, Worley S, Yared JP, Paganini EP: A clinical score to predict acute renal failure after cardiac surgery. *J Am Soc Nephrol* 2005, **16**:162–168.

43. Fortescue EB, Bates DW, Chertow GM: Predicting acute renal failure after coronary bypass surgery: cross-validation of two risk stratification algorithms. *Kidney Int* 2000, **57**:2594–2602.

44. Thakar CV, Liangos O, Yared J-P, Nelson DA, Hariachar S, Paganini EP: Validation and re-definition of a risk stratification algorithm. *Hemodial Int* 2003, **7**:143–147.

45. Eriksen BO, Hoff KRS, Solberg S: Prediction of acute renal failure after cardiac surgery: retrospective cross-validation of a clinical algorithm. *Nephrol Dial Transplant* 2003, **18**:77–81.

46. Brienza N, Giglio MT, Marucci M, Fiore T: Does perioperative hemodynamic optimization protect renal function in surgical patients? A meta-analytic study. *Crit Care Med* 2009, **37**:2079–2090.

47. Candela-Toha A, Elias-Martin E, Abraira V, Tenorio MT, Parise D, de Pablo A, Centella T, Liano F: Predicting acute renal failure after cardiac surgery: external validation of two new clinical scores. *Clin J Am Soc Neprhol* 2008, **3**:1260–1265.

48. Mayeux R: Biomarkers: potential uses and limitations. *NeuroRx* 2004, **1**:182–188.

49. Ray P, Yannick M, Riou B, Houle T: Statistical evaluation of a biomarker. *Anesthesiology* 2010, **112**:1023–1040.

50. Waiker SS, Betensky RA, Bonventre JV: Creatinine as the gold standard for kidney injury biomarker studies? *Nephrol Dial Transplant* 2009, **124**:3263–3265.

51. Mishra J, Dent C, Tarabishi R, Mitsnefes MM, Ma Q, Kelly C, Ruff SM, Zahedi K, Shao M, Bean J, Mori K, Barasch J, Devarajan P: Neutrophil gelatinase-associated lipocalin (NGAL) as a biomarker for acute renal failure after cardiac surgery. *Lancet* 2005, **365**:1231–1238.

52. Wagener G, Gubitosa G, Wang S, Borregaard N, Kim M, Lee HT: Urinary neutrophil gelatinase-associated lipocalin and acute kidney injury after cardiac surgery. *Am J Kidney Dis* 2008, **52**:425–433.

53. Hirch R, Dent C, Pfriem H, Allen J, Beekman RH, Ma Q, Bennett M, Mitsnefes M, Devarajan P: NGAL is an early predictive biomarker of contrast-induced nephropathy in children. *Pediatr Nephrol* 2007, **22**:2089–2095.

54. Mishra J, Ma Q, Prada A, Mitsnefes M, Zahedi K, Yang J, Barasch J, Devarajan P: Identification of neutrophil gelatinase-associated lipocalin as a novel early urinary biomarker for ischemic renal injury. *J Am Soc Nephrol* 2003, **14**:2534–2543.

55. Perry TE, Muehlschlegel JD, Liu KY, Fax AA, Collard CD, Shernan SK, Body SC for the CABG Genomics Investigators: Plasma neutrophil gelatinase-associated lipocalin and acute postoperative kidney injury in adult cardiac surgical patients. *Anesth Analg* 2010, **110**:1541–1547.

56. Koyner JL, Vaidya VS, Bennett MR, Ma Q, Worcester E, Akhtar SA, Raman J, Jeevanandam V, O'Connor MF, Devarajan P, Bonventre JV, Murray PT: Urinary biomarkers in the clinical prognosis and early detection of acute kidney injury. *Clin J Am Soc Nephrol* 2010, **5**:2154–2165.

57. McIlroy DR, Wagener G, Lee TH: Neutrophil gelatinase-associated lipocalin and acute kidney injury after cardiac surgery: the effect of baseline renal function on diagnostic performance. *Clin J Am Soc Nephrol* 2010, **5**:211–219.

58. Han WK, Bailly V, Abichandani R, Thadhani R, Bonventre JV: Kidney injury molecule-1 (KIM-1): a novel biomarker for human renal proximal tubule injury. *Kidney Int* 2002, **62**:237–244.

59. Han WK, Waikar SS, Johnson A, Betensky RA, Dent CL, Deverajan P, Bonventre JV: Urinary biomarkers in the early diagnosis of acute kidney injury. *Kidney Int* 2008, **73**:863–869.

60. Liangos O, Perianayagam MC, Vaidya VS, Han WK, Wald R, Tighiouart H, MacKinnon RW, Li L, Balakrishnan VS, Pereira BJG, Bonventre JV, Jaber BL: Urinary N-acetyl-β-(D)-glucosaminidase activity and kidney injury molecule-1 level are associated with adverse outcomes in acute renal failure. *J Am Soc Nephrol* 2007, **18**:904–912.

61. Parikh CR, Mishra J, Thiessen-Philbrook H, Dursun B, Ma Q, Kelly C, Dent C, Deverajan P, Edelstein CL: Urinary IL-18 is an early predictive biomarker of acute kidney injury after cardiac surgery. *Kidney Int* 2006, **70**:199–203.

62. Parikh CR, Jani A, Melnikov VY, Faubel S, Edelstein CL: Urinary interleukin-18 is a marker of human acute tubular necrosis. *Am J Kidney Dis* 2004, **43**:405–414.

63. Parikh CR, Abraham E, Ancukiewicz M, Edelstein CL: Urine IL-18 is an early diagnostic marker for acute kidney injury and predicts mortality in the intensive care unit. *J Am Soc Nephrol* 2005, **16**:3046–3052.

64. Washburn KK, Zappitelli M, Arikan AA, Lofis L, Yalavarthy R, Parikh CR, Edelstein CL, Goldstein SL: Urinary interleukin-18 is an acute kidney injury biomarker in critically ill children. *Nephrol Dial Transplant* 2008, **23**:566–572.

65. Parikh CR, Jani A, Mishra J, Ma Q, Kelly C, Barasch J, Edelsteinn CL, Deverajan P: Urine NGAL and IL-18 are predictive biomarkers for delayed graft

function following kidney transplantation. *Am J Transplant* 2006, 6:1639–1645.

66. Wald R, Liangos O, Perianayagam MC, Kolyada A, Herget-Rosenthal S, Mazer CD, Jaber BL: **Plasma cystatin C and acute kidney injury after cardiopulmonary bypass.** *Clin J Am Soc Nephrol* 2010, 5:1373–1379.

67. Koyner JL, Bennet MR, Worcester EM, Ma Q, Raman J, Jeevanadam V, Kasza KE, O'Connor MF, Konczal DJ, Trevino S, Devarajan P, Murray PT: **Urinary cystatin C as an early biomarker of acute kidney injury following adult cardiothoracic surgery.** *Kidney Int* 2008, 74:1059–1069.

68. Dharnidharka VR, Kown C, Stevens G: **Serum cystatin C is superior to serum creatinine as a marker of kidney function: a meta-analysis.** *Am J Kidney Disease* 2002, 40:221–226.

69. Redfors B, Bragadottir G, Sellgren J, Sward K, Rickstein SE: **Acute renal failure is NOT an "acute renal success" – a clinical study on the renal oxygen supply/demand relationship in acute kidney injury.** *Crit Care Med* 2010, 38:1695–1701.

70. Brezis M, Rosen S, Silva P, Epstein FH: **Renal ischemia: a new perspective.** *Kidney Int* 1984, 26:375–383.

71. Bonventre JV, Weinberg JM: **Recent advances in the pathophysiology of ischemic acute renal failure.** *J Am Soc Nephrol* 2003, 14:2199–2210.

72. Callister MEJ, Evans TW: **Pulmonary vs extra-pulmonary ARDS: different disease or just a useful concept.** *Curr Opin Crit Care* 2002, 8:21–25.

73. Okusa MD: **The inflammatory cascade in acute ischemic renal failure.** *Nephron* 2002, 90:133–138.

74. Wan L, Bellomo R, Giantomasso DD, Ronco C: **The pathogenesis of septic acute renal failure.** *Curr Opin Crit Care* 2003, 9:496–502.

75. Fink MP: **Cytopathic hypoxia. Is oxygen use impaired in sepsis as a result of an acquired intrinsic derangement in cellular respiration?** *Crit Care Clin* 2002, 18:165–175.

76. Rahbari NN, Zimmermann JB, Schmidt T, Koch M, Weigand MA, Weitz J: **Meta-analysis of standard, restrictive and supplemental fluid administration in colorectal surgery.** *Br J Surg* 2009, 96:331–341.

77. Prowle JR, Echeverri JE, Ligabo EV, Ronco C, Bellomo R: **Fluid balance and acute kidney injury.** *Nat Rev Nephrol* 2010, 6:107–115.

78. Sugrue M, Jones F, Deane SAG, Bauman A, Hillman K: **Intra-abdominal hypertension is an independent cause of post-operative renal impairment.** *Arch Surg* 1999, 134:1082–1085.

79. McNelis J, Marini CP, Jurkiwicz A, Fields S, Caplin D, Stein D, Ritter G, Nathan I, Simms H: **Predictive factors associated with the development of abdominal compartment syndrome in the surgical intensive care unit.** *Arch Surg* 2002, 137:133–136.

80. Joannidis M, Druml W, Forni LG, Groeneveld ABJ, Honore P, Oudemas-van Straaten HM, Ronco C, Schetz MRC, Wottiez AJ: **Prevention of acute kidney injury and protection of renal function in ITU.** *Intensive Care Med* 2010, 36:392–411.

81. Chappell D, Matthias J, Hofmann-Kiefer K, Conzen P, Rehm M: **A rational approach to perioperative fluid management.** *Anesthesiology* 2008, 109:723–740.

82. Pearse R, Dawson D, Fawcett J, Rhodes A, Grounds RM, Bennett EDI: **Early goal-directed therapy after major surgery reduces complications and duration of hospital stay. A randomized controlled trial.** *Crit Care* 2005, 9: R687–R693.

83. Shoemaker WC, Appel PL, Kram HB: **Hemodynamic and oxygen transport responses in survivors and non-survivors of high-risk surgery.** *Crit Care Med* 1993, 21:977–990.

84. Rhodes A, Cecconi M, Hamilton M, Poloniecki J, Woods J, Boyd O, Bennett D, Grounds RM: **Goal-directed therapy in high-risk surgical patients: a 15-year follow-up study.** *Intensive Care Med* 2010, 36:1327–1332.

85. Haase M, Haase-Fielitz A, Bellomo R, Devararjan P, Story D, Matalanis G, Reade MC, Bagshaw SM, Seevanayagam N, Seevanayagam S, Doolan L, Buxton B, Dragun D: **Sodium bicarbonate to prevent increases in serum creatinine after cardiac surgery: a pilot double-blind, randomized controlled trial.** *Crit Care Med* 2009, 37:39–47.

86. Zacharias M, Conlon NP, Herbison GP, Sivalingam P, Hovhannisyan K: **Interventions for preventing renal function in the perioperative period.** *Cochrane Database Syst Rev* 2008, 8(4) CD003590.

87. *Medicines and Healthcare Products Regulatory Agency: Non-steroidal anti-inflammatory drugs: reminder on renal failure and impairment.* www.mhra. gov.uk/Publications/Safetyguidance/DrugSafetyUpdate/CON088004.

88. McCullough PA, Soman SS: **Contrast induced nephropathy.** *Crit Care Clin* 2005, 21:261–280.

89. Aspelin P, Aubry P, Fransson SG, Strasser R, Willenbrock R, Berg KJ, NEPHRIC Study Investigators: **Nephrotoxic effects in high-risk patients undergoing angiography.** *N Engl J Med* 2003, 348:491–499.

90. Brigouri C, Colombo A, Violante A, Balastrieri P, Manganelli F, Paolo Elia P, Golia B, Lepore S, Riviezzo G, Scarpato P, Focaccio A, Librera M, Bonizzoni E, Ricciardelli B: **Standard vs double dose of N-acetylcysteine to prevent contrast agent associated nephrotoxicity.** *Eur Heart J* 2004, 25:206–211.

91. Habib RH, Zacharias A, Schwann TA: **Role of hemodilutional anemia and transfusion during cardiopulmonary bypass in renal injury after coronary revascularization: implications on operative outcomes.** *Crit Care Med* 2005, 33:1749–1756.

92. Kartouki K, Wijeysundera DN, Yau TM, Callum JL, Cheng DC, Crowther M, Dupuis JY, Fremes SE, Kent B, Laflamme C, Lamy A, Legare JF, Mazer CD, McCLuskey SA, Rubens FD, Sawchuk C, Beattie WS: **Acute kidney injury after cardiac surgery: focus on modifiable risk factors.** *Circulation* 2009, 119:495–502.

93. Murphy GJ, Reeves BC, Rogers CA, Rizvi SI, Culliford L, Angelini GD: **Increased mortality, postoperative morbidity, and cost after red blood cell transfusion in patients having cardiac surgery.** *Circulation* 2007, 116:2544–2552.

94. Kartouki K, Wijeysundera DN, Beattie WS: **Risk associated with preoperative anemia in cardiac surgery: a multicenter cohort study.** *Circulation* 2008, 117:478–484.

95. Kartouki K, Wijeysundera DN, Yau TM, McCluskey SA, Chan CT, Wony PY, Beattie WS: **Influence of erythrocyte transfusion on the risk of acute kidney injury after cardiac surgery differs in anemic and nonanemic patients.** *Anesthesiology* 2011, 115:523–530.

96. Song YR, Lee T, You SJ, Chin HJ, Chae DW, Lim C, Park KH, Han S, Kim JH, Na KY: **Prevention of acute kidney injury by erythropoietin in patients undergoing coronary artery bypass gratfing: a pilot study.** *Am J Nephrol* 2009, 30:253–260.

97. Swaminathan M, Phillips-Bute BG, Conlon PJ, Smith PK, Newman MF, Stafford-Smith M: **The association of lowest hematocrit during cardiopulmonary bypass surgery with acute renal failure after coronary artery bypass surgery.** *Ann Thorac Surg* 2003, 76:784–792.

98. Karkouti K, Beattie WS, Wijeysundera DN, Rao V, Chan C, Dattilo KM, Djaiani G, Ivanon J, Karski J, David TE: **Hemodilution during cardiopulmonary bypass is an independent risk factor for acute renal failure in adult cardiac surgery.** *J Thorac Cardiovasc Surg* 2005, 129:391–400.

99. Society of Thoracic Surgeons Blood Conservation Guideline Task Force, Ferraris VA, Ferraris SP, Saha SP, Hessel EA, Haan CK, Royston BD, Bridges CR, Higgins RS, Despotis G, Brown JR, Society of Cardiovascular Anaesthesiologists Special Task Force on Blood Transfusion, Spiess BD, Shore-Lesserson L, Stafford-Smith M, Mazer CD, Bennett-Guerrero E, Hill E, Body S: **Perioperative blood transfusion and blood conservation in cardiac surgery: the Society of Thoracic Surgeons and The Society of Cardiovascular Anesthesiologists clinical practice guideline.** *Ann Thorac Surg* 2007, 83:S27–S86.

100. Vretzakis G, Kleitsaki A, Stamoulis K, Bareka M, Georgopoulou S, Karanikolas M, Giannoulas A: **Intra-operative intravenous fluid restriction reduces perioperative red blood cell transfusion in elective cardiac surgery, especially in transfusion-prone patients: a prospective, randomized controlled trial.** *J Cardiothorac Surg* 2010, 5:7.

101. Lassnigg A, Donner E, Grubhofer G, Presterl E, Druml W, Hiesmayr M: **Lack of renoprotective effects of dopamine and furosemide during cardiac surgery.** *J Am Soc Nephrol* 2000, 11:97–104.

102. Carcoana OV, Hines RL: **Is renal dose dopamine protective or therapeutic? Yes.** *Crit Care Clin* 1996, 12:677–685.

103. Kellum JA, Decker JM: **Use of dopamine in acute renal failure: A meta-analysis.** *Crit Care Med* 2001, 29:1526–1531.

104. Landoni G, Biondi-Zoccai GG, Marino G, Bove T, Fochi O, Maj G, Calabro MG, Sheiban I, Tumlin JA, Ranucci M, Zangrillo A: **Fenoldopam reduces the need for renal replacement therapy and in-hospital death in cardiovascular surgery: a meta-analysis.** *J Cardiothorac Vasc Anesth* 2008, 22:27–33.

105. Ng MK, Tremmel J, Fitzgerald PJ, Fearon WF: **Selective renal arterial infusion of fenoldopam for the prevention of contrast-induced nephropathy.** *J Interv Cardiol* 2006, 19:75–79.

106. Carcoana OV, Mathew JP, David E, Byrne DW, Hayslett JP, Hines RL, Garwood S: **Mannitol and dopamine in patients undergoing cardiopulmonary bypass: A randomized clinical trial.** *Anesth Analg* 2003, 97:1222–1229.

107. Sirivella S, Gielchinsky I, Parsonnet V: **Mannitol, furosemide, and dopamine infusion in postoperative renal failure complicating cardiac surgery.** *Ann Thorac Surg* 2000, **69**:501–506.

108. Van der Voort PHJ, Boerma EC, Koopmans M, Zandberg M, de Ruiter J, Gerritsen RT, Egbers PH, Kingma WP, Kuiper MA: **Furosemide does not improve renal recovery after hemofiltration for acute renal failure: a double blind randomized controlled trial.** *Crit Care Med* 2009, **37**:533–538.

109. Rigden SP, Dillon MJ, Kind PR, de Leval M, Stark J, Barratt TM: **The beneficial effect of mannitol on postoperative renal function in children undergoing cardiopulmonary bypass surgery.** *Clin Nephrol* 1984, **21**:148–151.

110. Allgren RL, Marbury TC, Rahman SN, Weisberg LS, Fenves AZ, Lafayette RA, Sweet RM, Genter FC, Kurnik BR, Conger JD, Sayegh MH: **Anaritide in acute tubular necrosis: Auriculin Anaritide Acute Renal Failure Study Group.** *N Engl J Med* 1997, **336**:828–834.

111. Lewis J, Salem MM, Chertow GM, Weidberg LS, McGrew F, Marbury TC, Allgren RL: **Atrial natriuretic factor in oliguric acute renal failure. Anaritide Acute Renal Failure Study Group.** *Am J Kidney Dis* 2000, **36**:767–774.

112. Rahman SN, Kim GE, Mathew AS, Goldberg CA, Allgren R, Schrier RW, Conger JD: **Effects of atrial natriuretic peptide in clinical acute renal failure.** *Kidney Int* 1994, **45**:1731–1738.

113. Sward K, Valsson F, Odencrants P, Samuelsson O, Ricksten SE: **Recombinant human atrial natriuretic peptide in ischemic acute renal failure: a randomized placebo-controlled trial.** *Crit Care Med* 2004, **32**:1310–1315.

114. Nigewaker SU, Navaneethan SD, Parikh CR, Hix JK: **Atrial natriuretic peptide for management of acute kidney injury: a systematic review and meta-analysis.** *Clin J Am Soc Nephrol* 2009, **4**:261–272.

115. Mentzer RM, Oz MC, Sladen RC, Graeve AH, Hebeler RF Jr, Luber JM Jr, Smedira NG, NAPA Investigators: **Effects of perioperative nesiritide in patients with left ventricular dysfunction undergoing cardiac surgery: The NAPA trial.** *J Am Coll Cardiol* 2007, **49**:716–726.

116. Sackner-Bernstein JD, Kowalski M, Fox M, Aaronson K: **Short-term risk of death after treatment with nesiritide for decompensated heart failure: a pooled analysis of randomized controlled trials.** *JAMA* 2005, **293**:1900–1905.

117. Bagshaw SM, Ghali A: **Theophylline for prevention of contrast-induced nephrology.** *Arch Intern Med* 2005, **165**:1087–1093.

118. Kramer BK, Preuner J, Ebenburger A, Kaiser M, Bergner U, Eilles C, Kammerl MC, Riegger GAJ, Birnbaum DE: **Lack of renoprotective effect of theophylline during aortocoronary bypass surgery.** *Nephrol Dial Transplant* 2002, **17**:910–915.

119. Adabag AS, Ishani A, Bloomfoeld HE, Ngo AK, Wilt TJ: **Efficacy of N-acetylcysteine in preventing renal injury after heart surgery: a systematic review of randomized trials.** *Eur Heart Journal* 2009, **30**:1910–1917.

120. Nigwekar SU, Kandula P: **N-acetylcysteine in cardiovascular-surgery-associated renal failure: a meta-analysis.** *Ann Thorac Surg* 2009, **87**:139–147.

121. Van de Berghe G, Wouters P, Weekers F, Verwaest C, Bruyninckx F, Schetz M, Vlasselaers D, Ferdinande P, Lauwers P, Bouillon R: **Intensive insulin therapy in critically ill patients.** *N Engl J Med* 2001, **345**:1359–1367.

122. Lena D, Kalfon P, Preiser JC, Ichai C: **Glycemic control in the Intensive Care Unit and during the postoperative period.** *Anesthesiology* 2011, **114**:438–444.

123. Duncan AE, Abd-Elsayed A, Maheshwari A, Xu M, Soltesz E, Koch CG: **Role of intraoperative and postoperative blood glucose concentrations in predicting outcomes after cardiac surgery.** *Anesthesiology* 2010, **112**:860–871.

124. Durmaz I, Yagdi T, Calkavur T, Mahmudiv R, Apaydon AZ, Posacioglu H, Atay Y, Engin C: **Prophylactic dialysis in patients with renal dysfunction undergoing on-pump coronary artery bypass surgery.** *Ann Thorac Surg* 2003, **75**:859–864.

125. Marenzi G, Marana I, Lauri G, Assanelli E, Grazi M, Campodonico J, Trabattoni D, Fabiocchi F, Montorsi P, Bartorelli AL: **The prevention of radiocontrast-agent-induced nephropathy by hemofiltration.** *N Eng J Med* 2003, **349**:1333–1340.

126. Ostermann M, Chang R: **Correlation between the AKI classification and outcome.** *Crit Care* 2008, **12**:R144.

127. Granado RC, Mehta RL: **Assessing and delivering dialysis dose in acute kidney injury.** *Semin Dial* 2011, **24**:157–163.

128. Ronco C, Bellomo R, Homel P, Brendolan A, Dan M, Piccinni P, La Greca G: **Effects of different doses in continuous veno-venous haemofiltration on outcomes of acute renal failure: A prospective randomised trial.** *Lancet* 2000, **356**:26–30.

129. Tolwani AJ, Campbell RC, Stofan BS, Lai KR, Oster RA, Wille KM: **Standard versus high dose CVVHDF for ICU-related acute renal failure.** *J Am Soc Nephrol* 2008, **19**:1233–1238.

130. Bellomo R, Cass A, Cole L, Finfer S, Gallagher M, Lo S, McArthur C, McGuiness S, Myburgh J, Norton R, Scheinkestel C, Su S: **Intensity of continuous renal replacement therapy in critically ill patients.** *N Engl J Med* 2009, **361**:1627–1638.

131. Palevsky PM, Zhang JH, O'Connor TZ, Chertow GM, Crowley ST, Choudhury D, Finkel K, Kellum JA, Paganini E, Schein RM, Smith MW, Swanson KM, Thompson BT, Vijayan A, Watnick S, Star RA, Peduzzi P: **Intensity of renal support in critically ill patients with acute kidney injury.** *N Engl J Med* 2008, **359**:7–20.

23

Neither dynamic, static, nor volumetric variables can accurately predict fluid responsiveness early after abdominothoracic esophagectomy

Hironori Ishihara[*], Eiji Hashiba, Hirobumi Okawa, Junichi Saito, Toshinori Kasai and Toshihito Tsubo

Abstract

Background: Hypotension is common in the early postoperative stages after abdominothoracic esophagectomy for esophageal cancer. We examined the ability of stroke volume variation (SVV), pulse pressure variation (PPV), central venous pressure (CVP), intrathoracic blood volume (ITBV), and initial distribution volume of glucose (IDVG) to predict fluid responsiveness soon after esophagectomy under mechanical ventilation (tidal volume >8 mL/kg) without spontaneous respiratory activity.

Methods: Forty-three consecutive non-arrhythmic patients undergoing abdominothoracic esophagectomy were studied. SVV, PPV, cardiac index (CI), and indexed ITBV (ITBVI) were postoperatively measured by single transpulmonary thermodilution (PiCCO system) after patient admission to the intensive care unit (ICU) on the operative day. Indexed IDVG (IDVGI) was then determined using the incremental plasma glucose concentration 3 min after the intravenous administration of 5 g glucose. Fluid responsiveness was defined by an increase in CI >15% compared with pre-loading CI following fluid volume loading with 250 mL of 10% low molecular weight dextran.

Results: Twenty-three patients were responsive to fluids while 20 were not. The area under the receiver-operating characteristic (ROC) curve was the highest for CVP (0.690) and the lowest for ITBVI (0.584), but there was no statistical difference between tested variables. Pre-loading IDVGI (r = −0.523, P <0.001), SVV (r = 0.348, P = 0.026) and CVP (r = −0.307, P = 0.046), but not PPV or ITBVI, were correlated with a percentage increase in CI after fluid volume loading.

Conclusions: These results suggest that none of the tested variables can accurately predict fluid responsiveness early after abdominothoracic esophagectomy.

Keywords: Cardiac preload, Esophagectomy, Fluid responsiveness, Glucose, Intrathoracic blood volume, Stroke volume variation

Background

Abdominothoracic esophagectomy for esophageal cancer is a major surgical procedure with high rates of morbidity and mortality [1]. According to our experience, approximately 60% of patients who undergo esophagectomy develop hypotension requiring subsequent fluid volume loading during the first 15-h postoperative period, even though cardiovascular states immediately after surgery are relatively stable and/or postoperative bloody drainage is minimal [2].

Over the last decade, respiratory variations or dynamic preload variables such as stroke volume variation (SVV) and pulse pressure variation (PPV) have been reported to be better predictors of fluid responsiveness than commonly monitored static preload variables such as cardiac filling pressures [3,4], even though SVV or PPV measurements generally require mechanical ventilation (tidal volume >8 mL/kg) in the absence of spontaneous breathing and/or cardiac arrhythmias [4,5]. However, Cannesson *et al.* [6] recently showed that approximately 25% of patients undergoing prediction of fluid responsiveness are in the 'grey zone' of PPV and that a 'black-or-white' decision based on the receiver-operating characteristic

* Correspondence: concerto0328@yahoo.co.jp
Department of Anesthesiology, Hirosaki University Graduate School of Medicine, 5 Zaifu-Cho, Hirosaki-Shi 036-8562, Japan

(ROC) curve approach does not fit the reality of clinical or screening practice.

To our knowledge, only one study has measured SVV after esophagectomy, suggesting that SVV is clinically relevant as a guide of fluid volume management [7]. However, as this measurement was made in the presence of spontaneous respiratory activity (pressure support ventilation), it would be of limited use in evaluating fluid responsiveness. Abdominothoracic esophagectomy can lead to hemodynamic instability soon after the operation [8] and may also modify the original thoracic structure, decreasing the constraints of the chest wall imposed on the heart and the lungs and altering cyclic changes in intrathoracic pressure on heart-lung interactions. We therefore hypothesized that studies into fluid responsiveness would be of limited value during such hemodynamically unstable states.

The initial distribution volume of glucose (IDVG) has been proposed as a representative of the central extracellular fluid (ECF) volume status without significant modification of glucose metabolism [9,10], and can be measured simply and rapidly in any intensive care unit (ICU) by injecting a small amount of glucose (5 g) and determining plasma glucose changes 3 min post injection [11]. Measurements can also be repeated at 30-min intervals without sustained increases in plasma glucose [12]. We previously reported that IDVG, rather than intrathoracic blood volume (ITBV) or central venous pressure (CVP), is closely correlated with cardiac output (CO) during hypotension and subsequent fluid volume loading early after esophagectomy [8]. Moreover, IDVG was recently reported to predict hypovolemic hypotension early after abdominal aortic surgery [13] and to have an inverse correlation with PPV after the induction of anesthesia in neurosurgical patients [14]. Accordingly, IDVG has the potential to be a useful marker of fluid responsiveness.

This study aimed to evaluate the ability of currently available preload variables such as SVV, PPV, CVP, and ITBV as well as IDVG to predict fluid responsiveness early after admission to the ICU following abdominothoracic esophagectomy.

Methods

Ethical approval for this study was provided by the Ethical Committee of Hirosaki University Graduate School of Medicine, Hirosaki, Japan, and each patient gave written informed consent before surgery. The study was planned to consist of at least 31 hypotensive patients, since a sample size of 31 is required to detect differences of 0.10 between areas under the ROC curve (5% type I error rate, 80% power, two-tailed test) [15]. Patients with aortic aneurysms and/or sustained arrhythmias including atrial fibrillation were excluded from the study. Those with

diabetes mellitus and/or cardiovascular diseases such as hypertension without apparent ischemic heart disease were included. Preoperative echocardiographic measurements of left ventricular ejection fraction were required to exceed 60%.

Each patient underwent radical surgery for esophageal cancer that was performed using a right thoracoabdominal approach together with extensive resection of adjacent lymph nodes, subcarinal lymph nodes and/or cervical lymph nodes. Fluid and cardiovascular management decisions during anesthesia, including amounts of crystalloid solution and use of colloidal solutions, blood products or vasoactive drugs, were made by individual anesthesiologists. No patients received a continuous infusion of vasoactive drugs during anesthesia. Neither vasoactive drugs nor blood products were administered when patients arrived at the ICU. All patients postoperatively received controlled mechanical ventilation (tidal volume >8 mL/kg of ideal body weight), with peak airway pressure above positive end-expiratory pressure (10–15 cmH_2O, respiratory rate 12-15/min) with a low positive end-expiratory pressure (<5 cm H_2O) and continuous infusions of propofol (2–3 mg/kg/h) and morphine (0.4-0.8 mg/h) at least until the completion of the study. Supplemental midazolam (2–6 mg/h) was infused to achieve complete control of ventilation without spontaneous respiration during the study period. The infusion rate of these sedatives and analgesics was kept constant from at least 30 min before and during the study period. Although each patient had a thoracic epidural catheter for postoperative analgesia, epidural analgesia was only started after completion of the study.

Both 4.3% glucose solution with electrolytes and lactated Ringer's solution were infused simultaneously at a constant rate of 1.5 mL/kg/h and 1.0 mL/kg/h, respectively, for at least 12 h after surgery. No vasoactive drugs were administered throughout the study period. One patient required continuous infusion of insulin (1 U/h) throughout the study period.

Measurement of fluid volume loading

Measurements were made twice: the first was taken during the 90 min after postoperative admission to the ICU on the operative day in the absence of apparent hypotension (pre-loading) followed by fluid volume loading with 250 mL of 10% low molecular weight dextran 40 (Otsuka Pharmaceutical Factory Inc., Tokyo, Japan) over a period of 20 min. The second measurement was made 10 min after completion of fluid volume loading (post-loading).

A right subclavian venous catheter had been put in place before the operative day. A thermistor tipped catheter for thermodilution and pulse contour analysis (PV2015L20N, Pulsion, Munich, Germany) was inserted into a femoral artery and connected to the PiCCO monitoring system (PiCCO plus, Pulsion) in the ICU immediately after surgery as described elsewhere [16]. Transducers monitoring arterial pressure and CVP were positioned at the mid-axillary level with atmospheric pressure used as the zero reference level. Ten mL of cold isotonic saline solution (<8°C) was injected through the right subclavian venous line to determine CO and ITBV before and after fluid volume loading. A variation of ±10% within triplicate measurements of CO was defined as acceptable. Coefficients of variation for repeated CO measurements were ≤7.3%. SVV and PPV were recorded automatically as percentage changes using the PiCCO monitoring system [16].

Immediately after these measurements were taken, 10 mL of 50% glucose solution (Otsuka Pharmaceutical Factory Inc.) (5 g) was injected through the same central venous line to calculate the IDVG. Blood samples were obtained through a radial artery catheter immediately before and 3 min after the injection. Plasma was separated immediately, and measurements of glucose concentrations were performed within 5 min of sampling. Plasma glucose concentrations of all blood samples were measured using amperometry by a glucose oxidase immobilized membrane-H_2O_2 electrode (glucose analyzer GA-1150; Arkray Co, Ltd, Kyoto, Japan). IDVG was calculated using the difference between plasma glucose concentrations immediately before and 3 min after the glucose injection as described previously [11]. Measurements were made in duplicate. Coefficients of variation for repeated measurements were 1.0% or less for plasma glucose (range, 3.0-17.0 mmol/L). Routine hemodynamic and clinical variables including automated SVV and PPV were recorded immediately before each volume measurement.

Statistical analysis

Unless otherwise stated, data are presented as mean (SD) and median (interquartile range) values. ITBV, stroke volume, CO, and IDVG are indexed to body surface area based on the reported preoperative height and body weight. Statistical analysis was performed with SigmaPlot 12 (Systat Software Inc., San Jose, CA, USA). Pre- and post-volume loading variables were compared using a paired t-test for normally distributed data. The Wilcoxon signed rank test was used for data that were not normally distributed.

Fluid responsiveness was defined by an increase in cardiac index (CI) >15% as reported previously [17,18], since most reports using the percentage increase in CO or stroke volume (SV) for this purpose set the threshold value at 10% or 15% after a 250 or 500 mL fluid challenge [4]. The ability to predict fluid responsiveness was quantified for each preload variable by calculating the area under the ROC curve. The diagnostic value was

defined from this value as: excellent, >0.85; good, >0.75; and poor 0.50-0.75 [19]. The cutoff value was chosen to minimize the mathematical distance to the ideal point (sensitivity = specificity = 1). Pearson's linear correlation was performed to determine the relationship between each preloading variable and the percentage changes in CI after fluid volume loading (△CI), between each actual preloading and postloading variable and the corresponding CI, and between changes in each preloading and postloading variable and those in CI. P <0.05 was considered significant.

Results

Initially, 45 consecutive patients with no arrhythmias after esophagectomy were recruited to the study. Of these, two were excluded because of technical problems in measuring CO, and the development of hypotension soon after admission to the ICU, requiring fluid volume loading during the first measurement. Thus, 43 consecutive patients were finally enrolled into the study. Of these, 23 patients were responsive to fluids and 20 were not.

Table 1 shows patient demographics and fluid management during anesthesia and surgery. Only the amounts of administered lactated Ringer's solution and estimated intraoperative blood loss different between the groups (P = 0.030, respectively). During the study period, two patients had apparent continuous air leakage from the chest drainage tube so their SVV and PPV data were excluded to prevent inaccuracies [20]. Table 2 shows the comparison of cardiovascular variables and tidal volume between responders and non-responders. Only pre-loading CVP and IDVGI differed between these two groups (P = 0.033 and P = 0.043, respectively), and the remaining variables showed no differences (Table 3).

The area under the ROC curve for evaluation of the ability to predict fluid responsiveness was highest for CVP (0.690) and lowest for ITBVI (0.584), but this difference was not statistically significant (Figure 1, Table 4). Pre-loading IDVGI was inversely correlated with △CI (r = −0.523, P <0.001), and pre-loading SVV and CVP were slightly correlated with △CI (r = 0.348, P = 0.026 and r = −0.307, P = 0.046, respectively) (Figure 2). Neither preloading PPV nor ITBVI were correlated with △CI (r = 0.288, P = 0.068 and r = −0.148, P = 0.345, respectively).

Using all data before and after fluid volume loading, actual or changed IDVGI showed the highest correlation with actual and changed CI, respectively (Table 5).

Discussion

Most fluid responsiveness studies have been performed in the absence of severe hypotension. For ethical reasons, however, it is not appropriate to give fluid volume loading to normotensive patients, particularly non-responders in

Table 1 Patients demographics and fluid management during anesthesia and surgery

	Responders (n = 23)	Non-responders (n = 20)	P[z]
Gender (Male/Female)	22/1	20/0	1.000
Age (years)	65 ± 6 (66, 60–69)	65 ± 7 (65, 61–70)	0.815
Height (m)	1.65 ± 0.05 (1.67, 1.63-1.70)	1.66 ± 0.05 (1.67, 1.63-1.70)	0.279
Preoperative body weight (kg)	60.9 ± 8.6 (60.9, 56.9-64.8)	59.8 ± 7.9 (60.0, 54.1-67.6)	0.702
Body surface area (m^2)	1.67 ± 0.12 (1.68, 1.59-1.74)	1.67 ± 0.11(1.68, 1.60-1.75)	0.970
Duration of surgery (hrs)	6.9 ± 1.3, (6.6, 6.3- 7.6)	7.3 ± 1.1, (7.2, 6.8- 7.8)	0.090
Lactated Ringer's solution (L)	4.6 ± 1.0 (4.5, 3.9-5.0)	5.4 ± 1.3 (5.6, 4.5-6.0)	0.030
Patients receiving packed red cell (n)	5 (260–520)	3 (260–780)	0.704
Patients receiving colloids (n)	8 (250–750)	7 (250–1320)	1.000
Urine output (mL)	600 ± 390 (410, 310–770)	610 ± 390 (480, 330–790)	0.808
Estimated blood loss (g)	750 ± 400 (650, 470–1000)	810 ± 490 (680, 520–900)	0.030

Data are presented as mean ± SD (median, interquartile range) or as number of patients (range of administered volume).
[a]Between responders and non-responders.

this study who received a large fluid volume during anesthesia and surgery, unless some indication is present.

Major surgical procedures result in a shift of the ECF from the central to the peripheral compartment as well as generalized capillary protein and water leakage both intra- and postoperatively [21]. Indeed, two patients in the present study recorded decreased CI despite fluid volume loading. Furthermore, most patients in this study required additional volume loading and/or an infusion of noradrenaline to overcome repeated hypotension throughout the first postoperative day. As hypotension development can be affected by hypovolemia and changes in peripheral vascular resistance, we believe that our study is ethically appropriate even in the absence of severe hypotension early after abdominothoracic esophagectomy.

The present study demonstrates that none of the tested variables can accurately predict fluid responsiveness soon after abdominothoracic esophagectomy, as assessed by the area under the ROC curve, even though definitions of fluid responsiveness may have a major impact on the results of SVV or PPV validity [22]. Fluid responders in this study were defined by an increase in CI >15% after fluid volume loading as reported previously [17,18]. When CI or stroke volume index (SVI) for evaluating fluid responsiveness set the threshold value at 10%, the number of fluid responders and non-responders differed (31 versus 12 for CI at 10%, and 33 versus 10 for SVI at 10%) suggesting that ROC curve analysis is inadequate since it assumes an expected rate of fluid responsiveness of 50% [6,23]. When the threshold value for SVI was set at

Table 2 Comparison of routine cardiovascular variables and tidal volume between responders and non-responders

		Responders	Non-responders	P[a]
Heart rate (bpm)	Pre	74 ± 13 (73, 66–80)	69 ± 11 (69, 59–77)	0.143
	Post	75 ± 12 (73, 65–80)	69 ± 9 (68, 62–77)	0.066
Mean arterial pressure (mmHg)	Pre	82 ± 14 (82, 70–88)	86 ± 16 (83, 75–95)	0.301
	Post	93 ± 15 (90, 83–105)[b]	93 ± 14 (93, 82–100)[c]	0.91
Cardiac index (L/min/m^2)	Pre	2.6 ± 0.5 (2.6, 2.2-3.0)	2.9 ± 0.3 (2.9, 2.7-3.1)	0.063
	Post	3.4 ± 0.6 (3.4, 2.9-3.8)[b]	3.1 ± 0.3 (3.1, 2.9-3.4)[b]	0.095
Stoke volume index (mL/m^2)	Pre	36.4 ± 7.7 (34.5, 31.2-42.4)	42.5 ± 5.4 (42.8,38.6-47.5)	0.005
	Post	46.4 ± 7.6 (47.3, 39.8-52.2)[b]	45.6 ± 4.3 (46.4, 42.2-48.9)[b]	0.635
Hematocrit (%)	Pre	30.9 ± 4.4 (29.5, 27.4-32.7)	30.4 ± 4.0 (29.8, 27.7-32.1)	0.855
	Post	27.5 ± 4.1 (26.7, 24.5-29.6)[b]	27.9 ± 4.1 (27.6, 25.5-29.8)[b]	0.661
Tidal volume (mL/kg)[d]		9.0 ± 1.0 (8.8, 8.3-9.4)	8.8 ± 0.8 (8.5, 8.1-9.3)	0.342

Data are presented as mean ± SD (median, interquartile range).
[a]Between responders and non-responders.
[b]P <0.001 as compared with pre-fluid loading.
[c]P <0.05.
[d]Per kg of ideal body weight.
Pre, Immediately before volume loading; Post, 10 min after volume loading.

Table 3 Comparison of cardiac preload variables between responders and non-responders

		Responders	Non-responders	P^a
Stroke volume variation (%)	Pre	13.9 ± 4.6 (13.0, 11.0-16.3)	12.2 ± 4.1 (11.5, 9.0-15.5)	0.232
	Post	7.8 ± 4.1 (7.0, 4.8-10.3)[b]	6.4 ± 2.2 (6.0, 5.0-7.0)[b]	0.27
Pulse pressure variation (%)	Pre	10.6 ± 3.5 (9.0, 8.0-13.0)	8.7 ± 3.7 (8.5, 6.0-11.0)	0.107
	Post	4.9 ± 2.4 (4.0, 3.5-5.0)[b]	4.5 ± 1.4 (4.0, 3.5-5.0)[b]	0.862
Central venous pressure (mmHg)	Pre	5 ± 2 (5, 4–7)	7 ± 3 (7, 5–9)	0.033
	Post	7 ± 2 (8, 6–9)[b]	9 ± 2 (9, 8–11)[b]	0.008
ITBVI(L/m^2)	Pre	0.78 ± 0.1 (0.78, 0.72-0.85)	0.81 ± 0.09 (0.83, 0.75-0.87)	0.292
	Post	0.84 ± 0.09 (0.85, 0.77-0.91)[b]	0.84 ± 0.10 (0.84, 0.76-0.89)	0.964
IDVGI(L/m^2)	Pre	4.2 ± 0.7 (4.2, 3.9-4.8)	4.6 ± 0.5 (4.6, 4.3-4.8)	0.043
	Post	4.8 ± 0.7 (4.9, 4.4-5.3)[b]	4.9 ± 0.6 (5.0, 4.8-5.2)[b]	0.574

Data are presented as mean ± SD (median, interquartile range).
[a]Between responders and non-responders.
[b]P <0.001 as compared with pre-fluid volume loading values.
ITBVI, Indexed intrathoraci blood volume; IDVGI, Indexed initial distribution volume of glucose; Pre, Immediately before volume loading; Post, 10 min after volume loading.

15%, only SVV reached the lowest edge of a 'good' diagnostic value (0.757), but there was no statistical difference among tested variables indicating no obvious difference from the present results(Additional file 1: Figure S1). Accordingly, we believe that a threshold value of 15% for CI in this study was adequate, even though the 'grey zone' approach has been proposed to avoid the binary

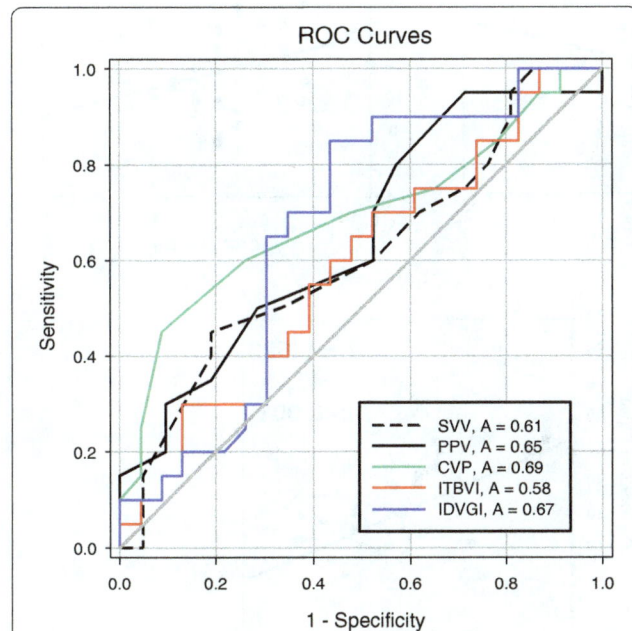

Figure 1 Receiver-operating characteristic (ROC) curves comparing the ability of various preload variables to discriminate responders and non-responders. CVP, Central venous pressure; IDVGI, Indexed initial distribution volume of glucose; ITBVI, Indexed intrathoracic blood volume; PPV, Pulse pressure variation; SVV, Stroke volume variation.

constraints of a 'black-or-white' decision of the ROC curve approach [6].

The open-chest surgical procedure was performed with a right thoracoabdominal approach and it is likely that the extensive resection of adjacent lymph nodes, subcarinal lymph nodes, cervical lymph nodes and esophageal substitution such as gastric advancement would modify the intrathoracic structure. Furthermore, postoperative left pleural effusion was common. Two of the 43 patients experienced continuous air leakage from the chest drainage tube, so were excluded from the SVV and PPV study to avoid potential inaccuracies [20]. Indeed, these two patients had a low SVV (both 7%) and PPV (11% and 7%), despite an obvious increase in △CI (71% and 34%). Although a closed-chest condition after open-chest coronary artery bypass graft surgery enables the assessment of fluid responsiveness [24], changes in these thoracic structures and reduction of the pericardial constraint may have abated the effects of cyclic changes in intrathoracic pressure to heart-lung interactions even in the absence of an open-chest condition after esophagectomy. Such pathophysiology may lead to inaccuracies in respiratory variation results.

Of the variables tested, only pre-loading IDVGI had an inverse correlation with △CI following fluid volume loading in this study (power = 0.956). We used 250 mL of 10% dextran 40 solution for fluid volume loading, which has an oncotic pressure of 40 mmHg. Subsequent increments in plasma volume can exceed its infusion volume by up to 1.5 times while depleting the interstitial fluid volume [25], which could have an important impact on IDVG after fluid volume loading since IDVG represents both intravascular volume and the interstitial fluid volume of highly perfused tissues [10]. An inconsistent increase in IDVG associated with

Table 4 Diagnostic parameters for predicting fluid responsiveness

	Area under ROC curve	95% CI	Best threshold	Sensitivity (%)	Specificity (%)	PPV (%)	NPV (%)
SVV (%)	0.609	0.433-0.785	10.5	45	81	70	60
PPVa (%)	0.651	0.481-0.821	8.5	50	71	64	59
CVP (mmHg)	0.69	0.524-0.856	6.5	60	74	70	65
ITBVI (L/m²)	0.584	0.410-0.758	0.78	65	48	55	58
IDVGI (L/m²)	0.666	0.497-0.835	4.23	85	57	66	79

CI, Confidence interval; CVP, Central venous pressure; IDVGI, Indexed initial distribution volume of glucose; ITBVI, Indexed intrathoracic blood volume; NPV, Negative predictive value; PPV, Positive predictive value; PPVa, Pulse pressure variation; SVV, Stroke volume variation.

unchanged mean arterial pressure after colloid loading has also been reported following cardiac surgery [26]. Additionally, Harvey *et al.* [27] showed that IDVG and systolic area variability could not predict fluid responsiveness following cardiac surgery. Presumably, the presence of hemodynamically unstable states caused by internal bleeding, temperature change, alteration in vasomotor tone, or fluid shifts between compartments during volume loading rather than methodological flaws of IDVG would also play a role in these inconsistent results [28].

Although this study showed the limited predictive value of tested variables for fluid responsiveness, measurement of IDVG is desirable when either hypotension or decreases in arterial blood pressure occur early after abdominothoracic esophagectomy since IDVG has the highest correlation with CO, as reported previously [8]. When a small IDVG (<110 mL/kg) is observed, fluid volume loading is indicated and *vice versa*. However, an infusion of noradrenaline is indicated when a large IDVG (>130 mL/kg) is observed.

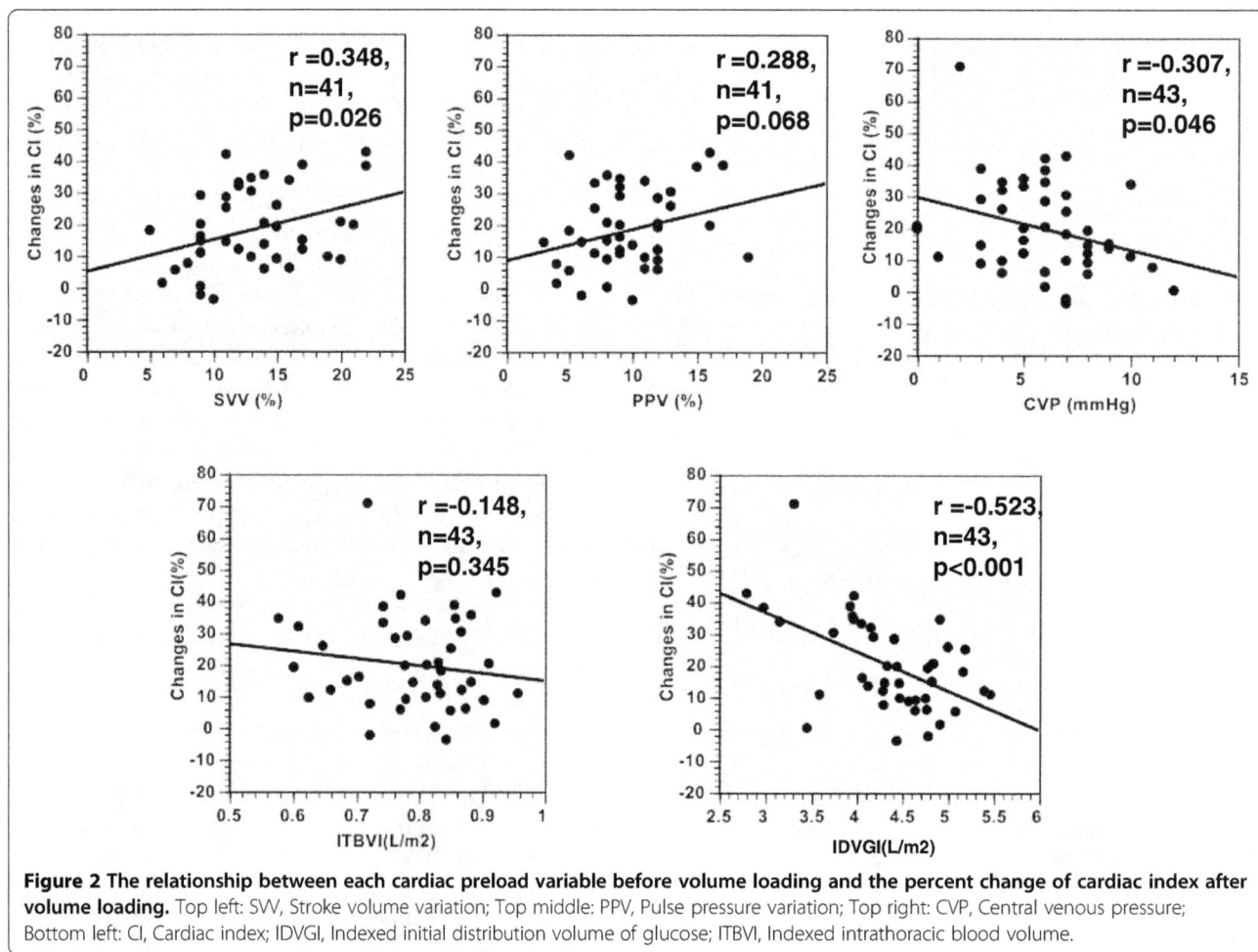

Figure 2 The relationship between each cardiac preload variable before volume loading and the percent change of cardiac index after volume loading. Top left: SVV, Stroke volume variation; Top middle: PPV, Pulse pressure variation; Top right: CVP, Central venous pressure; Bottom left: CI, Cardiac index; IDVGI, Indexed initial distribution volume of glucose; ITBVI, Indexed intrathoracic blood volume.

Table 5 Correlation coefficient with cardiac index using pre-and post-fluid volume loading data

	Actual values (r) (n = 86)	Changed values (r) (n = 43)
SVV (%)	−0.367 (P <0.001)[a]	−0.0445 (P = 0.782)[b]
PPV (%)	−0.414 (P <0.001)[a]	−0.0158 (P = 0.922)[b]
CVP (mmHg)	0.320 (P = 0.003)	−0.0530 (P = 0.736)
ITBVI (L/m²)	0.335 (P = 0.002)	0.215 (P = 0.165)
IDVGI (L/m²)	0.561 (P <0.001)	0.473 (P = 0.001)

[a]$n = 82$.
[b]$n = 41$.
CVP, Central venous pressure; IDVGI, Indexed initial distribution volume of glucose; ITBVI, Indexed intrathoracic blood volume; PPV, Pulse pressure variation; SVV, Stroke volume variation.

The present study has a number of limitations. First, most studies on fluid responsiveness evaluated post-fluid volume loading variables at the completion of fluid volume loading or soon after its completion [6,18,29]. In this study, however, its measurement was performed 10 min after completion of fluid volume loading as reported previously [8], since a minimum interval of 30 min is required for repeated IDVG measurements to avoid sustained hyperglycemia [12]. Consequently, many of the important signals may have been lost during this 10-min period, particularly during hemodynamic unstable states. However, the magnitude of an increase in CI after fluid volume loading in fluid responders of this study was comparable or even greater than other fluid responsive studies [6,30], supporting the idea that the poor predictive values of tested variables were not attributable to insufficient signals in post-fluid loading measurements.

Second, we used 10% low molecular weighted dextran for fluid volume loading as reported previously [8], although 6% hydroxyethyl starch (medium molecular weight: 200,000 Da) is now widely used for this purpose and may have been more desirable in our study. However, considering the almost equivalent effects of either colloid on plasma volume expansion [25], it is likely that we can extrapolate our results to studies using 6% hydroxyethyl starch.

Third, we administered a fixed amount of dextran rather than an amount based on body weight. However, as determined by preoperative body weight, its variability was lower than that of other fluid responsiveness studies [6,20,23], reflecting insufficient preoperative nutritional status. As a lower preoperative body weight was observed in the majority of patients prior to diagnosis of esophageal cancer, most were administered approximately 4 mL/kg dextran.

Fourth, we did not test fluid responsiveness in the presence of hypotension or cardiac compromised conditions. Nevertheless, preload variables might be useful during hemodynamically unstable states such as hypotension when either fluid volume loading or an infusion of vasoactive drugs is required. Further studies are therefore required to assess this. Finally, we did not evaluate simultaneous echocardiography so an adequate view of cardiac chambers could not be consistently obtained following surgery for esophageal cancer.

Conclusions

Our data demonstrate that none of the dynamic, static, or volumetric variables measured in this study can be accurately used as a predictor of fluid volume responsiveness early after abdominothoracic esophagectomy.

Abbreviations
CI: Cardiac index; CO: Cardiac output; CVP: Central venous pressure; ECF: Extracellular fluid; GEDV: Global end-diastolic volume; IDVG: Initial distribution volume of glucose; ITBV: Intrathoracic blood volume; MTT: Mean transit time; PEEP: Positive end-expiratory pressure; PPV: Pulse pressure variation; ROC: Receiver operating characteristic; SV: Stroke volume; SVI: Stroke volume index; SVV: Stroke volume variation.

Competing interests
The authors declare that they have no competing interests.

Authors' contributions
HI conceived of the study, designed the study, carried out data collection, statistical analysis, and drafted the manuscript. EH participated in its design and helped to draft the manuscript. JS, TK, HO, and TT participated in the data collection from the patients. All authors read and approved the final manuscript.

References
1. Brodner G, Pogatzki E, Van Aken H, Buerkle H, Goeters C, Schulzki C, Nottberg H, Mertes N: A multimodal approach to control postoperative pathophysiology and rehabilitation in patients undergoing abdominothoracic esophagectomy. *Anesth Analg* 1998, **86**:228–234.
2. Suzuki A, Ishihara H, Okawa H, Tsubo T, Matsuki A: Can initial distribution volume of glucose predict hypovolemic hypotension after radical surgery for esophageal cancer? *Anesth Analg* 2001, **92**:1146–1151.
3. Bendjelid K, Romand J-A: Fluid responsiveness in mechanically ventilated patients: a review of indices used in intensive care. *Intensive Care Med* 2003, **29**:352–360.
4. Marik PE, Cavallazzi R, Vasu T, Hirani A: Dynamic changes in arterial waveform derived variables and fluid responsiveness in mechanically ventilated patients: a systematic review of the literature. *Crit Care Med* 2009, **37**:2642–2647.
5. Maguire S, Rinehart J, Vakharia S, Cannesson M: Technical communication: respiratory variation in pulse pressure and plethysmographic waveforms: intraoperative applicability in a North American academic center. *Anesth Analg* 2011, **112**:94–96.
6. Cannesson M, Manach YL, Hofer CK, Goarin JP, Lehot J-J, Vallet B, Tavernier B: Assessing the diagnostic accuracy of pulse pressure variations for the prediction of fluid responsiveness. A "Gray Zone" Approach. *Anesthesiology* 2011, **135**:231–241.

7.   Kobayashi M, Koh M, Irinoda T, Meguro E, Hayakawa Y, Takagane A: **Stroke volume variation as a predictor of intravascular volume depression and possible hypotension during the early postoperative period after esophagectomy.** *Ann Surg Oncol* 2009, **16**:1371–1377.

8.   Ishihara H, Nakamura H, Okawa H, Yatsu Y, Tsubo T, Hirota K: **Comparison of initial distribution volume of glucose and intrathoracic blood volume during hemodynamically unstable states early after esophagectomy.** *Chest* 2005, **128**:1713–1719.

9.   Ishihara H, Suzuki A, Okawa H, Ebina T, Tsubo T, Matsuki A: **Comparison of the initial distribution volume of glucose and plasma volume in thoracic fluid-accumulated patients.** *Crit Care Med* 2001, **29**:1532–1538.

10. Iwakawa T, Ishihara H, Takamura K, Sakai I, Suzuki A: **Measurements of extracellular fluid volume in highly perfused organs and lung water in hypo- and hypervolaemic dogs.** *Eur J Anaesthesiol* 1998, **15**:414–421.

11. Ishihara H, Nakamura H, Okawa H, Takase H, Tsubo T, Hirota K: **Initial distribution volume of glucose can be approximated using a conventional glucose analyzer in the intensive care unit.** *Crit Care* 2005, **9**:R144–R149.

12. Rose BO, Ishihara H, Okawa H, Panning B, Piepenbrock S, Matsuki A: **Repeatability of measurements of the initial distribution volume of glucose in haemodynamically stable patients.** *J Clin Pharm Ther* 2004, **29**:317–323.

13. Orban JC, Blasin-Chadoutaud A, Zolfaghari P, Ishihara H, Grimaud D, Ichai C: **Hypovolaemic hypotension after abdominal aortic surgery is predicted by initial distribution volume of glucose.** *Eur J Anaesthesiol* 2010, **27**:364–368.

14. He Z, Qiao H, Zhou W, Wang Y, Xu Z, Che X, Zhang J, Liang W: **Assessment of cardiac preload status by pulse pressure variation in patients after anesthesia induction: comparison with central venous pressure and initial distribution volume of glucose.** *J Anesth* 2011, **25**:812–817.

15. Obuchowski NA: **Sample size tables for receiver operating characteristic studies.** *Am J Roentgenol* 2000, **175**:603–608.

16. Sakka SG, Rühl CC, Pfeiffer UJ, Beale R, McLuckie A, Reinhart K, Meier-Hellmann A: **Assessment of cardiac preload and extravascular lung water by single transpulmonary thermodilution.** *Intensive Care Med* 2000, **26**:180–187.

17. Huang C-C, Fu J-Y, Hu H-C, Kao K-C, Chen N-H, Hsieh M-J, Tsai Y-H: **Prediction of fluid responsiveness in acute respiratory distress syndrome patients ventilated with low tidal volume and high positive end-expiratory pressure.** *Crit Care Med* 2008, **36**:2810–2816.

18. De Backer D, Heenen S, Piagnerelli S, Koch M, Vincent JL: **Pulse pressure variations to predict fluid responsiveness: influence of tidal volume.** *Intensive Care Med* 2005, **31**:517–523.

19. Ray P, Le Manach Y, Riou B, Houle TT: **Statistical evaluation of a biomarker.** *Anesthesiology* 2010, **112**:1023–1040.

20. de Waal EE, Rex S, Kruitwagen CL, Kalkman CJ, Buhre WF: **Dynamic preload indicators fail to predict fluid responsiveness in open-chest conditions.** *Crit Care Med* 2009, **37**:510–515.

21. Gold MS: **Perioperative fluid management.** *Crit Care Clin* 1992, **8**:409–421.

22. Michard F, Teboul JL: **Predicting fluid responsiveness in ICU patients: A critical analysis of the evidence.** *Chest* 2002, **121**:2000–2008.

23. Muller L, Louart G, Bengler C, Fabbro-Peray P, Carr J, Ripart J, de La Coussaye J-E, Lefrant J-Y: **The intrathoracic blood volume index as an indicator of fluid responsiveness in critically ill patients with acute circulatory failure: a comparison with central venous pressure.** *Anesth Analg* 2008, **107**:607–613.

24. Reuter DA, Goepfert MSG, Gorsch T, Schmoeckel M, Kilger E, Goetz AE: **Assessing fluid responsiveness during open chest conditions.** *Br J Anaesth* 2005, **94**:318–323.

25. Marino PL: **Colloid and crystalloid resuscitation.** In *The ICU Book*. 3rd edition. Edited by Marino PL, Sutin KM. Philadelphia, PA: Lippincott Williams & Wilkins; 2007:233–253.

26. van Tulder L, Michaeli B, Chioléro R, Berger MM, Revelly JP: **An evaluation of the initial distribution volume of glucose to assess plasma volume during a fluid challenge.** *Anesth Analg* 2005, **101**:1089–1093.

27. Harvey M, Voss L, Sleigh J: **Preload response in patients after cardiac surgery: a comparison of systolic pressure and systolic area variability and initial distribution volume of glucose.** *Crit Care Resusc* 2003, **5**:171–176.

28. Ishihara H: **Initial distribution volume of glucose early after cardiac surgery (Letter to the Editor).** *Anesth Analg* 1904, **2005**:102.

29. Hofer CK, Muller SM, Furrer L, Klaghofer R, Genoni M, Zollinger A: **Stroke volume and pulse pressure variation for prediction of fluid responsiveness in patients undergoing off-pump coronary artery bypass grafting.** *Chest* 2005, **128**:848–854.

30. Solus-Biguenet H, Fleyfel M, Tavernier B, Kipnis E, Onimus J, Robin E, Lebuffe G, Decoene C, Pruvot FR, Vallet B: **Non-invasive prediction of fluid responsiveness during major hapatic surgery.** *Br J Anaesth* 2006, **97**:808–816.

The cost-effectiveness of an outpatient anesthesia consultation clinic before surgery

Anna Lee*, Po Tong Chui, Chun Hung Chiu, Tony Gin and Anthony MH Ho

Abstract

Background: Outpatient anesthesia clinics are well established in North America, Europe and Australia, but few economic evaluations have been published. The Perioperative Systems in Hong Kong are best described as a hybrid model of the new and old systems of surgical care. In this matched cohort study, we compared the costs and effects of an outpatient anesthesia clinic (OPAC) with the conventional system of admitting patients to the ward a day before surgery for their pre-anesthesia consultation. A second objective of the study was to determine the patient's median Willingness To Pay (WTP) value for an OPAC.

Methods: A total of 352 patients were matched (1:1) on their elective surgical procedure to either the clinic group or to the conventional group. The primary outcome was quality of recovery score and overall perioperative treatment cost (US$). To detect a difference in the joint cost-effect relationship between groups, a cost-effectiveness acceptability curve (CEAC) was drawn. A modified Poisson regression model was used to examine the factors associated with patients willing to pay more than the median WTP value for an OPAC.

Results: The quality of recovery scores on the first day after surgery between the clinic and conventional groups were similar (mean difference, -0.1; 95% confidence interval (CI), -0.6 to 0.3; $P = 0.57$). Although the preoperative costs were less in the clinic group (mean difference, -$463, 95% CI, -$648 to -$278 per patient; $P < 0.001$), the total perioperative cost was similar between groups (mean difference, -$172; 95% CI, -$684 to $340 per patient; $P = 0.51$). The CEAC showed that we could not be 95% confident that the clinic was cost-effective. Compared to the conventional group, clinic patients were three times more likely to prefer OPAC care (relative risk (RR) 2.75, 95% CI, 2.13 to 3.55; $P < 0.001$) and pay more than the median WTP (US$13) for a clinic consultation (RR 3.27, 95% CI, 2.32 to 4.64; $P < 0.001$).

Conclusions: There is uncertainty about the cost-effectiveness of an OPAC in the Hong Kong setting. Most clinic patients were willing to pay a small amount for an anesthesia clinic consultation.

Keywords: Cost-effectiveness analysis, Outpatient anesthesia clinic, Perioperative system, Patient satisfaction

Background

Healthcare systems of today place much emphasis on patient-centered quality outcomes and cost effectiveness. Compared to a conventional system of admitting patients at least a day before surgery, Perioperative Systems with outpatient anesthesia consultation clinics are well established in North America [1-3], Europe [4] and Australia [5,6]. While there are significant variations in

the development of these Perioperative Systems between hospitals and health systems both within individual countries and between countries, this model of care involves a multidisciplinary team that provides integrated patient-focused evidence-based care from the time a decision is made that a patient should have an operation until the patient has recovered to their stable preoperative health status [7].

The benefits of establishing an outpatient anesthesia clinic (OPAC) include increasing hospital efficiency by a rapid shift from inpatient to same day admission surgery,

* Correspondence: annalee@cuhk.edu.hk
Department of Anaesthesia and Intensive Care, Prince of Wales Hospital, The Chinese University of Hong Kong, Shatin, New Territories, Hong Kong

reduction in length of hospital stay, fewer cancellations of surgery and fewer preoperative investigations [1,2,4]. While it is intuitive that re-engineering of the surgical care system should result in a substantial reduction of healthcare costs from the benefits described, there is a paucity of economic evaluations [7]. Two previous studies [8,9] suggested that the greatest gain in cost savings in the Perioperative System come from costs associated with shorter length of stay rather than from fewer preoperative investigations, but neither were formal cost-effectiveness studies.

Despite the apparent benefits associated with a Perioperative System, most Hong Kong patients are admitted to public hospitals a day before surgery and then visited by an anesthesiologist for preoperative consultation on the ward. Among the few hospitals in Hong Kong with a co-existing conventional surgical system and an OPAC in place (Figure 1), the Prince of Wales Hospital established an OPAC in January 2006. From 1 January to 31 December 2009, the percentage of elective operations performed as an outpatient surgery admission and same day admission surgery were 7% and 16%, respectively (unpublished observations).

As data were required to justify any expansion of the OPAC, we performed a cost-effectiveness study on patients undergoing selective surgical procedures for which patients could be seen at either an OPAC (Perioperative System) or through the conventional system, whichever was acceptable to the surgeons. A randomized controlled trial was not possible because many surgeons were unwilling to change their admission practices and there were established clinical pathways for preoperative care for many surgical procedures in place at the time of developing the study proposal. The main objective of the matched cohort study was to compare the costs and effects of the OPAC care with the conventional approach from the perspective of the Hospital Authority (a government body funding public health services in Hong Kong). The secondary objective was to determine the patient's Willingness To Pay (WTP) value for an OPAC.

Methods

The study was conducted at the Prince of Wales Hospital in Hong Kong, a large university hospital. The study was approved by the local Clinical Research Ethics Committee. After written informed consent, adult patients were enrolled from 20 March 2007 to 25 November 2009. The anesthesiologist-led OPAC began operation in January 2006 but did not have its own designated office space until July 2008. It is staffed by 0.5 anesthesiologist full-time equivalent and one nurse full-time equivalent to provide the service five afternoons a week, serving an average of 8 to 10 patients per day (unpublished observations for 2010). Patients were seen in the OPAC up to three months before their surgery.

Patients

We prospectively identified patients who underwent the following elective surgical procedures: orthopedic (total knee replacement, knee arthroscopy, anterior cruciate ligament reconstruction, total hip replacement, arthroscopic

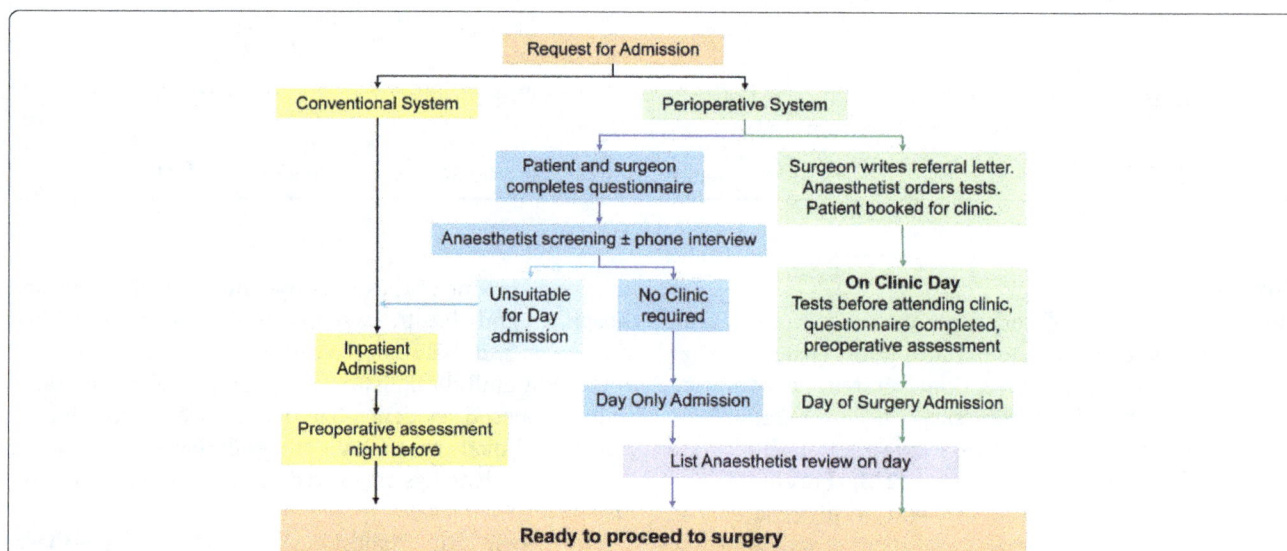

Figure 1 Conventional and Perioperative System preprocedural processes at Prince of Wales Hospital, Hong Kong. There are three types of patient groups: Day only admissions (patients admitted and discharged on the same day after elective surgery), Day of surgery admissions (patients admitted on the day of elective surgery and then stay in hospital for at least one night) and Inpatients (patients admitted before the day of surgery and then discharged on the same day or afterwards following surgery). The Perioperative System was operational in 2006 but a dedicated pre-anesthetic clinic space was not available until July 2008.

shoulder repair), gynecological (hysterectomy, salpingo-oophorectomy, cone biopsy), general (laparoscopic cholecystectomy, ligation and stripping of varicose vein, inguinal hernia repair), urological (transurethral resection of the prostate) and other (tonsillectomy, functional endoscopic sinus surgery). For these procedures, the surgeons had the option of referring their patients to the OPAC (clinic group) or through the conventional system of admitting the patient into the hospital one day before surgery (conventional group). Each clinic patient was matched by the same surgical procedure to a conventional patient on a 1:1 ratio. Selection bias could influence the association between OPAC and outcomes because high risk patients were more likely to be referred to the clinic for 'work up' [10]. In the design of this study, we addressed this issue by matching patients on their type of surgical procedure and adjusting for American Society of Anesthesiologists (ASA) Physical Status in statistical analyses when necessary.

Patients were expected to receive general anesthesia with or without regional anesthesia supplement. All patients received the usual care from surgeons and nursing staff in the surgical ward. Patients were excluded if they were younger than 18 years of age, undergoing emergency or obstetric surgery, or were unable to give consent. To ensure that the type of anesthesia given to patients was comparable between groups, those receiving regional or local anesthesia were not matched and were excluded from the study after reviewing their anesthetic records. Patients were also excluded from the study if they had their elective surgery cancelled before being matched to a suitable case. Data were not collected in patients who had another surgical procedure within the study period.

Data collection

Patients in both groups were interviewed by an investigator (CHC) with a standardized questionnaire before surgery in the OPAC (clinic group) or on the ward (conventional group). We collected data on patient's demographics, ASA physical status, cancellation of surgery on the day of intended surgery and length of hospital stay. The level of surgical invasiveness was classified as 'minor' (for example, hysteroscopy), 'intermediate' (for example, inguinal hernia repair), 'major' (for example, cholecystectomy) and 'ultra-major' (for example, total knee replacement) using the Hong Kong Government Gazette [11].

We measured the anxiety levels by asking patients to mark the visual analogue scale (VAS) on a 100 mm horizontal line with 'not anxious at all' at the left and 'extremely anxious' at the right; one for their level of anxiety about their surgical procedure and another for their level of anxiety about anesthesia. The anxiety scores were the distance in millimeters from the left side of the scales to the marks. The use of VAS to measure preoperative anxiety has been shown to be valid [12].

To measure a patient's satisfaction with the anesthetic consultation at the OPAC or on the ward, a validated and reliable questionnaire was used [13]. The questionnaire contained five specific questions about various aspects of the anesthesia consultation and one global question on the patient's satisfaction using a 6-point Likert scale (1 = strongly disagree to 6 = strongly agree) [13]. The total patient satisfaction score ranged from 6 to 30 and was converted to a score out of 100 for the purposes of this study. Patient satisfaction was collected immediately after the anesthesia consultation at the OPAC or on the ward. On the first day after surgery, a global measure of patient satisfaction with anesthesia care was obtained by asking patients to 'Circle the one number that describes how satisfied you are with the overall anesthetic care (before and after surgery) provided to you' using a 5-point Likert scale (1 = insufficient, 2 = fair, 3 = appropriate, 4 = very good and 5 = excellent) [14].

Outcomes

The primary outcome was the nine-item Quality of Recovery (QoR) score [15] used to measure the patient's health-related quality of life after anesthesia on the first day after surgery. The QoR score ranged from 0 to 18 and is a valid and reliable patient-centered outcome.

Willingness To Pay (WTP) was examined to establish how patients value the different approaches to anesthetic consultation before surgery. We asked patients about their preference for the location of the anesthesia consultation (Table 1) and the maximum amount of money they were willing to pay using an open ended question format [16] for their preferred care after their consultation with an anesthesiologist. Both groups were presented with a comparison of the major differences between the two forms of anesthesia consultation during the face-to-face interview using a standardized WTP questionnaire before surgery. The likelihood of having the same anesthesiologist at both the anesthesia consultation visit and at induction, and the risk of cancellation of the surgery was based upon our empirical unpublished data. The risk of wound infection was estimated from a published study [6]. Patients were aware that HK$100 was charged for attendance at all outpatient specialist clinics in Hong Kong public hospitals. They were also aware that they were charged for admission and hospital stay (HK$50 and HK$100/day, respectively) in the public hospital system.

Costs

To perform the cost-analysis from the hospital's perspective, the following direct costs related to anesthesia consultation were identified and summated to estimate the total direct perioperative treatment cost. First, preoperative drugs prescribed for optimizing the patient's condition

Table 1 Preference for clinic and conventional pre-anesthetic consultation

Outpatient pre-anesthetic clinic	Standard inpatient surgical ward (conventional)
See anesthesiologist up to one month before surgery as an outpatient. Less chance (10 in 100, 10%) that the clinic anesthesiologist will be the same anesthesiologist who will give you the anesthesia on the day of surgery.	See anesthesiologist one day before surgery as an inpatient. More chance (90 in 100, 90%) that this anesthesiologist will be the same anesthesiologist who will give you the anesthesia on the day of surgery.
Two visits to hospital (clinic and for surgery).	One visit to hospital for surgery.
Admission to hospital on the day of surgery.	Admission to hospital one day before surgery
Less chance (5 in 100, 5%) of surgical wound infections because overall hospital stay is shorter.	Higher chance (16 in 100, 16%) of surgical wound infections because overall hospital stay is longer.
Less chance (1 in 100, 1%) of cancellation of surgery on the day of surgery due to medical reasons.	Higher chance (5 in 100, 5%) of cancellation of surgery on the day of surgery due to medical reasons.

There are two locations in the Prince of Wales Hospital where patients can see an anesthesiologist before their surgery. One is the Outpatient Preanesthetic Clinic and the other is an Inpatient Surgical Ward. The discussion about the risks of complications and processes of anesthesia is the same at each location. The descriptions above concentrate only on the differences between these two locations.

before anesthesia were extracted from the drug chart in the patient's medical records. The unit cost was obtained from the hospital's pharmacy. Second, the laboratory investigations ordered by the anesthesiologist before surgery during the consultation were noted in the patient's medical records. The cost of a laboratory investigation was estimated by the unit cost from the hospital's pathology and radiology departments. Third, the OPAC cost (HK $840) was obtained from the Hospital Authority 2008/2009 annual report [17]. Finally, we assumed the ward costs for the clinic and conventional groups on the surgical ward were the same for each day as all patients received the same care on the designated surgical wards before and after surgery. Thus, the ward cost for each patient was estimated by calculating the average hospital bed cost (HK $3,650) from the Hospital Authority 2008/2009 annual report [17]. At the time of reporting the study results, 1US $ = HK$7.78. Cancellation costs and length of hospital stay, related to a previous admission to hospital for the intended surgical procedure, were also included in the present analysis.

Statistical analysis

We calculated that a sample size of 280 patients per group would provide 80% power to detect a difference in cost and QoR of US$128 and 0.3, respectively; the expected standard deviations of cost and QoR of US$643 and 1.2, respectively; an expected correlation of the differences of 0.1 and the maximum WTP of US$1,285 at two-tailed alpha level of 0.05 [18]. However, due to slow recruitment resulting from unexpected cancellation of elective surgery (62 working days) and lack of financial support for many surgical procedures to be admitted through the Perioperative System as planned during the study period, we recruited 176 patients per group.

Values are reported as mean and standard deviation (SD) or median and interquartile range (IQR). The mean difference and 95% confidence interval (95% CI) was defined as the OPAC variable of interest minus conventional variable

of interest. We used matched paired t-test, Wilcoxon signed ranked test and McNemar's test to compare preoperative patient characteristics between the matched groups. A multivariate analysis of variance was used to examine differences among the five components of the patient satisfaction with anesthesia consultation questionnaire [13] with a Bonferroni correction for multiple pairwise comparisons.

We assumed that the OPAC was cost-effective if there was a reduction in the overall perioperative treatment cost per gain in QoR. Using similar methodology to our previous paper on the cost-effectiveness of an Acute Pain Service [19], a cost-effectiveness acceptability curve (CEAC) was constructed from a net benefit regression [20] to examine the probability of cost-effectiveness of an OPAC over a conventional anesthesia consultation on the ward. The CEAC is a graphical transformation from a cost-effectiveness plane, where the joint density of incremental costs and effects may straddle the northwest, northeast, southwest and southeast quadrants of the plane [21]. The construction of the CEAC was performed using the macro 'iprogs' available from the University of Pennsylvania (www.uphs.upenn.edu/dgimhsr/stat-cicer. htm; accessed May 25, 2010). A *post-hoc* sensitivity CEAC was used to determine if the OPAC was cost-effective if only preoperative costs were considered.

A Poisson regression model [22] was used to examine the factors associated with patients willing to pay more than the median WTP value for an OPAC after adjusting for the patient's level of income, age, gender, ASA physical status and matching. We considered a two-sided $P < 0.05$ to be statistically significant. All analyses were performed using STATA software version 10.1 (StataCorp, College Station, TX, USA).

Results

Of the 676 patients screened for the study, 352 patients were matched on the type of surgical procedure in the final analysis. The remaining patients were all seen at the

OPAC but not in the ward (for example, inguinal hernia repair, joint replacement, hysterectomy), or all in the ward but not at the OPAC (for example, coronary artery bypass graft surgery) during the latter half of the study.

The preoperative characteristics of the 176 matched pairs were similar (Table 2). The number of matched patients undergoing orthopaedic, general, gynaecology and urology/other procedures were 133 (76%), 24 (14%), 11 (6%) and 8 (4%), respectively.

Patients in the clinic group had similar rates of surgery being cancelled on the scheduled date compared to the conventional group (2.3% versus 3.4% respectively, $P = 0.75$). Of the 10 cancellations of surgery, 9 (4 in clinic

group, 5 in conventional group) were due to no available operating room time from the overrun of previous surgical procedures. Surgery was cancelled due to a respiratory infection in a patient belonging to the conventional group.

There was no difference between clinic and conventional groups for median levels of anxiety for surgery (26 versus 25 respectively, $P = 0.12$) or for anesthesia (20 versus 19 respectively, $P = 0.60$). Patients in the OPAC group were more satisfied with the consultation taking place without time pressure and felt more informed about their procedure than conventional patients (Table 3). When the individual components of the patient satisfaction score were summated in Table 3, the score was higher in the OPAC group (mean difference 2.10%, 95% CI: 0.51% to 3.70%). After surgery, the mean patient satisfaction with perioperative anesthesia care score out of 5 was similar between the OPAC (3.88 ± 0.73) and conventional (3.89 ± 0.74) groups ($P = 0.94$).

The median length of stay in the hospital was shorter in the OPAC group than in the conventional group (three versus five days, $P < 0.001$). This was due to shorter median duration of stay before surgery in the OPAC group (1, IQR zero to one day) than in the conventional group (1, IQR one to three days) ($P < 0.001$). There was no difference in the median duration of stay after surgery between OPAC and conventional groups (three versus two and a half days, $P = 0.67$).

Cost-effectiveness

The mean QoR score on the first day after surgery was similar between OPAC (13.17 ± 2.73) and conventional (13.31 ± 2.65) groups ($P = 0.57$). Table 4 shows the mean perioperative treatment costs (in $US) per patient. Of the 176 patients in the OPAC group, 81 (46%) were admitted on the day of surgery. Although the OPAC group had a significantly lower total preoperative cost than the conventional group (mean difference -$463,

Table 2 Patient characteristics

Characteristics	Clinic group (n = 176)	Conventional group (n = 176)	P-value
Age, median (IQR), years	44 (28 to 59)	45 (26 to 59)	0.87
Women, number (%)	63 (35.8)	67 (38.1)	0.68
Education level, number (%)			0.20
No formal education	16 (9.1)	10 (5.7)	
Primary	36 (20.5)	42 (23.9)	
Secondary	74 (42.0)	67 (38.1)	
College	18 (10.2)	14 (7.9)	
University	32 (18.2)	43 (24.4)	
Work status, number (%)			0.54
Student	16 (9.1)	20 (11.4)	
Retired	35 (19.9)	44 (25.0)	
Employed	87 (49.4)	75 (42.6)	
Self-employed	9 (5.1)	9 (5.1)	
Unemployed	7 (4.0)	11 (6.3)	
Housewife	22 (12.5)	17 (9.7)	
Income level (US$ per month), number (%)			0.06
<$1,285	103 (58.9)	123 (70.3)	
$1,286 to $3,856	65 (37.1)	44 (25.1)	
>$3,857	7 (4.0)	8 (4.6)	
Magnitude of surgery, number. (%)			0.29
Minor	8 (4.5)	12 (6.8)	
Intermediate	26 (14.8)	21 (11.9)	
Major	48 (27.3)	44 (25.0)	
Ultramajor	94 (53.4)	99 (56.3)	
ASA physical status grade, number (%)			0.15
I	114 (64.8)	105 (59.7)	
II	56 (31.8)	60 (34.0)	
III/IV	6 (3.4)	11 (6.3)	
Duration of anesthesia, mean (SD), minutes	114 (45)	115 (44)	0.88

Table 3 Comparison of patient satisfaction with anesthesia consultation

	Clinic group (n = 176)	Conventional group(n = 176)	P-value
a. Consultation took place without time pressure (mean, SD)	4.94 ± 0.69	4.76 ± 0.84	0.03
b. Explanations were easily understood (mean, SD)	5.01 ± 0.48	4.99 ± 0.53	0.67
c. Questions were clarified (mean, SD)	4.95 ± 0.70	4.89 ± 0.75	0.42
d. More informed about procedure (mean, SD)	5.05 ± 0.56	4.80 ± 0.83	<0.01
e. Process of consultation was clear (mean, SD)	4.70 ± 0.97	4.58 ± 1.01	0.26
Global satisfaction score	5.05 ± 0.44	5.00 ± 0.47	0.27
Summated score (a to e) (%)	82.16 ± 6.88	80.06 ± 8.27	0.01

95% CI: -$648 to -$278 per patient, P <0.01), the mean difference in the total perioperative treatment cost was not significant (-$172, 95% CI: -$684 to 340 per patient; $P = 0.51$) even after adjusting for cancellation on the day of surgery costs.

As there was no significant gain in QoR or significant reduction in perioperative cost in the OPAC group over the conventional group, we cannot be 95% confident that the OPAC is cost-effective. The CEAC for the observed data (Figure 2) represents the joint density (incremental cost and incremental effect) covering all four quadrants of the cost-effectiveness plane, with the curve suggesting that most densities fell within the southwest quadrant (less costly, less effective). As the CEAC did not cut the y-axis at 0, some of the density involved cost-savings (71% in the southeast or southwest quadrants). As the CEAC for the observed data did not asymptote to 100, only 42% of the density involved QoR gains.

When only preoperative costs were considered, the CEAC showed that the joint density fell within the southeast and southwest quadrants (less costly, more or less effective; that is, 100% cost-savings). The CEAC for preoperative cost also shows that we can be confident that the conventional system is not cost-effective compared to the OPAC when the decision maker is willing to pay less than US$596 for an extra unit gain in QoR per patient; if the decision maker is willing to pay above US$596 for an extra unit gain in QoR per patient, then we cannot be 95% confident that the two systems differ in value.

Willingness to pay

As expected, patients in the OPAC group preferred to have their consultation at the clinic (75%) than on the ward (11%), with 14% indicating no preference for either location. More patients in the conventional group preferred to have their consultation on the ward (37%) than at the clinic (27%), with 36% indicating no preference for either location. Thus, clinic patients were three times more likely

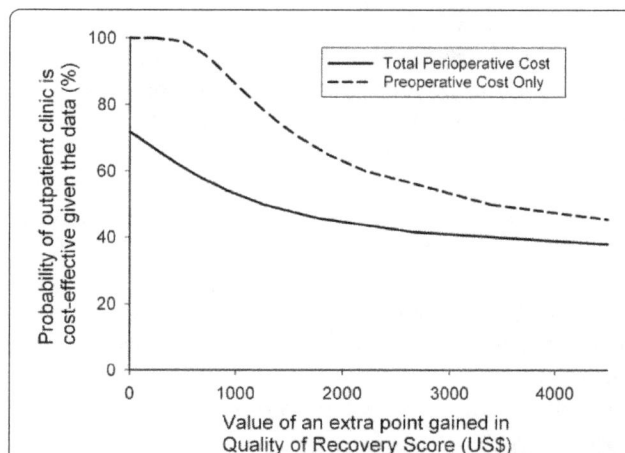

Figure 2 Cost-effectiveness acceptability curves. These were derived from comparing incremental total perioperative cost and incremental preoperative cost per incremental Quality of Recovery Score.

to prefer OPAC care (relative risk (RR) 2.75, 95% CI: 2.13 to 3.55; P <0.001) than conventional patients. The median (IQR) WTP for an OPAC and conventional ward anesthesia consultation were US$12.85 ($7.71 to $12.85) and US$12.85 ($0 to $25.71) respectively. However, compared to conventional patients, OPAC patients were more likely to pay more than US$12.85 for a clinic consultation (RR 3.27, 95% CI: 2.32 to 4.64; P <0.001) after adjusting for income, gender, age and ASA Physical Status score.

Discussion

We conducted a formal cost-effectiveness study using matched patients undergoing elective surgery through the conventional and Perioperative Systems running concurrently. Previous cost-analysis studies [8,9] have quantified the cost savings associated with establishing a Perioperative System but were likely to be biased because of the before-after study design used.

Table 4 Mean preoperative and overall perioperative costs ($US) per patient

Cost category	Clinic group (n = 176)	Conventional group (n = 176)	Mean difference (95% CI)[a]	P-value
a. Outpatient clinic	109.20	0	109.20	<0.001
b. Medication prescribed by anesthesiologist	0.48	0.15	0.33 (−0.18 to 0.85)	0.20
c. Investigations ordered by anesthesiologist	36.14	24.74	11.40 (0.59 to 22.19)	0.04
d. Cancellation of surgery	15.99	58.64	−42.65 (−126.49 to 41.13)	0.32
e. Inpatient bed before surgery[b]	335.87	876.99	−541.12 (−656.58 to −425.67)	<0.001
Total preoperative cost (a to d)	497.68	960.52	−462.84 (−648.12 to −277.58)	<0.001
f. Inpatient bed on day of surgery and afterwards	2,247.13	1,956.58	290.55 (−187.01 to 768.12)	0.23
Total perioperative cost (a to f)	2,744.81	2,917.10	−172.29 (−684.48 to 339.89)	0.51

[a]Negative value implies that outpatient anesthesia consultation clinic is less expensive than conventional approach; positive value implies that outpatient anesthesia consultation clinic is more expensive than conventional approach. [b]95 patients in the clinic group were admitted at least one day before surgery into hospital.

Although the length of stay was shorter in the OPAC group, this did not translate to significant cost savings in favor of the Perioperative System. Even after the patients had their anesthesia consultation at the OPAC, surgeons continued to admit more than half the group into hospital at least one day before surgery to occupy a hospital bed and a place on the operating list. In many developed Perioperative Systems, this practice would be obsolete unless the patient was at very high risk of postoperative complications.

It should be noted that postoperative bed cost accounts for approximately 75% of the total perioperative cost. This explains why we failed to find the OPAC to be cost-effective when all direct costs before and after surgery were summated. However, if all patients in the OPAC group were admitted on the day of surgery, the total perioperative cost-savings of US$525 (95% CI: $18 to $1,033) per patient would be significantly in favor of the Perioperative System ($P = 0.04$). Compared to the conventional system, this would translate to an 18% reduction in overall perioperative treatment costs, a similar finding to Boothe and Finegan's study (18% reduction) [8]. The implication of this analysis suggests that there are some barriers to adopting the OPAC approach in some of our surgeons. These may include their traditional belief that OPAC patients are 'not ready' on the day of surgery and their prevailing practice of admitting an OPAC patient overnight before surgery [23]. Continued efforts are ongoing by anesthesiologists and surgeons to promote appropriate referral of patients to the OPAC and timely hospital admission on the day of surgery of OPAC patients. We believe that a 10% to 20% reduction in the total perioperative cost per patient associated with our Perioperative System is highly feasible in this setting in line with overseas experience [7].

Caution is needed in the interpretation of our sensitivity analysis (Figure 2) that included only the preoperative cost as it made up a small proportion (approximately 25%) of the overall perioperative cost. The implication of these results highlights the need for financial incentives to be put in place to encourage shorter length of stay, especially after surgery. This may include the Pay for Performance diagnosis-related case-mix model that has recently been introduced into the Hong Kong public hospital funding allocation scheme [24].

The surgical system at the Prince of Wales Hospital in Hong Kong is unique with a hybrid model of the new and old systems of surgical care (Figure 1). This has been due in part to a number of factors. First, the incentive to maximize the bed occupancy in Hong Kong public hospitals is less than in similar Australian hospitals as the number of acute hospital beds per population is higher (2.9 [25] versus 2.6 [26] per 1,000, respectively). Also the lack of a centralized preoperative holding area has impeded the use of 'hot bedding' whereby patients do not require a ward bed until the latter part of the morning, enabling the bed to be fully utilized overnight. Second, the role of the community primary healthcare team in Hong Kong [27] for supporting the patient before and after surgery is less defined than in the Australian setting. Despite favorable patient attitudes towards day case surgery in Hong Kong [28], most elective surgery cases are booked and performed under individual surgical specialty teams who look after their own operating room lists rather than through a centrally organized and integrated Perioperative Service. These unique factors produce particular challenges to implementing the complete Perioperative model in Hong Kong and potentially limit the stakeholders from deriving the benefits associated with such a system.

From the patient's perspective, both groups valued the two approaches to anesthesia consultation equally at an average WTP value of US$13. Despite careful wording of the WTP question, the low WTP value may reflect the actual charge that patients currently pay for specialist-based outpatient clinics in Hong Kong and a high patient expectation of the government to heavily subsidize public health services. Nevertheless, those who were seen at the OPAC were three times more likely to both prefer it and pay more than US$13 for this type of care over the conventional approach. Irrespective of where anesthesia consultation takes place, patients in a German study were found to value a close relationship with an anesthesiologist without waiting too long to see them [29]. Of the €100 available to spend, patients were willing to pay €36 for a pre-anesthetic visit performed by the anesthesiologist who would give anesthesia, €26 to wait less than two hours, €16 for preferred location of pre-anaesthetic visit, €12 for multimedia information and €10 for ambience [29].

The strong preference for an OPAC may be associated with a marginally higher preoperative patient satisfaction level in clinic patients than those in the conventional system. OPAC patients were more informed about the risks and processes of anesthesia without constraints on the length of their consultation. Our findings are consistent with high levels of patient satisfaction with the information from, and sufficient time with, an anesthesiologist at an OPAC [13,30]. As in a previous study [14], we found no difference in the overall perioperative patient satisfaction ratings for anesthesia care between groups.

Previous studies [1,4,31,32] have consistently shown a significant decrease in the rate of cancellation of surgery associated with a Perioperative System. However, as our rate of surgery cancellations was already low in OPAC patients, we did not find a significant difference between groups. The majority of these cancellations were related to operating room lists overrun rather than inadequately prepared patients, a similar finding to a recent study [33]. Many surgeons scheduled their OPAC patients in the later part of the operation list to allow more time for pre-procedural processes to occur but often underestimated the length and/or complexity of the procedures of other patients at the start of the operating list. Strategies to reduce the rate of cancellations from cases running over the allocated time may improve the overall operating room efficiency and reduce healthcare costs.

There are several limitations to this study. In calculating the direct costs of both approaches to anesthesia consultation, the net costs related to better prepared patients and perioperative complications costs were not accounted for. Previous studies have shown that patients in the Perioperative System are better prepared for surgery [10] and may have less risk of wound infections [6], implying that our CEAC may be imprecise. Despite the lack of randomization in this study, the ASA physical status was similar between matched patients; indirect evidence (median postoperative length of hospital stay) suggests that OPAC patients were at no greater risk of complications after surgery than conventional patients.

The results of this study may not be generalizable to different organizational structures of OPAC outside Hong Kong. However, it highlights the difficulties in changing hospital organization culture, clinical practice and behaviors when implementing a new Perioperative System. In many centers elsewhere, a nurse-led OPAC can provide a similar service without affecting patient satisfaction levels [30] and patient safety [34] but we are unaware of any published formal cost-effectiveness analysis using this model.

Conclusions

In conclusion, the cost-effectiveness of the OPAC in Hong Kong remains uncertain because significant reductions in the preoperative costs make up a small proportion of the overall perioperative treatment cost. Nevertheless, OPAC patients had a strong preference for where the anesthesia consultation should take place, were willing to pay a small amount for it, and were more informed about the risks and processes of anesthesia. Encouraging more surgeons to use our OPAC may help address the expected growth in the number and complexity of surgical procedures being performed on older and sicker patients, with increasing awareness of and demand for high quality and safe care, in a setting of limited healthcare resources.

Abbreviations
ASA: American Society of Anesthesiologists; CEAC: cost-effectiveness acceptability curve; CI: confidence interval; IQR: interquartile range; OPAC: outpatient anaesthesia clinic; QoR: quality of recovery; RR: relative risk; SD: standard deviation; VAS: visual analogue scale; WTP: willingness to pay.

Competing interests
The authors declare that they have no competing interests.

Acknowledgements
The work described in this paper was fully supported by a grant from the Central Policy Unit of the Government of HKSAR and the Research Grants Council of the HKSAR, China (Project reference: CUHK4003-PPR-3). The funding body had no role in the design, collection, analysis and interpretation of the data; in writing of the manuscript; or decision to submit the manuscript for publication.

Authors' contributions
AL conceived of the study, designed the study, analyzed and interpreted the data, and drafted the manuscript. PTC, TG and AMHH participated in the study design and interpretation of the data. CHC collected the data. PTC, CHC, TG and AMHH helped revise the manuscript. All authors read and approved the final manuscript.

References
1. Fischer SP: Development and effectiveness of an anesthesia preoperative evaluation clinic in a teaching hospital. Anesthesiology 1996, 85:196–206.
2. Pollard JB, Garnerin P: Outpatient preoperative evaluation clinic can lead to a rapid shift from inpatient to outpatient surgery: a retrospective review of perioperative setting and outcome. J Clin Anesth 1999, 11:39–45.
3. Wijeysundera DN, Austin PC, Beattie WS, Hux JE, Laupacis A: A population-based study of anesthesia consultation before major noncardiac surgery. Arch Intern Med 2009, 169:595–602.
4. van Klei WA, Moons KG, Rutten CL, Schuurhuis A, Knape JT, Kalkman CJ, Grobbee DE: The effect of outpatient preoperative evaluation of hospital inpatients on cancellation of surgery and length of hospital stay. Anesth Analg 2002, 94:644–649.
5. Kerridge R, Lee A, Latchford E, Beehan SJ, Hillman KM: The perioperative system: a new approach to managing elective surgery. Anaesth Intensive Care 1995, 23:591–596.
6. Caplan GA, Brown A, Crowe PJ, Yap SJ, Noble S: Re-engineering the elective surgical service of a tertiary hospital: a historical controlled trial. Med J Aust 1998, 169:247–251.
7. Lee A, Kerridge R, Chui PT, Chiu CH, Gin T: Perioperative Systems as a quality model of perioperative medicine and surgical care. Health Policy 2011, 102:214–222.
8. Boothe P, Finegan BA: Changing the admission process for elective surgery: an economic analysis. Can J Anaesth 1995, 42:391–394.
9. Caplan G, Board N, Paten A, Tazelaar-Molinia J, Crowe P, Yap SJ, Brown A: Decreasing lengths of stay: the cost to the community. Aust N Z J Surg 1999, 69:433–437.
10. Lee A, Lum ME, Perry M, Beehan SJ, Hillman KM, Bauman A: Risk of unanticipated intraoperative events in patients assessed at a preanaesthetic clinic. Can J Anaesth 1997, 44:946–954.
11. Hong Kong Government: Hong Kong Government Gazette No 13/2003 Special Supplement No 4 Annex IV.; 2003:D4668–D4704. 2003.
12. Kindler CH, Harms C, Amsler F, Ihde-Scholl T, Scheidegger D: The visual analog scale allows effective measurement of preoperative anxiety and detection of patients' anesthetic concerns. Anesth Analg 2000, 90:706–712.
13. Snyder-Ramos SA, Seintsch H, Bottiger BW, Motsch J, Martin E, Bauer M: Patient satisfaction and information gain after the preanesthetic visit: a comparison of face-to-face interview, brochure, and video. Anesth Analg 2005, 100:1753–1758.
14. Harms C, Nubling M, Langewitz W, Kindler CH: Patient satisfaction with continued versus divided anesthetic care. J Clin Anesth 2007, 19:9–14.
15. Myles PS, Hunt JO, Nightingale CE, Fletcher H, Beh T, Tanil D, Nagy A, Rubinstein A, Ponsford JL: Development and psychometric testing of a quality of recovery score after general anesthesia and surgery in adults. Anesth Analg 1999, 88:83–90.
16. Frew EJ, Whynes DK, Wolstenholme JL: Eliciting willingness to pay: comparing closed-ended with open-ended and payment scale formats. Med Decis Making 2003, 23:150–159.
17. Hospital Authority: Hospital Authority Annual Report 2008/09. Hong Kong: Hong Kong Hospital Authority; 2010.
18. Glick HA, Doshi JA, Sonnad SS, Polsky D: Economic Evaluation in Clinical Trials. New York: Oxford University Press; 2007.
19. Lee A, Chan SK, Chen PP, Gin T, Lau AS, Chiu CH: The costs and benefits of extending the role of the acute pain service on clinical outcomes after major elective surgery. Anesth Analg 2010, 111:1042–1050.

20. Hoch JS, Briggs AH, Willan AR: **Something old, something new, something borrowed, something blue: a framework for the marriage of health econometrics and cost-effectiveness analysis.** *Health Econ* 2002, **11**:415–430.

21. Fenwick E, O'Brien BJ, Briggs A: **Cost-effectiveness acceptability curves–facts, fallacies and frequently asked questions.** *Health Econ* 2004, **13**:405–415.

22. Zou G: **A modified Poisson regression approach to prospective studies with binary data.** *Am J Epidemiol* 2004, **159**:702–706.

23. Chan FW, Wong FY, Cheung YS, Chui PT, Lai PB: **Utility of a preoperative assessment clinic in a tertiary care hospital.** *Hong Kong Med J* 2011, **17**:441–445.

24. Lee KH, Gillett S: **Introducing pay-for-performance within Hong Kong's public hospitals.** *BMC Heal Serv Res* 2010, **10**(Suppl 2):A17.

25. Statistics and Research Section, Strategy and Planning Division: *Hospital Authority Statistical Report 2007–2008.* 2009th edition. Hong Kong:Hong Kong Hospital Authority; 2009.

26. Australian Institute of Health and Welfare: *Australian Hospital Statistics 2007–08: Australian Institute of Health and Welfare, Health Services Series No.33.* Canberra: Australian Institute of Health and Welfare; 2009.

27. Lee A: **The need for integrated primary health care to enhance the effectiveness of health services.** *Asia Pac J Public Health* 2003, **15**:62–67.

28. Lee YC, Chen PP, Yap J, Yeo P, Chu C: **Attitudes towards day-case surgery in Hong Kong Chinese patients.** *Hong Kong Med J* 2007, **13**:298–303.

29. Aust H, Eberhart LH, Kalmus G, Zoremba M, Rusch D: **Relevance of five core aspects of the pre-anesthesia visit: results of a patient survey.** *Anaesthesist* 2010, **60**:414–420.

30. Harnett MJ, Correll DJ, Hurwitz S, Bader AM, Hepner DL: **Improving efficiency and patient satisfaction in a tertiary teaching hospital preoperative clinic.** *Anesthesiology* 2010, **112**:66–72.

31. Macpherson DS, Lofgren RP: **Outpatient internal medicine preoperative evaluation: a randomized clinical trial.** *Med Care* 1994, **32**:498–507.

32. Ferschl MB, Tung A, Sweitzer B, Huo D, Glick DB: **Preoperative clinic visits reduce operating room cancellations and delays.** *Anesthesiology* 2005, **103**:855–859.

33. Chiu CH, Lee A, Chui PT: **Cancellation of elective operations on the day of intended surgery: prevalence and reasons in a Hong Kong hospital.** *Hong Kong Med J* 2012, **18**:5–10.

34. Varughese AM, Byczkowski TL, Wittkugel EP, Kotagal U, Dean KC: **Impact of a nurse practitioner-assisted preoperative assessment program on quality.** *Paediatr Anaesth* 2006, **16**:723–733.

Permissions

List of Contributors

Ronald P. Olson and Ishwori B. Dhakal
Department of Anesthesiology, Duke University Medical Center, Duke Medicine Circle Dr, Durham, NC 27710, USA

Frederic Michard
Department of Critical Care, Edwards Lifesciences, 1 Edwards Way, Irvine, CA, USA

William K. Mountford, Michelle R. Krukas and Frank R. Ernst
Premier Inc., Charlotte, NC, USA

William K. Mountford
Current address: Quintiles, Durham, NC, USA

Michelle R. Krukas
Quintiles, Cambridge, MA, USA

Frank R. Ernst
Current address: Indegene Total Therapeutic Management, Kennesaw, GA, USA

Sandy L. Fogel
Virginia Tech Carilion School of Medicine, Roanoke, VA, USA

Daniela C Ionescu, Simona Claudia D Margarit
Department of Anesthesia and Intensive Care I, 'Iuliu Hatieganu' University of Medicine and Pharmacy, Croitorilor, nr. 19-21, Cluj-Napoca 400162, Romania

Daniela C Ionescu
Outcomes Research Consortium, Cleveland, OH, USA

Adina Norica I Hadade
Department of Anaesthesia and Intensive Care, Regional Institute of Gastroenterology and Hepatology'O Fodor', Croitorilor, nr. 19-21, Cluj-Napoca 400162, Romania

Teodora N Mocan
Department of Physiology, 'Iuliu Hatieganu' University of Medicine and Pharmacy, Croitorilor, nr. 19-21, Cluj-Napoca 400162, Romania

Nicolae A Miron
Department of Clinical Immunology, 'Iuliu Hatieganu' University of Medicine and Pharmacy, Croitorilor, nr. 19-21, Cluj-Napoca 400162, Romania

Daniel I Sessler
Department of Outcomes Research, The Cleveland Clinic 9500 Euclid Ave -- P77, Cleveland, OH 44195, USA

Stephen J Goodyear, Heng Yow, Mahmud Saedon, Joanna Shakespeare, Christopher E Hill, Duncan Watson, Colette Marshall, Asif Mahmood, Daniel Higman and Christopher HE Imray
University Hospitals Coventry and Warwickshire NHS Trust, Clifford Bridge Road, Coventry CV2 2DX, UK

Mahmud Saedon and Christopher HE Imray
Warwick Medical School, University of Warwick, Coventry CV4 7AL, UK

Caroline Ulfsdotter Nilsson, and Peter Reinstrup
Department of Anaesthesia and Intensive Care, Skåne University Hospital, Lund University, Lund, Sweden

Karin Strandberg
Department of Laboratory Medicine, Skåne University Hospital Malmö, Lund University, Malmö, Sweden

Martin Engström
Department of Anaesthesia and Intensive Care, Lund University, Lund, Sweden

Navid Alem, Joseph Rinehart, Brian Lee, Doug Merrill, Safa Sobhanie and Kyle Ahn
Department of Anesthesiology and Perioperative Care, School of Medicine, University of California, Irvine, 333 City Boulevard West Side, Orange, CA 92868-3301, USA

Ran Schwarzkopf
Division of Adult Reconstruction, Department of Orthopedic Surgery, NYU Langone Medical Center, Hospital For Joint Diseases, New York, USA

Maxime Cannesson
Department of Anesthesiology and Perioperative Care, School of Medicine, University of California, Los Angeles, Los Angeles, USA

Zeev Kain
Center for Stress and Health and Department of Anesthesiology and Perioperative Care, School of Medicine, University of California, Irvine, Orange, USA

Marit Habicher, Felix Balzer, Viktor Mezger, Jennifer Niclas and Michael Krämer
Department of Anaesthesiology and Intensive Care Medicine, Charité University Hospital Berlin, Campus Charité Mitte and Campus Virchow-Klinikum, Berlin, Germany

Michael Müller and Carsten Perka
Centre for Musculoskeletal Surgery, Department of Orthopaedics, Charité University Hospital Berlin, Campus Charité Mitte and Campus Virchow-Klinikum, Berlin, Germany

Michael Sander
Department of Anaesthesiology, Intensive Care Medicine and Pain Therapy, Justus-Liebig-University, Giessen, Germany

Julie Sanders
St Bartholomew's Hospital, Barts Health NHS Trust, London, UK

Jackie A. Cooper
Centre for Cardiovascular Genetics, University College London, London, UK

Daniel Farrar
Department of Cardiac Anaesthesia and Critical Care, University College London Hospitals NHS Foundation Trust, London, UK

Simon Braithwaite and Updeshbir Sandhu
UCL Medical School, University College London, London, UK

Michael G. Mythen
University College London Hospitals NHS Trust, London, UK

Hugh E. Montgomery
Institute for Sport, Exercise and Health, University College London, 1st Floor 170 Tottenham Court Rd, London W1T 7HA, UK

Julie Sanders
St Bartholomew's Hospital, Barts Health NHS Trust, London, UK

Julie Sanders, Michael G. Mythen and Hugh E. Montgomery
Institute for Sport, Exercise and Health, University College London, 1st Floor 170 Tottenham Court Rd, London W1T 7HA, UK

Jackie Cooper
Centre for Cardiovascular Genetics, University College London, London, UK

Michael G. Mythen
Department of Anaesthesia, University College London Hospitals NHS Trust, London, UK

Kevin R. Riggs
Division of Preventive Medicine, University of Alabama at Birmingham, Birmingham, AL, USA

Zackary D. Berger, Eric B. Bass and Geetanjali Chander
Division of General Internal Medicine, Johns Hopkins University School of Medicine, 1830 E. Monument Street, Room 8060, Baltimore, MD 21287, USA

Martin A. Makary
Department of Surgery, Johns Hopkins University School of Medicine, Baltimore, MD, USA

S. Ulyett, G. Shahtahmassebi, S. Aroori, M. J. Bowles, C. D. Briggs, M. G. Wiggans, G. Minto and D. A. Stell
Derriford Hospital, Plymouth PL6 8DH, UK

S. Ulyett, G. Shahtahmassebi, G. Minto and D. A. Stell
Peninsula Schools of Medicine and Dentistry, Plymouth University, Plymouth PL6 8BU, UK

G. Shahtahmassebi
Nottingham Trent University, Nottingham NG1 4BU, UK

Ramon Abola, Jamie Romeiser, Suman Grewal, Sabeen Rizwan, Rishimani Adsumelli, Ellen Steinberg and Elliott Bennett-Guerrero
Stony Brook Medicine, Department of Anesthesiology, HSC-4-060, Stony Brook, NY 11794, USA

Clare M. Morkane, Helen McKenna and Daniel S. Martin
Division of Surgery and Interventional Science (University College London) and Royal Free Perioperative Research Group, Department of Anaesthesia, Royal Free Hospital, 3rd Floor, Pond Street, London NW3 2QG, UK

Andrew F. Cumpstey and Michael P. W. Grocott
University of Southampton/University Hospital Southampton and NIHR Biomedical Research Centre, Tremona Rd, Southampton SO16 6YD, UK

Alex H. Oldman
University Hospital Southampton, Tremona Rd, Southampton SO16 6YD, UK

Fintan Hughes, Monty Mythen and Hugh Montgomery
Institute for Sport, Exercise and Health, University College London, 170 Tottenham Court Road, London W1T 7HA, UK

Thomas Deiss
Department of Biochemistry and Biophysics, University of California San Francisco, 505 Parnassus Ave., San Francisco, CA 94143, USA

Lee-lynn Chen
Department of Anesthesia and Perioperative Medicine, University of California San Francisco, 1825 4th St., San Francisco, CA 94158, USA

Ankit Sarin
Department of Surgery, University of California San Francisco, 1825 4th St., San Francisco, CA 94158, USA

Ramana K. Naidu
California Orthopedics and Spine, Director of Pain Management at Marin General Hospital, 18 Bon Air Road, Larkspur, CA 94939, USA

Philip Spreadborough, Sarah Lort and Matthew Popplewell
West Midlands Research Collaborative, University of Birmingham, Edgbaston, Birmingham B15 2TH, UK

Sandro Pasquali and Olga Tucker
Department of Upper Gastro-Intestinal Surgery, Queen Elizabeth Hospital, Birmingham, UK

Andrew Owen
School of Immunity and Infection, University of Birmingham, Birmingham, UK

Irene Kreis
Clinical Effectiveness Unit, Royal College of Surgeons England, London, UK

Olga Tucker
Academic Department of Surgery, University of Birmingham, 4th Floor, (Old) Queen Elizabeth Hospital, Edgbaston, Birmingham B15 2TH, UK

Ravinder S Vohra
Nottingham Oesophagi-Gastric unit, Nottingham University Hospitals NHS Trust, Queens Medical Centre, Nottingham NG7 2UH, UK

N. Li
Department of Medicine, Växjö County Hospital, Växjö, Sweden

S. Statkevicius, B. Asgeirsson and U. Schött
Department of Anaesthesia and Intensive Care, Lund University and Skane University Hospital, Lund S-22185, Sweden

Eirik K Aahlin, Arthur Revhaug and Kristoffer Lassen
Department of GI and HPB Surgery, University Hospital Northern Norway, Breivika, Tromsø, Norway

Maarten von Meyenfeldt and Cornelius HC Dejong
Department of Surgery, University Hospital Maastricht and NUTRIM School for Nutrition, Toxicology and Metabolism, Maastricht, The Netherlands

Olle Ljungqvist
Department of Surgery, Örebro University Hospital, Örebro, Sweden
Department of Molecular Medicine and Surgery, Karolinska Institutet, Stockholm, Sweden

Kenneth C Fearon and Stephen J Wigmore
Clinical Surgery, University of Edinburgh, Royal Infirmary of Edinburgh, Edinburgh, UK

Dileep N Lobo
Division of Gastrointestinal Surgery, Nottingham Digestive Diseases Centre National Institute for Health Research, Biomedical Research Unit, Nottingham University Hospitals, Queen's Medical Centre, Nottingham, UK

Nicolas Demartines
Department of Visceral Surgery, University Hospital of Lausanne (CHUV), Lausanne, Switzerland

Eirik K Aahlin, Arthur Revhaug and Kristoffer Lassen
Institute of Clinical Medicine, University of Tromsø, Tromsø, Norway

Lee A Fleisher
Department of Anesthesiology and Critical Care, Perelman School of Medicine, Leonard Davis Institute of Health Economics, University of Pennsylvania, 3400 Spruce Street, Dulles 680, Philadelphia, PA 19104, USA

Walter T Linde-Zwirble
ZD Associates, Perkasie, PA, USA

Robert G. Hahn
Research Unit at Södertälje Hospital, 152 86 Södertälje, Sweden

Toby Reynolds and Amanda Vivian-Smith
Adult Critical Care Unit, Royal London Hospital, Barts Health NHS Trust, Whitechapel Rd, London E1 1BB, UK

Shaman Jhanji
Intensive Care Unit, Royal Marsden Hospital, Fulham Road, London SW3 6JJ, UK

Rupert M Pearse
Barts and The London School of Medicine and Dentistry, Queen Mary's University of London, Turner Street, London E1 2AD, UK

Stacey Calvert
St George's Hospital, London, SW17 0QT, UK

Andrew Shaw
Dept of Anesthesiology and Critical Care Medicine, Duke University Medical Center/Durham VAMC, Durham, USA

Hironori Ishihara, Eiji Hashiba, Hirobumi Okawa, Junichi Saito, Toshinori Kasai and Toshihito Tsubo
Department of Anesthesiology, Hirosaki University Graduate School of Medicine, 5 Zaifu-Cho, Hirosaki-Shi 036-8562, Japan

Anna Lee, Po Tong Chui, Chun Hung Chiu, Tony Gin and Anthony MH Ho
Department of Anaesthesia and Intensive Care, Prince of Wales Hospital, The Chinese University of Hong Kong, Shatin, New Territories, Hong Kong

Index

A

Abdominal Aortic Aneurysm, 12-13, 25-26, 31, 33-37, 100

Adenosine Triphosphate, 72

Albumin, 41, 74, 77, 80-84, 137-140, 142-146

Anaemia, 64-65, 68-73, 81, 84

Anesthesia, 2, 7-8, 14, 17-23, 27, 47, 55, 84, 89-91, 101-105, 111, 127-129, 160, 163, 184-186, 190-191, 193-199

Anesthesiology, 1-3, 7-8, 15, 24, 36, 47-49, 54-55, 63, 84-85, 87, 89-90, 93-94, 100-101, 104, 129, 146, 152, 158, 166, 172, 179-183, 189-190, 198-199

Aneurysm Surgery, 25-26, 36-37

Anti-inflammatory Interleukin, 17

B

Blood Glucose, 159, 182

Breastfeeding, 101-105

C

Cardiac Arrest, 107, 111, 152, 159, 166

Cardiac Arrhythmias, 183

Cardiac Surgery, 10, 13, 15, 23-24, 26, 45-46, 63-65, 70-75, 81, 83-84, 100, 130, 132-135, 146, 172, 174-175, 177, 179-182, 188, 190

Cardiopulmonary Exercise Test, 25

Cardiovascular Cause, 66, 76

Cell Adhesion Molecule, 17-18, 20, 22-24

Cesarean Delivery, 101-105

Charlson Comorbidity, 60, 94, 100

Chlorhexidine, 130-136

Chlorhexidine Gluconate, 131, 135

Circulating Haemoglobin, 64

Cirrhosis, 16, 95, 100, 167-171

Colloid Infusion, 139-141

Colorectal Surgery, 8, 16, 99-100, 124-125, 127-129, 150-151, 181

Craniotomy, 38-39, 42, 45-46, 137

Cytokine, 17-20, 22-24, 175

D

Dehydration, 113-115, 118, 120-123

Diabetes Mellitus, 36, 58, 60, 117, 121, 123, 167-170, 174

E

Electrolyte, 66, 69-70, 76, 123, 139, 162

Endocrine, 3, 64, 66, 69-70, 76, 86, 88, 90

Esophagectomy, 12-13, 183-190

Excessive Fibrinolysis, 38

F

Fibrinogen, 38-43, 45-46, 138, 142-144, 146

Fluid Responsiveness, 183-190

Functional Recovery, 147-149

G

Goal-directed Fluid Therapy, 9, 13, 15, 56, 62

H

Haemodynamic Monitoring, 56, 60, 145

Haemoglobin Concentration, 64, 73, 108-109, 140

Hip Revision Arthroplasty, 56-57, 62

Hip Surgery, 56-57, 59

Hydroxyethyl Starch, 38-39, 42, 45-46, 137-146, 189

Hyperoxaemia, 106-107, 110-111

Hyperoxia, 106, 110-112

Hypocoagulation, 38

I

Inhalation Anesthetics, 17

Interleukin, 17-18, 20-21, 23-24, 179-180

Intraoperative Oxygenation, 106, 109

Intrathoracic Blood, 183-184, 187-190

L

Laparoscopic Cholecystectomies, 17, 23

Liver Resection, 94-100

M

Major Surgery, 14-16, 36, 42, 57, 63, 73, 90, 107, 109, 135, 146, 170, 172, 178-179, 181

Metabolism, 64, 73, 151, 159, 163, 166, 184

Metabolism Glucose, 159

Microvascular Flow, 63, 167-170

Mitochondrial Oxidative, 64

Morbidity Burden, 64-65, 70, 72-75, 84

Myocardial Infarction, 11, 26, 60, 66, 76, 84, 107, 113, 123, 152, 154

N

Neurosurgery, 4, 38-39, 42-43, 45-46, 108, 137-145

Nosocomial Infection, 130-131, 133-135

Nurse Screening, 1-4, 7-8

O

Oral Chlorhexidine, 130-131, 133-134

Orthopaedic Surgery, 56, 59, 99

Osmoregulation, 113, 115, 122-123

P

Perioperative Medicine, 8, 47, 49, 55, 93, 111, 129, 170, 198

Perioperative Surgical Home, 7-8, 47-48, 54-55

Plasma Osmolality, 113-115, 117-118, 120-122

Platelet Aggregation, 137, 139, 143, 146

Pleural Effusion, 66, 76, 97, 152-153, 155, 187

Pneumonia, 48, 58, 130-136, 152-153, 155-158

Post Anesthesia Care Unit, 101-102, 104

Post-operative Morbidity, 64-66, 70, 72, 74-77, 81, 83

Postoperative Nausea, 18-19, 22, 24, 53, 101, 104-105

Postoperative Pain, 76, 101-102, 105, 124-125, 127-129

Postsurgical Complication, 15

Prelabor Cesarean Delivery, 101, 104

Preoperative Medical Evaluation, 85-86, 88, 90, 92

Propofol, 17-19, 21-22, 24, 39, 57, 138, 184

R

Readmission Reduction, 47

Red Blood Cell Transfusion, 39, 64, 69, 181

Risk Stratification, 32, 34, 47-48, 53, 83-84, 91, 172, 174-175, 179-180

S

Surgery Cancellation, 1, 8

Surgical Care Quality, 47

Surgical Procedure, 9-10, 13, 56-57, 95, 183, 187, 191, 193-194

Surgical Readmission, 55

T

Thromboelastography, 38-39, 45-46, 137, 145-146

Total Joint Arthroplasty, 47-48, 53-55

Tracheobronchitis, 152, 155

Tumour Neurosurgery, 137, 141-144

V

Vaginal Delivery, 103

Vasopressin Release, 113-114, 122-123

Volatile Anesthesia, 17-21